THE SOCIAL IMPACT OF
AIDS
IN THE UNITED STATES

Albert R. Jonsen and Jeff Stryker, editors

Panel on Monitoring the Social Impact of the AIDS Epidemic

Committee on AIDS Research and the Behavioral,
Social, and Statistical Sciences

Commission on Behavioral and Social Sciences and Education

National Research Council

NATIONAL ACADEMY PRESS
Washington, D.C. 1993

National Academy Press • 2101 Constitution Avenue, N.W. • Washington, D.C. 20418

NOTICE: The project that is the subject of this report was approved by the Governing Board of the National Research Council, whose members are drawn from the councils of the National Academy of Sciences, the National Academy of Engineering, and the Institute of Medicine. The members of the committee responsible for the report were chosen for their competences and with regard for the appropriate balance.

This report has been reviewed by a group other than the authors according to procedures approved by a Report Review Committee consisting of members of the National Academy of Sciences, the National Academy of Engineering, and the Institute of Medicine.

The project that is the subject of this report was supported by the Public Health Service, U.S. Department of Health and Human Services; the Lilly Endowment, Inc.; and the Sierra Foundation.

Library of Congress Cataloging-in-Publication Data

National Research Council (U.S.). Panel on Monitoring the Social
  Impact of the AIDS Epidemic.
    The social impact of AIDS in the United States / Panel on
  Monitoring the Social Impact of the AIDS Epidemic ; Committee on
  AIDS Research and the Behavioral, Social, and Statistical Sciences,
  Commission on Behavioral and Social Sciences and Education, National
  Research Council.
       p.   cm.
    Includes bibliographical references and index.
    ISBN 0-309-04628-9
    1. AIDS (Disease)—Social aspects—United States. I. National
  Research Council (U.S.). Committee on AIDS Research and the
  Behavioral, Social, and Statistical Sciences. II. Title
  RA644.A25N27   1993
  362.1'969792'00973—dc20   92-38885
                                          CIP

PANEL ON MONITORING THE SOCIAL IMPACT OF THE AIDS EPIDEMIC

ALBERT R. JONSEN (*Chair*), Department of Medical History and Ethics, School of Medicine, University of Washington

RONALD BAYER, School of Public Health, Columbia University

RICHARD A. BERK,* Department of Sociology, University of California, Los Angeles

ALLAN M. BRANDT, Departments of Social Medicine and History of Science, Harvard University, and Harvard Medical School

DAVID L. CHAMBERS, School of Law, University of Michigan

DEBORAH COTTON, School of Public Health, Harvard University

JOHN H. GAGNON, Department of Sociology, State University of New York, Stony Brook

SHIRLEY LINDENBAUM, The Graduate Center, City University of New York

EARL E. SHELP, Foundation for Interfaith Research and Ministry, Houston, Texas

MARK D. SMITH, Kaiser Family Foundation, Menlo Park, California

JAMES TRUSSELL, Office of Population Research, Princeton University

JEFF STRYKER, *Study Director* (through June 1991)

---

*Did not participate after spring 1991.

The National Academy of Sciences is a private, nonprofit, self-perpetuating society of distinguished scholars engaged in scientific and engineering research, dedicated to the furtherance of science and technology and to their use for the general welfare. Upon the authority of the charter granted to it by the Congress in 1863, the Academy has a mandate that requires it to advise the federal government on scientific and technical matters. Dr. Frank Press is president of the National Academy of Sciences.

The National Academy of Engineering was established in 1964, under the charter of the National Academy of Sciences, as a parallel organization of outstanding engineers. It is autonomous in its administration and in the selection of its members, sharing with the National Academy of Sciences the responsibility for advising the federal government. The National Academy of Engineering also sponsors engineering programs aimed at meeting national needs, encourages education and research, and recognizes the superior achievements of engineers. Dr. Robert M. White is president of the National Academy of Engineering.

The Institute of Medicine was established in 1970 by the National Academy of Sciences to secure the services of eminent members of appropriate professions in the examination of policy matters pertaining to the health of the public. The Institute acts under responsibility given to the National Academy of Sciences by its congressional charter to be an advisor to the federal government and, upon its own initiative, to identify issues of medical care, research, and education. Dr. Kenneth I. Shine is president of the Institute of Medicine.

The National Research Council was organized by the National Academy of Sciences in 1916 to associate the broad community of science and technology with the Academy's purposes of furthering knowledge and advising the federal government. Functioning in accordance with general policies determined by the Academy, the Council has become the principal operating agency of both the National Academy of Sciences and the National Academy of Engineering in providing services to the government, the public, and the scientific and engineering communities. The Council is administered jointly by both Academies and the Institute of Medicine. Dr. Frank Press and Dr. Robert M. White are chairman and vice chairman, respectively, of the National Research Council.

COMMITTEE ON AIDS RESEARCH AND THE BEHAVIORAL, SOCIAL, AND STATISTICAL SCIENCES

LIAISON REPRESENTATIVES TO THE PANEL FROM THE PUBLIC HEALTH SERVICE

CONSULTANTS TO THE PANEL

GREGORY HEREK, Department of Psychology, University of California, Davis

MARTIN LEVINE, Department of Sociology and Social Psychology, Florida Atlantic University

HARRY MARKS, Institute of the History of Medicine, Johns Hopkins University

CATHERINE O'NEILL, Legal Action Center, New York

RONALD STALL, Center for AIDS Prevention, San Francisco

RAND STONEBURNER, New York City Department of Health

BARBARA VAUGHAN, Office of Population Studies, Princeton University

Acknowledgments

The panel's work was supported primarily by the Public Health Service, U.S. Department of Health and Human Services. We thank the Centers for Disease Control (CDC) for coordinating this support. The Lilly Endowment, Inc., and the Sierra Health Foundation provided funding that enabled the panel to undertake the study of religion and religious groups. We are very grateful to these private foundations for their assistance.

First and foremost I thank my fellow panel members, without whose untiring work and much tried patience this book would not have been possible (see Appendix A for biographical sketches). The list below identifies the panel and staff members who prepared the first drafts of each chapter— and sometimes uncounted subsequent drafts—and those who collaborated with ideas. The first authors wrote the substance of the chapters; the collaborators contributed some language and important ideas. The purpose of this list is to give credit to individuals, but of course the responsibility for the entire text rests with the panel.

1: Albert Jonsen and James Trussell, in collaboration with John Gagnon and Shirley Lindenbaum
2: Ronald Bayer, in collaboration with Mark Smith
3: Mark Smith, in collaboration with Deborah Cotton and Jeff Stryker
4: Deborah Cotton and Allan Brandt
5: Albert Jonsen and Earl Shelp
6: Jeff Stryker, Mark Smith, and Earl Shelp

7: Jeff Stryker

8: David Chambers, in collaboration with Shirley Lindenbaum

9: John Gagnon and Shirley Lindenbaum, in collaboration with Albert Jonsen, Jeff Stryker, and James Trussell

The panel benefited from the collaboration and the advice of many scholars and other people deeply involved in the HIV/AIDS epidemic (see Appendix B). We wish to thank all of them for their generous help.

The panel appreciates the hard work of the staff of the National Research Council. They were indispensable to the administration, research, and editing that went into this report. We thank Charles F. Turner, who was the parent committee's study director, and Jeff Stryker, the panel study director. Heather G. Miller and Susan L. Coyle of the committee staff provided helpful research assistance in the first phase of the panel's activities. Kirsten Johnson and Tracy Brandt were most efficient research and administrative assistants. In the final drafting of the report, Elaine McGarraugh coordinated everyone else as well as managing innumerable manuscript drafts. Eugenia Grohman and consultant Jean Shirhall were excellent editors, and Susanne Stoiber oversaw the completion of the panel's work. On behalf of the panel, I express my sincere gratitude for the staff's work.

Albert R. Jonsen, *Chair*
Panel on Monitoring the
Social Impact of the AIDS Epidemic

Contents

THE SOCIAL IMPACT OF
AIDS
IN THE UNITED STATES

1

Introduction and Summary

An epidemic is both a medical and a social occurrence. Medically, it is the appearance of a serious, often fatal, disease in numbers far greater than normal. Socially, it is an event that disrupts the life of a community and causes uncertainty, fear, blame, and flight. The etymology of the word itself suggests the broader, social meaning: *epi demos*, in ancient Greek, means "upon the people or the community."

The epidemic of acquired immune deficiency syndrome (AIDS)—which was recognized in the United States in 1981, continues today, and will continue into the foreseeable future—mirrors epidemics of the past. The medical meaning of the epidemic has been revealed in the sobering numbers reported in epidemiologic studies. During 1991, 45,506 new AIDS cases were reported to the Centers for Disease Control (CDC), which brought the cumulative total of cases in the United States to 206,392; 133,233 (65 percent) deaths have been tallied (Centers for Disease Control, 1992). It is estimated that 1 million people are currently infected with the human immunodeficiency virus (HIV), which causes AIDS (Centers for Disease Control, 1990), but this number is very uncertain (see Technical Note at the end of this chapter).

These numbers identify the first and most obvious impact of the HIV/AIDS epidemic on American society: the large population of infected, sick, and dying persons attacked by a previously unknown disease. Behind the epidemiologic reports and the statistical estimates lies the social disruption of the epidemic: the destroyed life for which each of the numbers stands and the changed lives of many others touched by the disease. And behind the individual lives are the manifold ways in which a variety of institutions and practices have been affected by the epidemic.

In 1987 the National Research Council of the National Academy of Sciences established the Committee on AIDS Research in the Social, Behavioral, and Statistical Sciences. Two of the committee's reports, *AIDS: Sexual Behavior and Intravenous Drug Use* (Turner, Miller, and Moses, 1989) and *AIDS: The Second Decade* (Miller, Turner, and Moses, 1990), reviewed and evaluated a wide range of social and behavioral science research relevant to HIV/AIDS prevention, education, and intervention. In the course of preparing those reports, the committee noted that many of the social consequences of the epidemic were not being studied in any systematic way. It judged that systematic study would be beneficial in predicting the course of the epidemic's path through U.S. society and in formulating policies to deal with it. Thus, in 1989 the committee established the Panel on Monitoring the Social Impact of the AIDS Epidemic, with the general mandate to study the social impact of the epidemic and to recommend how it could be monitored in order to contribute to the formulation of policies that might effectively deal with it. In the course of its work, the panel, with the agreement of the parent committee and the several federal agencies that were sponsoring its work, modified this mandate and deleted the plan to recommend systems for monitoring.

This report is an unusual undertaking for the National Research Council. Its objective is to form a picture of the effects of the AIDS epidemic on selected social and cultural institutions in the United States and to describe how those institutions have responded to the impact of the epidemic. No attempt has been made to write a comprehensive history—there are not yet adequate studies of the epidemic upon which to base such an effort. Instead we have been selective in looking at those institutions for which sufficient information is available to describe impact and response. These descriptions cannot be considered complete and authoritative; but we do believe they suggest a pattern that should be of concern to the country and command the attention of policy makers attempting to deal with the epidemic over the next decade.

EPIDEMICS, IMPACTS, AND RESPONSES

The impact of AIDS has many dimensions, only a few of which are captured in official statistics or analysis by the research community. The numbers of AIDS cases and HIV infection count as an impact: cumulatively, they state the effect on the population of the United States and on particular subpopulations. Each case has many dimensions—personal, professional, and institutional—through the many social organizations that touch the life of each infected person. Each set of interactions creates an impact, and the diverse impacts have generated equally diverse responses by individuals, groups, and communities.

The panel set out to study these impacts, and it immediately confronted the problem of defining the terms of reference. "Impact" is an overused word that in common parlance has become a synonym for "effect." In this sense, it indicates that one action or state of affairs is caused or influenced by some other action or state of affairs and is used to describe both major and minor effects. Reaching deeper into the language, however, impact has a more powerful meaning—*collision*. In this use of the word, an impact is an effect that radically changes the previous state of affairs or even destroys it.

After much discussion, the panel adopted a definition of impact that fits somewhere between these two meanings. "Impact" as used by the panel describes a concentrated force producing change, a compelling effect. We adopted this hybrid meaning not only because it more accurately describes the impact of AIDS on contemporary America—social institutions have not been destroyed—but because we quickly realized that social impact does not merely destroy; it evokes a reaction or a response. It is more organic than physical. Persons and societies do not merely feel the impact of an event; they remake their lives and institutions to accommodate, negate, or preserve its effects. In this report, we attempt to capture and describe the process of impact and response of selected social institutions to the HIV/AIDS epidemic.

The task of this panel was to go beyond, to the extent possible to limited human vision, the impression of the extraordinary impacts of AIDS on individual lives and on social institutions. We have tried to sort out those that will endure in such a way as to force, or to invite, Americans to take them into account in the next decade. This epidemic is not ordinary in one quite specific way: it can be determined many years in advance of the onset of actual illness in a patient that the illness will come. This epidemic is not, like many historical epidemics, an invasion of morbidity and mortality that rapidly sweeps through a population. It comes and will stay for years, not only in the population, but in the individual people infected, and its presence will often be known to them and to others long before they suffer the disabling, lethal effects. Similarly, rough estimates can be made of the numbers of people who will begin to experience those disabling, lethal effects years from now. Thus, Americans must think about this epidemic for many years into the future.

The institutions we studied appear to have absorbed the impact of AIDS and accommodated to it in a very limited way. However, even a response that is partial and apparently transitory may mark the beginning of more fundamental change. Several of the institutions we studied may follow this trajectory of limited initial response, followed some years later by very significant changes. These longer term responses would be interesting to follow, and we hope that researchers will attempt to do so. However, the panel did not attempt to suggest a methodology for longer term monitoring: the data needs and methods of observation would be very different for the individual institutions studied.

After extensive deliberation, the panel determined that it had sufficient information and understanding to describe social impact and response for six institutions (broadly defined):

- the public health system
- health care finance and delivery
- clinical research and drug regulation
- religion
- voluntary organizations
- the correctional system

These institutions were selected for several reasons: the panel members had the competence to study and evaluate them, we judged that sufficient empirical data and informed opinion existed to formulate our own assessment of impact and response, and they had not been treated in previous reports of the parent committee. The six institutions chosen are very different in structure, degree of centralization, and other dimensions. Such differences affect the level of generalization appropriate to each area.

In the course of our work we also began to see another kind of impact and response—on public policies not necessarily connected to institutions. The HIV/AIDS epidemic has clearly had an impact on policies related to families, and we thus decided to add to our study an examination of two policy areas: issues related to newborns and children and issues related to intimate nonmarital relationships.

Finally, in addition to examining institutional systems as a whole and selected family policies, the panel wanted to look at the impact of HIV/AIDS on communities, where several institutions converge and where the synergy resulting from that convergence is most clearly seen. Originally, three case studies were envisioned: New York, Miami, and Sacramento. We were able to complete only New York—a city that could never be described as typical, but one that does vividly illustrate the impact and response to AIDS among major social institutions.

It is common to find references to the impact of AIDS and HIV. It is also rather common to find such references expressed in quite strong terms. For example, *Milbank Quarterly's* two-volume study, *A Disease of Society: Cultural Responses to AIDS*, opens with these words (Nelkin et al., 1991:1):

> AIDS is no "ordinary" epidemic. More than a devastating disease, it is freighted with profound social and cultural meaning. More than a passing tragedy, it will have long-term, broad-ranging effects on personal relation-

ships, social institutions, and cultural configurations. AIDS is clearly affecting mortality—though in some communities more than others. It is also costly in terms of the resources—both people and money—required for research and medical care. But the effects of the epidemic extend far beyond their medical and economic costs to shape the very ways we organize our individual and collective lives.

It is not clear what an "ordinary" epidemic would be. No epidemic seems ordinary to those who experience it. The AIDS epidemic has invoked comparison with many epidemics of the past. Most commonly, the bubonic plague (the Black Death) that devastated Europe in the fourteenth century is recalled: between 1348 and 1350, some 20 million people, one-third of the population of Europe, died. (Additional tens of millions had died in Asia during the preceding decade [McNeil, 1976].) This epidemic had unquestionable impacts. Historians attribute to it, at least in part, the emergence of nation states, the rise of mercantile economies, and the religious movements that led to the Reformation (Campbell, 1931; McNeil 1976; Tuchman, 1978). As Anna Campbell (1931) noted, the Black Death "changed the minds of men" bringing new ways of understanding God, the meaning of death, the place of tradition, and the role of authority in religious and social life. Changes in the collective mind of a society might be the most profound of all impacts, for the new ideas generated by a major social tragedy can propel institutional change and outlast immediate changes to affect lives far in the future. Difficult though it might be to predict the future import of the present impact of the HIV/AIDS epidemic, one should not shrink from the task, especially when one must plan for that future.

AIDS has been compared with other epidemics, too: the resurgence of bubonic plague in England in the mid-seventeenth century, the cholera epidemics of the nineteenth century, the venereal disease epidemics of the sixteenth century and the early twentieth centuries, and the polio epidemics of the twentieth century (Brandt, 1988; Risse, 1988; Slack, 1988). AIDS has its analogies to each of these epidemics—number of deaths, methods of prevention, stigmatization of sufferers and presumed carriers, and responses of authorities—all can be compared in general or in detail. The comparisons are often illuminating, but sometimes misleading (Fee and Fox, 1988). It can be said with some assurance, however, that none of the historical epidemics was "ordinary." Each had impacts that struck its sufferers and subsequent commentators as "extraordinary."

The comparison with epidemics of the past invokes the features that are remembered about those plagues. They have, in this respect, had an impact on history or, as Campbell wrote (1931), "on the minds of men." They also left social institutions that sometimes affect present-day thinking about the AIDS epidemic: cholera, for example, left a public health approach to epidemic disease that stressed quarantine; venereal diseases gave rise to the public health approach of contact tracing. These established public health practices have had to be reconsidered in the current epidemic. Many of the prominent, even dramatic impacts of past epidemics, however, have so melded into the social fabric that people are often astonished to hear of them today, and some, interesting though they be, seem of little relevance to the current problem. For example, to attribute the existence of Protestant Christianity to the effects of the Black Death on religious ideas and sentiments has little influence on the ways in which people today think about religion or about epidemics. Similarly, to attribute the existence of Canada as an independent nation to the fact that British troops had been vaccinated against smallpox before the Battle of Quebec, but American troops were decimated by the disease, is certainly to point to an effect of epidemic and, indeed, an impact. Yet that impact has been of little relevance to subsequent citizens and governments, except that "some Canadians to this day worship smallpox as the deliverer from United States citizenship" (Foege, 1988:332).

Many features of epidemics are no longer remembered and have left little imprint on the societies that they ravished for a time. Indeed, one of the greatest of epidemics, the influenza of 1918-1920, has been called by its historian "the forgotten epidemic" (Crosby, 1989). Worldwide, perhaps 30 million people died; in the United States, 675,000 people died, most of whom were not the usual victims of influenza (the very old, infants, and children), but men and women in their 20s and 30s. This terrible scourge might have had a great impact, but it passed and left almost no mark on the social institutions and practices of the time. Many people were mourned, but life quickly returned to normal. Even the absence of impact has a lesson for this study: it is possible that many of the effects currently taken as important and lasting will pass or be absorbed into the course of American life and culture. It is not entirely clear how confidently one should accept the words of *Milbank* editors Nelkin, Willis, and Parris (1991:1,2):

> More than a passing tragedy, it [AIDS] will have long-term, broad-ranging effects on personal relationships, social institutions, and cultural configurations . . . AIDS will reshape many aspects of society, its norms and values, its interpersonal relationships and its cultural representations . . . the future will be different from both the past and the present.

Our report suggests that, in some respects, the AIDS epidemic may be more like the influenza of 1918 than the bubonic plague of 1348: many of its most striking features will be absorbed in the flow of American life, but, hidden beneath the surface, its worst effects will continue to devastate the lives and cultures of certain communities.

GENERAL FINDINGS AND CONCLUSIONS

Historically, certain epidemics have done great damage to social institutions: the Black Death in a 3-year sweep through Europe wiped out enough laborers to cause a major restructuring of the economy of the continent. The HIV/AIDS epidemic, although often compared to the Black Death, has not affected U.S. social institutions to any such extent. Although it had by the end of 1991 infected perhaps 1 million people, brought devastating sickness to 206,392, and death to 133,233, it had not significantly altered the structures or directions of the social institutions that we studied. Many of the responses have been ad hoc and may be reversed when pressures subside. Others may be more lasting, but only because they reinforced or accelerated changes already latent or budding within the institutions.

It is the panel's opinion that the limited responsiveness of institutions can in part be explained because the absolute numbers of the epidemic, relative to the U.S. population, are not overwhelming, and because U.S. social institutions are strong, complex, and resilient. However, we believe that another major reason for this limited response is the concentration of the epidemic in socially marginalized groups. The convergence of evidence shows that the HIV/AIDS epidemic is settling into spatially and socially isolated groups and possibly becoming endemic within them. Many observers have recently commented that, instead of spreading out to the broad American population, as was once feared, HIV is concentrating in pools of persons who are also caught in the "synergism of plagues" (see Wallace, 1988): poverty, poor health and lack of health care, inadequate education, joblessness, hopelessness, and social disintegration converge to ravage personal and social life. These coexisting conditions foster and aggravate HIV infection and AIDS. Our study of New York City (see Chapter 9) illustrates this dramatically for one epicenter of the epidemic. We believe that the patterns shown there are repeated throughout the country: many geographical areas and strata of the population are virtually untouched by the epidemic and probably never will be; certain confined areas and populations have been devastated and are likely to continue to be.

This epidemiological direction reveals the disconcerting implications of our major conclusion. The institutions that we studied are particularly weak at those points at which the epidemic is likely to be most destructive. For example, the health care system, which responded to the appearance of a new disease with some alacrity, is weakest organizationally and economically in those places where the affected populations are concentrated. The problems of caring for those who are infected are magnified by the particular configuration of the U.S. health care system, which emphasizes to a greater extent than other developed countries private insurance and ability-to-pay criteria. Providers, hospitals, and public health mechanisms can and have responded to a flood of patients with AIDS, but those responses were most successful where health care was better organized and financed and where the populations to be served had sufficient knowledge to understand the disease and its modes of transmission and were capable of organizing themselves in ways that supported and supplemented the health care system.

Thus, our most general conclusion about the epidemic is that its impact has hit institutions hardest where they are weakest: serving the most disadvantaged people in U.S. society. Predictions of the imminent collapse of the health care system due to the epidemic, for example, now look shrill, but, conversely, hopes that the epidemic would force the country toward more rational and equitable reform of the system now also seem unrealistic. In the panel's judgment, the HIV/AIDS epidemic has effected many transient changes in the institutions that we studied and relatively few changes that we expect to be permanent. Among the more permanent, however, two are particularly noteworthy.

First, the institutions of public health, of health care delivery, and of scientific research have become more responsive to cooperation and collaboration with "outsiders." Policies and practices have been modified in these three institutions under pressure from and in collaboration with those who are affected by the epidemic and their advocates. Many of these changes are positive and will contribute to the efficiency and efficacy of the institutions. Similarly, volunteer organizations stimulated by the challenge of the epidemic have discovered ways not only of supplying help where extant institutions were lacking, they have also influenced the policies and practices of those institutions.

Second, even in institutions with very defined purposes and strong constraints—institutions as different as religious groups and correctional agencies—the response to the epidemic has reflected awareness of the scientific realities, as well as the social implications, of HIV/AIDS. Traditionally based doctrinal constraints in the case of religious groups and the stringent requirements of civil punishment in the case of correctional agencies are powerful forces that could and did dictate rigid and narrow response. Yet, powerful as those forces were, they did not negate more reflective responses that contributed to containment of the epidemic and respected the rights of individuals. We are concerned, however, that as the epidemic strikes with greater force in socially and economically deprived communities, the directions toward more communal involvement and respect for civil and personal liberties might be constricted and diverted.

The panel believes that a failure by scientists and policy makers to appreciate the interaction between social, economic, and cultural conditions and the propagation of HIV/AIDS disease has often led to public misunderstanding and policy mistakes about the epidemic. Although in the beginning of the epidemic, gay life and behavior were certainly at the center of attention, even then they were noted primarily as "modes of transmission" and not as social contexts in which the disease had particular meanings around which strong forces for care, prevention, and political action could rally. Similarly, intravenous drug use was understood as a social behavior that could transmit infection, but its place in a matrix of social, cultural, and economic conditions was ignored.

A constant theme of this report and of the AIDS literature is the stigma, discrimination, and inequalities of the AIDS epidemic. At its outset, HIV disease settled among socially disvalued groups, and as the epidemic has progressed, AIDS has increasingly been an affliction of people who have little economic, political, and social power. In this sense, AIDS is an undemocratic affliction. In "democratic epidemics" (Arras, 1988), communicable illnesses cut across class, racial, and ethnic lines and threatens the community at large. In traditional societies with limited medical knowledge and technology, epidemics fall on most, if not all, of the people. In the modern world, particularly in industrial societies, inequalities in morbidity and mortality are often more social than biological phenomena. With HIV/AIDS, the concentration of the epidemic from its beginnings was among those who were, for a variety of reasons, members of marginalized social groups. In this case, the biology of viral transmission matched existing social inequalities and resulted in an unequal concentration of HIV/AIDS in certain regions and among certain populations (see Grmek, 1990). This pattern has created tension between the social and geographical localization of the epidemic and the need to mobilize resources to deal with the epidemic from among individuals, groups, and institutions that are removed from the social groups that are at the epicenter of the epidemic. As the epidemic becomes endemic in already deprived and segregated populations, this tension will be intensified.

If the current pattern of the epidemic holds, U.S. society at large will have been able to wait out the primary impact of the epidemic even though the crisis period will have stretched out over 15 years. HIV/AIDS will "disappear," not because, like smallpox, it has been eliminated, but because those who continue to be affected by it are socially invisible, beyond the sight and attention of the majority population.

SPECIFIC FINDINGS AND CONCLUSIONS

Public Health

The public health systems of the country—federal, state and local—absorbed the first shock of the AIDS epidemic and have remained at the forefront of research and policy development. Because of the increasing concentration of the epidemic in low-income and minority communities, the public health system at the local level has become the primary service provider for a large proportion of people with HIV disease or AIDS. Nowhere is this more apparent than in New York City.

HIV/AIDS challenged the public health community to set aside many of its traditional policies and practices for the containment of infectious disease. Quarantine, mass mandatory testing, and contact tracing all had notable disadvantages in dealing with a disease with a long latency period, that was spread chiefly through sexual activity or intravenous drug use, and that largely affected already stigmatized groups. Spokesmen for the affected groups, particularly the gay community, advanced other methods of containment that relied on community education and voluntary anonymous testing. This came to be know as an "exceptionalist" approach since it differed from responses to prior epidemics. However, mass education and other approaches to behavior modification were already emerging as the public health strategy of choice for substance abuse prevention, smoking, and behavioral disorders. Thus, HIV/AIDS accelerated the adoption of these approaches and invited their intensive application to an infectious disease. It also created a political environment that compelled the public health community to negotiate containment strategies with the population that was initially primarily infected—gay men.

As the second decade of the epidemic begins, some aspects of the exceptionalist approach are being reexamined and abandoned. More traditional public health methods are being reintroduced, although in forms modified by the experience of the first decade. The change is due in part to the availability of early treatment, which to infected individuals makes early identification more useful. It may also be the result of the steady shift of the epidemic itself into populations that are less politically potent than the gay community, primarily intravenous drug users and their sexual partners.

Overall, the impact of the epidemic on the public health system has been pervasive: it has prompted a critical examination of traditional responses to epidemics of infectious disease, challenged the public health community to devise more effective strategies for promoting behavioral change, and, because of the sheer size of the HIV/AIDS-related activities profoundly influenced the public's perception of the public health systems. HIV/AIDS has also increased the range of clinical responsibilities of public health agencies and further strained already burdened resources. In many cities, this has resulted in the neglect of traditional areas of public health activities such as sexually transmitted disease and tuberculosis.

The inextricable link between HIV disease and other diseases and conditions prevalent in poor populations (e.g., drug addiction, tuberculosis, and sexually transmitted diseases) means that public health providers will face even greater challenges as the HIV/AIDS epidemic unfolds in the 1990s. The newer views and practices of public health may revert into more traditional ways as the epidemic settles in communities where the newer techniques are more difficult to implement. The epidemic thus presents an opportunity and a challenge for the revitalization of the practice of public health, both with regard to infectious conditions and the chronic disorders that represent so much of the task of public health in the United States today.

Health Care

The HIV/AIDS epidemic has sent more than 200,000 patients into that system over the last decade and may, in this decade, send up to 1 million more. A substantial proportion of these patients are drawn from the pool of the uninsured or patients who rapidly exhaust their insurance benefits due to job loss or benefit restrictions. The people who became HIV/AIDS patients challenged the provider community on a number of fronts: they were generally young and previously healthy people who engaged in life styles that affronted many in the provider community. Before the modes of transmission were well understood, many health care personnel feared contact with AIDS patients, and both hospitals and private physicians struggled with unfamiliar problems of how to provide sensitive and responsive care while preserving the privacy of AIDS patients and protecting staff and other patients from infection. These problems have been complicated by the fact that many AIDS patients cannot pay for care, and thus the subset of the health care delivery system that provides care to indigent patients has absorbed the brunt of the epidemic. In the handful of cities that are the focus of the epidemic, there is a serious strain on the provider community, particularly public and voluntary teaching hospitals; in other cities, the capacity of hospitals to absorb AIDS inpatients is not as pressing a concern as are the stigma and inadequate reimbursement associated with AIDS care.

The complexity of the disease remains another major challenge for the provision of services. HIV disease attacks virtually every organ system of the body. The diverse and uncoordinated nature of the U.S. health system—reinforced by the reimbursement practices of the multiple plans that pay for care—has been often criticized for its failure to provide comprehensive, coordinated primary care and for too great a reliance on specialists and subspecialists. And it is just such comprehensive, primary care that is necessary to cope with a disease that is chronic and disabling and not limited to any one organ system. The urgent need for coordinated community-based care for AIDS patients has pushed the development of improved case management approaches.

AIDS has influenced health care providers in both direct and subtle ways. The specialty of infectious disease has enjoyed a renaissance and is now viewed as one of the few shortage medical specialties. Concern is growing, however, that the burden of the epidemic may further dissuade young physicians from entering specialties such as internal medicine or from practicing in a geographic location where the burden of caring for patients with HIV disease is perceived to be high. The care of AIDS patients in terminal stages of the disease falls very heavily on hospital-based nurses. Like the practice of oncology nursing, it is an emotionally as well as professionally demanding experience. It is impossible to assess the extent to which the HIV/AIDS epidemic has exacerbated staffing problems in hospitals and other institutional settings that care for AIDS patients; however, a shortage of nurses has been identified as a major obstacle to improved care of AIDS patients.

All health professionals are at risk of HIV infection through exposure by accidental cuts or punctures incurred while caring for HIV-infected patients. Procedures adopted to protect health care workers from accidental infection (universal precautions) are designed to avoid exposure to blood and body fluids regardless of whether patients or health care workers are believed to be infected. The techniques and behaviors in the health care setting that must be modified to reduce HIV transmission risks, however, may be as difficult to change as risky sexual behavior and drug-use habits. Health care procedures are learned behaviors and habits of years duration. The risk of transmission from patients to providers has been overshadowed in public attention by the extremely minor risk of transmission from providers to patients.

These and other considerations have made AIDS the most profound challenge to the care of patients that has faced the health care provider community in modern times. A substantial proportion of physicians avoid caring for patients with HIV disease or AIDS. This avoidance or outright refusal may result in a broad range of harm: in addition to leaving some patients without needed care, it stigmatizes patients and adds to the considerable psychological burdens of living with the disease. The avoidance or refusal also increases the risk for health care professionals who remain willing to treat patients and hence assume a disproportionate burden of the HIV/AIDS epidemic.

AIDS has challenged the economic arrangements of the health care system in many ways. Most visible, perhaps, has been the conflict over access to new drugs and a "fair price" for new therapeutic agents. The introduction of universal precautions in hospitals has significantly increased the demand for barrier protection and hence the cost of hospitalization for all patients. The HIV/AIDS epidemic has also expanded fissures already present in the health insurance system: the expense of the disease has caused insurance firms to use all available markers to avoid enrolling AIDS patients; and group plans have in many cases been modified to exclude the cost of AIDS treatments. As providers struggle to cope with uninsured patients, and patients struggle to pay for drugs and services they need, another voice has been added to the call for a comprehensive solution to the problem of health care financing.

Clinical Research and Drug Regulation

In perhaps no other area has the impact of the HIV/AIDS epidemic been more clear than in the identification, clinical testing, and regulation of new drugs and in the conduct of clinical research. The most profound change wrought by AIDS in drug development is simply the dramatic increase in public awareness of the nature, structure, and purpose of clinical trials. Debate about the ethics and scientific validity of clinical trials occurs not only among physicians, statisticians, and ethicists, but also among patients, activists, and politicians. AIDS has to a large degree publicized and politicized the aspects of clinical investigation that were heretofore largely within the private purview of the scientific community.

The modern history of clinical research and drug development shows that the interplay of politics, science, and ethics must be recognized as an ongoing dynamic during the twentieth century. The systems have been influenced by AIDS, but the effect has been more to accelerate change that was building in the system rather than to introduce fundamentally new concepts. The introduction of a parallel track model in clinical research and drug regulation in clinical trials is perhaps the most disquieting of the AIDS-related changes to the scientific community, since both the purposes and the procedures lack clarity or consensus. Pressure to expand clinical trials into community-based physicians' practices has similarly posed difficult questions of how to organize and support such trials, what results can realistically be expected from them, and how to distinguish between ad hoc extensions of experimental therapies into community practice and clinical research that produces replicable results. Although these questions were thrust on the research community by the HIV/AIDS epidemic, they will quickly become relevant to many other fields of research as increasing numbers of patients and their advocates seek access to the newest therapies.

HIV/AIDS has similarly challenged the traditional mode of scientific communication through peer-reviewed journals. That review process by scientific peers is time consuming, and the combination of review time and queuing for a place in the journals may result in long lag times between submission of a manuscript and publication. The cumbersome nature of the system has been accepted until now because of the safeguards it offers for objective assessment of the accuracy and relevance of research findings. AIDS, however, surfaced widespread objections to the delayed publication of research that appears to show a significant therapeutic benefit for serious diseases or that demonstrates a previously unknown toxicity of an accepted therapy. HIV/AIDS studies have not been the only ones in which disclosure before publication has occurred, but the intervention of AIDS activists has thrust the dilemma more squarely into the spotlight. The scientific community is grappling with the difficult problems of how to implement a more pragmatic yet still responsible approach to traditional peer review.

Although it is impossible at this time in the epidemic to reach any definitive conclusions about the impact of AIDS on clinical research and the regulation of new drugs, it is apparent that patient activism and the exigencies of the AIDS epidemic have generated the most significant re-evaluation of the research and regulation process to occur since World War II.

Voluntary and Community-Based Organizations

Government at all levels was slow to respond to the HIV/AIDS epidemic. The slow response was due partly to a general reduction in the growth of public spending on health care and social welfare and partly to a unique attribute of AIDS: its early association with two highly stigmatized minorities—gay men and intravenous drug users. When governments did respond, their flexibility and capacity to reach the groups in greatest need were limited, especially in regard to prevention education, for which there were constraints on how public monies could be used.

The vacuum was filled very early by an outpouring of volunteer activity. This was in part the result of the pulling together of the gay community in the belief that its members could best care for their own. The movement is also illustrative, however, of collective behavior in a period of social change and the forces that motivate individuals to volunteer their time. The response and mobilization of AIDS volunteers sheds light on the commitments individuals are willing to make to different kinds of social causes and it also points to new directions for understanding the meaning of volunteer work. In both San Francisco and New York, the AIDS crisis catalyzed volunteer movements that spanned both individual helping activities and strategic political campaigns. Particularly in San Francisco, the movement was innovative, effective, and enormously important in helping the gay community come to terms with the epidemic, as well as in shaping the response of the city's institutions to it.

Throughout the country, volunteer movements have carried a surprisingly large share of the burden of caring for AIDS patients, particularly outside hospitals. The cost of the epidemic for public agencies and private insurance has been significantly reduced by the extensive contributions of time and resources from volunteers. In addition, advocacy for appropriate social policies that would both contain the epidemic and protect the rights of affected individuals came from community-based organizations. At present, this powerful force has been weakened somewhat by financial constraints, burnout, and bureaucratization. There is also doubt that the ethos of volunteering will provide the same benefits to the economically and socially deprived communities, in which the epidemic is increasingly centered, as it has to the gay communities in which it was first identified.

Religion and Religious Groups

Religion, manifested in personal belief and in organized denominations, is a large part of American life. The responses of major religious denominations and of religiously identified individuals to HIV/AIDS have been an important feature of the epidemic: from the beginning, HIV/AIDS has evoked a response from religious groups and from persons who identify themselves with the beliefs of those groups. Some adherents of Christianity linked early church traditions that saw plague as a divine punishment for sinfulness in general with the single sin of male homosexuality. Even though the roots of this association in early Christian doctrine have been forgotten by most modern Christians, this ancient association seems to echo in the collective memory of those who are ready to view AIDS as divine punishment visited on homosexuals. As it became evident that the infection touched others as well, that position became more difficult to maintain, but it has not been wholly abandoned.

From time immemorial, religious tradition and teaching have had a place for pestilential disease. This new pestilence, however, arrives at a time when religious and theological beliefs and practices are different in many ways from what they were in the past. They are more diverse, for religious traditions have separated into many branches. In addition, the relation between theological and scientific understanding is more complex; even those who believe that divine causality stands behind the events of the world do not always see that relationship in a direct, unambiguous way. Thus, today, religions have reacted to the HIV/AIDS epidemic in a complex way. They have almost inevitably done so with some reference to the powerful beliefs of the past, but also with the more subtle and nuanced interpretations of the present.

The religious response has generally involved censure of the behaviors, particularly the sexual behaviors, that were implicated in the spread of the disease and, to some extent, also criticized the degree of frankness that public health educators and activists have advocated in education. On these grounds, religion has been indicated as obstructionist about the epidemic. Yet many churches have engaged in extensive programs for the care and support of persons with AIDS and have, within their doctrinal limits, become active educators about the epidemic with regard to both discrimination and prevention. The response of religious groups to the epidemic is, of course, defined by the doctrinal commitments of the various faiths, as well as by the attitudes of their congregations.

Because of the role of religious institutions in U.S. society, as well as the large number of people who identify with some religious group in the United States, it is important to elucidate the role that religious organizations have played in the epidemic and to understand the importance of taking their response into account in efforts to understand the impact of AIDS in American society. Overall, as the second decade of the epidemic begins, religious organizations have only begun to contribute to efforts to contain the epidemic or to deal with some of the social issues that surround it.

Correctional Systems

Approximately 1 million individuals are currently confined in prisons and local jails in the United States—426 out of every 100,000 residents. They are disproportionately black men, for whom the rate is 3,109 per 100,000. Since the beginning of the HIV/AIDS epidemic, the population in federal prisons and in prisons in the District of Columbia and 18 states has doubled. In California and New Jersey, two states hit particularly hard by the epidemic, the number of inmates tripled during the same period. The incarcerated population in the United States comprises in large part impoverished individuals from urban areas. Almost one-half of all prisoners are black. Not only are the majority of prisoners members of racial and ethnic minority groups, they are also overwhelmingly poor.

As the nation's prison population has burgeoned, so too has the population of inmates with HIV disease. The seroprevalence status of all inmates is not known, but it is certainly highly variable by region. In New York State prisons, approximately 17-20 percent of prisoners are HIV positive, which is probably the high end of the distribution. The question of whether to screen inmates for HIV antibodies has arisen with particular urgency in the prison setting, with no general resolution.

The question of whether to segregate HIV-positive inmates has been answered variously in different prison systems. In addition to concerns about transmission through forced or consensual sex, much attention has been paid to highly unlikely modes of transmission—casual contact or assaultive behaviors by HIV-positive inmates. Other potential mechanisms of disease spread are unique to prison culture and difficult to evaluate. At least 20 state prisons segregate all prisoners with AIDS, 8 segregate those with AIDS-related complex, and 6 segregate inmates who are HIV positive but not symptomatic. Segregation decisions have been justified on the grounds of inmate security, reducing the risk of transmission, or availability of specialized services. However, there is also widespread evidence that segregation is harmful, denying prisoners access to a range of services and exposing them to additional stigma and likelihood of assault. Most prison systems have instituted HIV prevention education programs for inmates and staff.

Prisons have found it difficult to respond to the health care needs of inmates with AIDS. In most cases, funds for HIV care in prisons must come from corrections systems budgets that are already strained almost beyond the breaking point. In New York State, for example, two thirds of the correctional system's health care budget of approximately $100 million is earmarked for HIV/AIDS care. AIDS tests the limits of prison health care because treatments tend to be expensive and difficult to deliver. In some jurisdictions the impact of AIDS is causing prison officials to reconsider how prison health care is delivered and paid for and to look at new ways to attract and retain quality medical staff.

One of the most significant impacts of HIV disease in correctional facilities may be a sea change in the way epidemiological and clinical research involving prisoners is viewed. Regulations adopted to protect prisoners from exploitation at the hands of drug companies or clinical investigators are now being looked at in an entirely different light when they may block prisoners from receiving experimental treatments.

Public Policies on Children and Families

When the HIV/AIDS epidemic began, law and policy about families and intimate relationships were in transition, as they still are, and the epidemic has raised difficult questions. For example, because AIDS can be transmitted perinatally, public policies regarding the relationships between mothers and their fetuses and the care of sick children without maternal or family support had to be reconsidered. Because HIV/AIDS often affects people living in unconventional relationships, issues of health insurance, inheritance, and housing and health decisions—which are usually linked to conventional family structures—called for reexamination.

Social policy regarding family relationships is complex: specific law encodes certain features of policy, but much is embedded in practices formulated by public agencies, employers, and insurers—practices that sometimes lead to litigation. Convinced of the importance of examining the impact of the epidemic on policies regarding families and children, yet aware of their extreme complexity, the panel undertook two case studies of the interaction between the epidemic, law, and public policy. The first study examined issues of parental authority and foster parenting in Miami and New York. The second study examined how the legal definition of familial relationships evolved in two political and legislative controversies, in San Francisco and New York.

Proposals for the mandatory testing of all newborns or of all pregnant women have raised long-standing disputes about public health needs and individual privacy and about the needs or rights of children as they may conflict with the rights of parents. Similarly, issues involved in caring for HIV-infected children or enrolling them in clinical trials of experimental therapies has starkly highlighted continuing arguments over the rights of biological parents versus the rights of foster parents or the state. In both cases, our study showed that there has as yet been no fundamental changes in broad policies, only changes in the clinical care and social services in certain communities. The rights of biological parents—regardless of their own degree of illness or ability to care for their children—have rarely been overridden in deciding on what will happen to their children.

There have been significant changes in the legal recognition of unmarried couples in some communities in recent years, but those changes were under way before the HIV/AIDS epidemic began, and it is impossible to determine exactly what role the epidemic played in bringing them about. In San Francisco, a domestic partnership ordinance was enacted in 1990, after failures in 1982 and 1989. It seems likely that the epidemic—and the increased organization among the gay and lesbian community in its wake—contributed to its passage. Similarly in New York, changes in the definition of "family" in relation to housing rights were, similarly, probably in part a result of effects of the HIV/AIDS epidemic.

In general, as the epidemic begins to center on economically and socially deprived communities, children will be increasingly affected. Born to infected mothers, they will be in need of special care and attention from their births. Some mothers die soon after their children's births, and many others are unable or unwilling, for financial and health reasons, to care for their children. In several cities where the problems are already noticeable, serious efforts have been made to meet those challenges. Still, those efforts reveal the basic tensions, inconsistencies, and anomalies in family policies that will need to be resolved as the epidemic becomes more endemic in those cities.

The epidemic first attacked the population of gay men. Such men have had to live outside the range of social policies that favored heterosexual couples joined in legal marriage and thus were often deprived of insurance, tax and inheritance benefits, and other legal rights and protections accorded to married couples. At the same time, gay men often are joined in enduring relationships and, in those relationships, often provide support and care to their ill partners. The effort to gain some social and legal recognition of those partnerships, already growing before the HIV/AIDS epidemic, was given some impetus by the epidemic. Questions about appropriate legal definitions of familial relationships will continue to be raised at least as long as the epidemic continues.

New York City

The panel examined the case of New York City—recognizing its atypicality—for the purpose of examining how the institutions we examined in the national context have been affected by and responded to the epidemic in a specific place. The objective was to improve understanding as well as call attention to the localized dimensions of the HIV/AIDS epidemic.

Much of the attention given to the epidemic has focused on national estimates and national needs. Ultimately, however, the epidemic and its impacts and the responses to it are experienced in specific locales, and responses are shaped by the resources, traditions, and leadership of the specific communities. The New York City study makes particularly clear the panel's major findings and conclusions in the context of specific local institutions and their management of issues presented by the epidemic. HIV disease in New York City occurs increasingly in the context of socioeconomic and ethnic deprivation, as well as among populations already suffering high levels of morbidity and mortality. The panel believes that this is a preview of the future of the epidemic in the country as a whole.

TECHNICAL NOTE

It is instructive to review briefly the procedures for estimating HIV incidence and prevalence to gain an understanding of the basis for the current uncertainty regarding the size of the epidemic and its prevalence among specific population groups. Given that there are no nationally representative seroprevalence surveys, the incidence and prevalence of HIV infection must be inferred from the reported cases of AIDS. New AIDS cases at time t result from infections acquired over a considerable period before that time. Suppose that the incubation distribution of duration from infection to AIDS is denoted by $I(d)$ and that the number of new HIV infections at time t is denoted by $H(t)$. Then the number of new AIDS cases at time t, $A(t)$, is given by the equation

$$A(t) = \int_0^{\omega} H(t - d) \times I(d)\, dd \tag{1}$$

where ω is the maximum incubation period. Although this equation may appear complicated to those without training in mathematics, the concept underlying it is quite simple: the number of new AIDS cases in the current year, for example, is the sum of the number of new infections last year times the fraction of infections that are manifested in AIDS 1 year later, the number of new infections 2 years ago times the fraction of infections that are manifested in AIDS 2 years later, and so forth.

What one observes, of course, is only the time series $A(t)$. One needs to invert the equation to estimate $H(t)$, the time series of new infections. It is well known that without knowledge of $I(d)$—the fraction of infections that progress to AIDS at each duration d since infection—there is no unique solution for $H(t)$; in fact, there are infinitely many combinations of $H(t)$ and $I(t)$ that satisfy equation (1). Therefore, to make progress, one must obtain external knowledge of $I(d)$. Estimates of the incubation distribution can be derived only from individuals whose date of infection is known. The most reliable data come from cohort studies of hemophiliacs and homosexual men (Brookmeyer, 1991). Note that these data provide information only on the waiting time from *seroconversion* to AIDS. The time from infection to seroconversion is assumed to be from 3 to 6 months, although seroconversion in some individuals is apparently much longer. The result is that if $I(d)$ is taken from these studies, then the resulting estimates of $H(t)$ pertain to seroconversions, not infections. In any event, one clear source of uncertainty in the estimates of $H(t)$ is the degree to which the $I(d)$ distribution obtained from either of these sources is applicable to the larger population of infected persons.

Assume that $I(d)$ is known. A very simple model will illustrate both the principles and the problems involved in recovering $H(t)$ through a procedure known as back-projection. Suppose it is known that of all HIV infections acquired in year t, 20 percent will progress to AIDS in year $t+2$, 30 percent in year $t+3$, and 50 percent in year $t+4$. Suppose that 1980 is the first year in which AIDS cases appear. It follows that these can have resulted only from infections in 1978, since if there had been infections in 1977, there would have been AIDS cases in 1979. Suppose that one observes 100 AIDS cases in 1980, 400 in 1981, and 1,000 in 1982. One can then solve the following three equations for the three unknowns,

$$
\begin{aligned}
100 &= A_{80} = .2H_{78} \, , \\
400 &= A_{81} = .2H_{79} + .3H_{78} \, , \text{ and} \\
1{,}000 &= A_{82} = .2H_{80} + .3H_{79} + .5H_{78} \, ,
\end{aligned}
\tag{2}
$$

to obtain $H_{78} = 500$, $H_{79} = 1{,}250$, and $H_{80} = 1{,}875$. Thus, the prevalence of HIV infection in 1978 is 500, in 1979 is 1,750 (500 + 1,250) (minus any who have died of AIDS), and in 1980 is 3,625 (500 + 1,250 + 1,875) (minus any who have died of AIDS). Note that even at the end of 1982, one cannot obtain any estimate of the number of new infections in 1981 or 1982 since there is at least a 2-year delay between infection and AIDS. In order to get an estimate of H_{81} and H_{82} before the end of 1984, one must forecast A_{83} and A_{84} by extrapolating the prior time series of new AIDS cases or directly forecast H_{81} and H_{82} by extrapolating the estimated prior time series of new HIV infections.

This simple model can be used to identify three sources of uncertainty in the estimates of HIV incidence and prevalence (Centers for Disease Control, 1990):

(1) Estimates of new HIV infections for very recent periods are less likely to be accurate than estimates for the more distant past.

(2) It is likely that the incubation distribution $I(d)$ has changed over time as new therapies have been introduced for people who are HIV positive but are asymptomatic. In addition, changes over time in the stage of infection at which infected peole are diagnosed would include changes in $I(d)$. Furthermore, there is uncertainty about whether the $I(d)$ distributions obtained from cohort studies of homosexual men or hemophiliacs accurately reflect the $I(d)$ distribution for all infected people.

(3) The time series of CDC counts of AIDS cases is not the time series of new AIDS cases, for two reasons. First, the case definition of AIDS has been expanded twice (in 1985 and 1987); consequently, the growth in AIDS cases is exaggerated. Second, there are delays from the time of diagnosis to the time a case is reported to the CDC. These delays would result in counts of diagnosed cases that are increasingly less complete as one moves from the past to the present. Some cases are never reported; these can be regarded as cases with infinite delays in reporting. The CDC estimates that its surveillance system identifies 70-90 percent of HIV-infection-related deaths and that it therefore provides a minimum estimate of HIV-infection-related mortality (Centers for Disease Control, 1991). Consequently, CDC counts must first be corrected for the changes in the case definition and for reporting delays before they can be used. Reporting delays may have changed over time, imparting further uncertainty into the corrected series, A_t (Harris, 1990).

REFERENCES

Arras, J.D. (1988) The fragile web of responsibility: AIDS and the duty to treat. *Hastings Center Report* 8(Suppl.):10-20.

Brandt, A.M. (1988) AIDS and metaphor: toward the social meaning of epidemic disease. *Social Research* 55:413-432.

Brookmeyer, R. (1991) Reconstriuction and future trends of the AIDS epidemic in the United States. *Science* 253:37-42.

Campbell, A.M. (1931) *The Black Death and Men of Learning.* New York: Columbia University Press.

Centers for Disease Control (CDC) (1990) HIV prevalence and AIDS case projections for the United States: report based on a workshop. *Morbidity and Mortality Weekly Report* 39:(RR-16):1-31.

Centers for Disease Control (CDC) (1991) Mortality attributable to HIV infection/AIDS— United States, 1981-1990. *Morbidity and Mortality Weekly Report* 40:41-46.

Centers for Disease Control (CDC) (1992) *HIV/AIDS Surveillance Report.* Atlanta, Ga.: Centers for Disease Control.

Crosby, A.W. (1989) *Epidemic and Peace, 1918: America's Forgotten Pandemic.* New York: Cambridge University Press.

Fee, E., and D. Fox (1988) *AIDS: The Burdens of History.* Berkeley, Calif.: University of California Press.

Foege, W.H. (1988) Plagues: perceptions of risk and social responses. *Social Research* 55:331-342.

Grmek, M.D. (1990) *The History of AIDS: Emergence and Origin of a Modern Pandemic.* Princeton, N.J.: Princeton University Press.

Harris, J. (1990) Reporting delays and the incidence of AIDS. *Journal of the American Statistical Association* 85:915-924.

McNeil, W.H. (1976) *Plagues and Peoples.* New York: Doubleday.

Miller, H.G., C.F. Turner, and L.E. Moses, eds. (1990) *AIDS: The Second Decade.* Committee on AIDS Research and the Behavioral, Social, and Statistical Sciences, Commission on Behavior and Social Sciences and Education, National Research Council. Washington, D.C.: National Academy Press.

Nelkin, D., D.P. Willis, and S.V. Parris (1991) Introduction. In D. Nelkin, D.P. Willis, and S.V. Parris, eds., *A Disease of Society: Cultural Responses to AIDS.* New York: Cambridge University Press.

Risse, G.B. (1988) Epidemics and history: ecological perspectives and social responses. In E. Fee and D.M. Fox, eds., *AIDS: The Burdens of History.* Berkeley, Calif.: University of California Press.

Slack, P. (1988) Responses to plague in early modern Europe: the implications of public health. *Social Research* 55:433-453.

Tuchman, B. (1978) *A Distant Mirror. The Calamitous 14th Century.* New York: Knopf.

Turner, C.F., H.G. Miller, and L.E. Moses, eds. (1989) *AIDS: Sexual Behavior and Intravenous Drug Use.* Committee on AIDS Research and the Behavioral, Social, and Statistical Sciences, Commission on Behavioral and Social Sciences and Education, National Research Council. Washington, D.C.: National Academy Press.

Wallace, R. (1988) A synergism of plagues: "planned shrinkage," contagious housing destruction and AIDS in the Bronx. *Environmental Research* 47:1-33.

2

The Practice of Public Health

The practice of public health in the United States is more strongly influenced by the federal character of the U.S. system than is almost any other aspect of the health care system. State governments have the primary responsibility for public health: each state and territory has a chief public health officer, a public health department, and a system of county and city health departments with links to the state system. The authorities and responsibilities of the state and territorial health officers vary, but all share a common mission of protecting the public against various types of infectious or communicable diseases. A number of states have strong traditions of providing primary health care services to low-income populations through county and city health facilities. At the federal level, the Centers for Disease Control (CDC, part of the U.S. Department of Health and Human Services) has responsibility for monitoring communicable diseases, many chronic diseases, and occupational disorders, as well as threats to public health that have been only recently recognized as being in the domain of the health care system, such as prevention of violence and accidents. CDC maintains strong working relationships with state and territorial health officers, frequently sending epidemiologists and other personnel to work at the state or local level and providing sophisticated surveillance and technical assistance programs to assist state and local health departments in dealing with novel or emergency situations.

It was therefore logical that in the early and mid-1980s, as the United States began to confront the public health challenge posed by the AIDS epidemic, the CDC became the focal point for developing a strategy of prevention and public health response. As a result of significant increases in funding for AIDS since the early 1980s, AIDS-related programs constitute more than 40 percent of the current CDC budget. In addition, the highly visible role that CDC epidemiologists played in linking AIDS to particular life-styles and in engaging the discussion of how to prevent the spread of the epidemic by public health measures has significantly defined the public perception of the public health profession.

Public health practitioners have long been responsible for surveillance of the spread of communicable diseases and for population-based interventions to alter the course of epidemics. Over the course of the AIDS epidemic, public health providers increasingly have been drawn into supplying primary care services for HIV-infected individuals. Especially since therapies have become available to treat HIV disease before symptoms appear, public health providers are not only implementing programs to offer individual counseling and education, but also providing diagnostic services and medical care.

This chapter considers both the public health response to the needs for surveillance and prevention of HIV/AIDS and the role that public health departments play in delivering health services related to the epidemic. It begins with the debate that has raged around whether HIV and AIDS should be treated as a condition that is exceptional or as one subject to traditional public health measures to stem the spread of infection. This controversy centers around the question of whether the history of responses to lethal infectious disease provides relevant lessons for containing the spread of HIV infection and whether policies developed for the control of sexually transmitted disease (STDs) or other communicable conditions can and should be applied to AIDS, a disease of marginalized, already stigmatized, groups.

Public health policies and practices are determined and implemented at all levels of government—federal, state, and local. This chapter does not attempt to cover all of these; it focuses primarily on national issues and actions. Nor does it try to review all policy decisions and controversies; rather, it considers those concerning HIV antibody testing and screening, contact tracing of the sexual and needle-sharing partners of infected individuals, and the isolation and quarantining of infectious individuals. The chapter concludes by considering the role of public health departments in delivering medical care, planning for health services, and reacting to political controversy.

HISTORICAL APPROACHES TO DISEASE CONTROL
AND "EXCEPTIONALISM"

The conventional approaches to public health threats were largely codified in the late nineteenth and early twentieth centuries. Public health law tended to provide a warrant for compulsory examination and screening and for breaching the confidentiality of the clinical relationship through requiring physicians to report to public health registries the names of people diagnosed with "dangerous diseases." It also established conditions for the imposition of treatment, and, in the most extreme cases, permitted confinement through the power of isolation and quarantine. Although the statutes were revised over the decades, they retained the imprint of their genesis (Merritt, 1986; Burris, 1989).

The most coercive elements of this public health tradition were rarely brought to bear in the mid-twentieth century because of changing patterns of morbidity and mortality, the development of effective clinical alternatives, and limitations imposed by changing conceptions of the police power of the state. As chronic diseases linked to smoking, alcohol consumption, and diet began to displace infectious diseases as the major concern of public health officials, a new approach emerged, one that centered on health promotion campaigns designed to foster the modification of personal behaviors. Major and widespread life-style changes, not the traditional repertoire of public health interventions, are central to the vision of such documents as *Healthy People 2000* (U.S. Department of Health and Human Services, 1991). In some contexts, coercion is still deemed effective and justifiable from a public health perspective (e.g., laws mandating use of motorcycle helmets and automobile seat belts; Moreno and Bayer, 1985), and elements of the restrictive tradition play a significant role in the assault on public smoking and the efforts to apply economic sanctions to behaviors deemed detrimental to public well-being (e.g., cigarette and alcohol tax policies), but mass persuasion is the core feature of the "new public health."

In its spread, HIV/AIDS resembles the infectious conditions and stigmatized sexually transmitted diseases that shaped early public health statutes and practices. But the HIV/AIDS epidemic also resembles the conditions that have become the major threats to public health in the post-antibiotic era—linked to patterns of behavior that are rooted in the normative structures of the communities at risk. Some public health traditionalists, supported by some conservative political forces, argued in favor of the similarities of AIDS to all other communicable diseases and pressed to have AIDS and HIV infection brought under the standing of broad statutory provisions for control of communicable and sexually transmitted diseases, but they were in the minority. Out of the often bitter controversies that surfaced in the epidemic's early years, people who argued that the new public health perspective, founded on education, should inform efforts to contain the spread of HIV infection, came to dominate public discourse. Against the tradition of infectious disease control, this perspective represented the determination to treat AIDS fundamentally different, thus necessitating "exceptionalist" policies (Bayer, 1991b).

The exceptionalist approach dominated in part because some important features of AIDS set it apart from most other infectious diseases. AIDS is incurable with present therapies. It largely afflicts marginalized or threatened populations who have historically rooted fears about the state and antagonism to its institutions. It is primarily transmitted in contexts that involve consenting adults engaging in specific sexual acts or drug-using activities. Containing the spread of HIV infection, then, requires modification in intimate behaviors that would presumably be difficult to make and maintain. Hence, it was believed that the strategy of prevention ought to eschew all appearance of coercion and threats to privacy. Failure to adopt a course that would win the cooperation of those most at risk, it was asserted, would "drive the epidemic underground."

The specter of the coercive tradition and the threat to privacy and modern understanding of civil liberties and individual rights most concerned proponents of civil liberties and advocates of gay rights as they considered the potential direction of public health policy in the face of AIDS (Bayer, 1991b). Would there be wide-scale compulsory testing? Would the names of the infected be recorded in central registries? How would such registries be used to restrict those with HIV infection? Would the power of quarantine be used, if not against all infected persons, then against those whose behavior, it was assumed, could result in the further transmission of infection? In answering these questions, an alliance of gay leaders, proponents of civil liberties, physicians, and public health officials began to shape a policy for dealing with AIDS. Education, it was broadly agreed, had to be the centerpiece of the effort. Sharp disagreements emerged, however, when political pressure was brought to bear to "sanitize" the campaigns through the imposition of restrictions on the language that could be used and the pictorial material that could be displayed (Barnes, 1989). Testing for HIV infection was to be undertaken only after obtaining the informed consent of those to be tested. The tradition of compulsory or routine mass public health screening in the face of epidemic threats was rejected. The reporting of those with HIV infection to public health registries was to be avoided because it might discourage individuals from voluntarily coming forward for HIV testing. Confidentiality of HIV-related medical records was to be rigorously protected, sometimes at the cost of warning intimates who could unknowingly be subjected to the threat of infection. The use of the power of quarantine was to be avoided even when it was found that in specific cases an individual was behaving in ways that posed a threat of infection to others.

Several critical questions were inevitably provoked by this set of policies: Were they an artifact of the early uncertainties that surrounded AIDS? Would the unique political alliance that made possible the exceptionalist perspective be sustained over time? Would policy toward AIDS provide an impetus for the reformulation of the standard approach to other sexually transmitted and communicable diseases?

As the epidemic's second decade begins, it is clear that the strength of the alliance that developed and defended the perspective of HIV exceptionalism has begun to wane (Bayer, 1991b). AIDS increasingly affects groups that are less articulate and lacking the political organization of the gay population that helped forge that alliance. In addition, there is little evidence that the response to AIDS has shaped the course of public health policy more generally. The erosion of the exceptionalist perspective and the lack of influence on broader public health policy related to disease surveillance and behavioral interventions are clear from an analysis of policy and practice with regard to HIV testing, reporting, partner notification, and quarantine and isolation. The extent to which these changes are attributable to the changing opportunities for treatment remains a matter of debate.

HIV TESTING

No issue has consumed more attention in the controversies over public policy and AIDS than the use of the antibody test to identify people infected with HIV. In the period following the test's development and licensing in 1985, controversy centered on the role of testing in supporting the radical modifications of behavior that were universally deemed to be critical to altering the epidemic's course. Proponents of aggressive but voluntary testing believed that knowledge of HIV status could be an important motivator of behavioral change, but gay leaders and their allies were skeptical. They suggested that the required changes could best be produced by aggressive education and by appropriately targeted strategies of individualized counseling even if individuals did not know their status. This debate was framed by the fears of gay men and those who spoke on their behalf that the putative benefits that testing could produce could not outweigh the negative psychological and social consequences of being identified as infected—loss of jobs, insurance, and housing. "Don't take the test" became their rallying cry (Bayer, 1991a).

Out of the testing debates emerged a broad consensus, often codified in state statutes, that testing should be conducted only with the informed, voluntary, and specific consent of individuals and that any testing that did occur should be preceded by counseling that would make explicit the risks and benefits of testing and followed by counseling that would explain the test's significance. However, there were a number of carefully defined, although always contested, exceptions to voluntary, individualized testing. The Defense Department initiated screening of all new recruits and students at service academies and in the college Reserve Officers' Training Corps (ROTC) program: people who test HIV positive are not eligible for military service. The State Department, Peace Corps, and Job Corps also routinely screen employees. These screening programs have withstood court challenges (Gostin, 1990). In addition, many clinicians and hospitals undertook surreptitious testing of patients, justifying their actions by the belief that the protection of health care workers and sound diagnostic work required such screening. In a survey of HIV testing policies in 561 nonfederal, acute care hospitals (Lewis and Montgomery (1990:2767) found:

> [T]he current state of policy adoption related to HIV testing provides no guarantee that [patients] rights will be protected. For example, one of four hospitals surveyed does not require patients' informed consent prior to testing, and one in three does not require pretesting counseling. Moreover, one in four hospitals surveyed does not require a patient to be notified if a test result is positive.

With the announcement in mid-1989 that clinical trials had revealed the efficacy of early therapeutic intervention in slowing the course of illness in asymptomatic but infected persons and in preventing the occurrence of *Pneumocystis carinii* pneumonia, the political debate about testing underwent a fundamental change. Gay groups such as Project Inform in San Francisco and the Gay Men's Health Crisis in New York (Lambert, 1989) began to encourage people whom they had formerly warned against testing to determine whether they were infected. Physicians pressed more vigorously for the return of AIDS to the medical mainstream so that testing might be routinely done under conditions of informed consent (Rhame and Maki, 1989). And state and federal public health officials launched more aggressive testing campaigns.

Physicians and public health officials have typically avoided the language of compulsion, stressing instead routine HIV testing, testing that would be initiated by doctors caring for people they believed to be at risk. Thus, in the fall of 1990, the House of Delegates of the American Medical Association voted to declare AIDS a sexually transmitted disease, a designation that would give physicians much greater latitude to determine the conditions under which HIV testing should be undertaken.

Nowhere has the shifting perspective on testing been clearer than in the emergence of a powerful movement, supported by obstetricians and pediatricians, for the routine screening of pregnant women, who can transmit HIV infection to their offspring, and the mandatory screening of infants at high risk for infection. For pregnant women, the public health practice of testing for syphilis and hepatitis B provided a model. For newborns, the wide-scale and broadly accepted tradition of screening for congenital conditions, such as phenylketonuria (PKU), served as the standard.[1] The promise—although based on only minimal clinical evidence—that early intervention might protect the fetus or at least enhance the life prospects of babies at risk for HIV infection was used to argue against ethical concerns about the coercive identification of infected women, most of whom were black or Hispanic, and the related dangers of exclusion from housing, social services, and health care itself that might be imposed on women and infants so identified. In the spring of 1991, evidence of the effectiveness of initiation of prophylaxis against *Pneumocystis carinii* pneumonia in HIV-positive infants who had yet to develop symptoms but had CD4 cell counts of fewer than 1,500 further fueled the arguments by pediatricians for newborn testing (Centers for Disease Control, 1991). However, none of the arguments overcame the opposition to mandatory testing by many health and other experts. In the words of a special committee of the Institute of Medicine (Hardy, 1991:1-2):

> History has revealed that mandatory screening programs are frequently inflexible, often because they are legislated, and that program modification over time proves difficult. . . . Voluntary HIV screening (with specific informed consent) permits greater flexibility than mandatory screening in accommodating change. The committee opposes any mandatory newborn or prenatal screening program (other than anonymous screening for surveillance purposes).

In 1991 the controversy over the risk posed to patients by HIV-infected health care workers who undertake invasive procedures reopened the question of testing medical personnel (Barnes et al., 1991). Some people argued that testing was not an issue because the risk of HIV transmission is extremely small. However, others believed that infected clinicians had a duty to inform their patients about their own HIV status or to seek advice from colleagues about withdrawing from the practice of invasive procedures; for them, testing was an issue that had to be confronted. Although some believed that mandatory screening of health care workers was not called for, most who believed that infected clinicians had a moral and professional duty either to inform their patients regarding their serologic status or to desist from invasive procedures held that the "duty to inform or withdraw" imposed a correlative responsibility on institutions to identify. Hovering over the entire debate has been the recognition that any policy of screening for health care workers would inevitably produce pressure for the mandatory testing of patients as well. (For further discussion of this subject, see "Confronting Occupational Risks" and "HIV-Infected Practitioners and Risks to Patients" in Chapter 3).

REPORTING AND CONTACT TRACING

Reporting Cases of AIDS and HIV Infection

A diagnosis of full-blown AIDS has been a reportable condition in every state since 1983. The names of people who meet specified diagnostic criteria are reported to confidential public health department registries, and the addition of AIDS to the list of reported conditions provoked little controversy. But all moves to extend such reporting requirements to HIV infection have been fiercely resisted by gay groups, civil liberties organizations, and others because of concerns about privacy and confidentiality. Public health officials in areas with a large number of AIDS cases also tended to oppose reporting because of the potential negative impact on the willingness of individuals to seek voluntary HIV testing and counseling. Such concerns also informed the recommendations of the Institute of Medicine (1988a) in its report, *Confronting AIDS*. As a consequence, the reporting of HIV infection had become policy in only a handful of states by the mid-1980s (Intergovernmental Health Policy Project, 1989). A major change in the reporting debate was signalled when the Presidential Commission on the HIV Epidemic (1988)—authorized by President Reagan and chaired by Admiral James D. Watkins—urged in its final report the universal adoption of a policy of mandatory HIV reporting.

More significant than the commission report, however, were the fissures that had begun to appear in the alliance among groups that had opposed named reporting in those states where the prevalence of HIV infection was high and where gay communities were well organized. In New York, for example, the same suit that sought to compel the commissioner of health to declare AIDS a sexually transmitted disease demanded that HIV infection be made a reportable condition,[2] a position that was echoed in 1990 by the American Medical Association. What made the suit so remarkable was the positions of the opposing sides. Historically, clinicians have resisted efforts by public health officials to require the reporting by name of individuals with infectious diseases, arguing that such policies represented an intrusion on the doctor-patient relationship (Fox, 1986). In this instance the representatives of clinical medicine were asserting that reporting was critical to the public health but the state's chief health official did not agree. That apparent paradox can be explained by the unique political alliances that had been created early in the epidemic among gay organizations, civil liberties groups, and public health officials. But by June 1989, even that feature of the political landscape of public health had begun to change.

In an address that was met with cries of protest, Stephen Joseph, commissioner of health in New York City, told the Fifth International Conference on AIDS that the prospect of early clinical intervention necessitated "a shift toward a disease control approach to HIV infection along the lines of classic tuberculosis practices" (Joseph, 1989:10). A central feature of such an approach would be the "reporting of seropositives" to ensure effective clinical follow-up and the initiation of "more aggressive contact tracing." Joseph's proposals opened a debate that was only temporarily settled by the defeat of New York's Mayor Edward Koch in his bid for reelection. When newly elected Mayor David Dinkins selected Woodrow Myers, former commissioner of health in Indiana, to replace Joseph, his appointment was almost aborted in part because he had supported the reporting of individuals with HIV infection (Lambert, 1990). The acrimonious debate was ended only by a political decision on the part of the mayor, who had drawn heavily on support within the gay community in his campaign, to stand by Myers' appointment while promising that there would be no named reporting in New York City.

In New Jersey, which shares with New York State a relatively high level of HIV infection, the commissioner of health also came to support named reporting, but the politics that surrounded the issue in New Jersey were very different. There, both houses of the state legislature endorsed without dissent a confidentiality statute that included named reporting of cases of HIV infection. New Jersey simply exemplified a national trend: although only nine states at the end of 1989 required named reporting without any provision for anonymity, states increasingly were adopting policies that required reporting in at least some circumstances (Intergovernmental Health Policy Project, 1989). At the end of 1990, the Centers for Disease Control (1990) also endorsed named reporting of those with HIV infection.

At the state and federal levels, the arguments for such a shift tended to stress that new therapeutic possibilities warranted reestablishing traditional public health practice. At the same time, there was pressure to extend the provision of Medicaid coverage for early HIV treatment and to expand government-funded clinics to treat those with HIV infection (Arno et al., 1989; Francis et al., 1989), which would inevitably result in the creation of records on a growing number of infected individuals, regardless of whether states adopted mandatory reporting requirements. Although reporting of HIV-infected individuals is still not widespread in the United States, the move toward early clinical intervention may be ultimately incompatible with the preservation of anonymity, so crucial to testing programs in the epidemic's early years.

Partner Notification and Contact Tracing

The move toward named reporting was only partly based on the argument that state health departments needed the names of individuals to ensure adequate clinical follow-up. Equally important was the assertion from public health officials that effective contact tracing, now more critical than ever because of the potential of early clinical intervention, could be undertaken only if those with HIV infection, but who were not yet diagnosed as having AIDS, could be encouraged to identify their sexual and needle-sharing partners. Despite the central and well-established role of contact tracing in venereal disease control, the notification of sexual and needle-sharing partners in the context of AIDS had been a source of ongoing conflict between gay groups and civil liberties organizations, on one hand, and many public health officials, on the other hand (Potterat et al., 1989).

Contact tracing was always predicated on the willingness of those with sexually transmitted diseases to provide public health workers with the names of their partners in exchange for a promise of anonymity, and it had been viewed by AIDS activists as a threat to confidentiality and as a potentially coercive intervention. Indeed, opponents of contact tracing, some of whom were deeply involved in AIDS policy formulation, typically denounced it as "mandatory." The debate over partner notification also led some officials and others to challenge the conventional wisdom that had dominated public health thinking for four decades: Was contact tracing an effective way of trying to control the spread of sexually transmitted diseases? Did changing patterns of sexuality, in particular, the increase among some populations of anonymous sexual encounters with a relatively large number of partners, render such efforts ineffective (Andrus et al., 1990)?

With time and a better understanding of how contact tracing functioned in the context of sexually transmitted diseases, some of the most vocal opponents of tracing raised fewer concerns about it in principle and more concerns about the cost of so labor intensive an activity. In the late 1980s, support for voluntary contact tracing came from the Institute of Medicine (1988a), the Presidential Commission on the HIV Epidemic (1988), the American Medical Association (Abraham, 1988), and the American Bar Association (1989). The American Medical Association's support for tracing was justified by its executive director, James Sammons, as having "the potential in the heterosexual society to substantially reduce the proliferation and spread of AIDS" (quoted in Abraham, 1988:4). Most striking, however, was the fact that in 1990 a panel charged by the commissioner of health of New York City with the responsibility of making recommendations on partner notification endorsed such efforts as part of the city's overall AIDS strategy. It supported (without dissent) the use of public health workers to notify individuals placed at risk for HIV infection by their sexual and needle-sharing partners, despite the fact that the panel included representatives of a number of community-based gay organizations (*New York Times*, 1991).

The CDC has been the most important organization in pressing for the adoption of contact-tracing programs at the state level, where all such programs are organized and funded (Toomey and Cates, 198¢ involved in the training of venereal disease workers and in tl local venereal disease programs, the CDC had from the outs adoption of this standard public health approach to AIDS and tion. In February 1988 the federal agency assumed a more aggressive posture, making the adoption of partner notification by the states a condition for the receipt of funds from its HIV Prevention Program (Centers for Disease Control, 1988).

Despite such pressure, the response on the part of the states was variable. Those that were most heavily burdened by AIDS continued to favor programs that encouraged infected individuals to notify their partners themselves. Of the states that stressed the role of professional public health workers—the "provider referral" model—most tended to have relatively modest numbers of AIDS cases (Toomey and Cates, 1989). Thus, local epidemiologic factors as well as political forces continued to influence the course of public health policy.

Confidentiality Versus the Physician's "Duty to Warn"

Both the early and lingering resistance to partner notification can in part be explained by the confusion between the standard public health approach to controlling sexually transmitted diseases and policies and practices that are rooted in a very different tradition, one entailing a "duty to warn" or protect those who might be threatened by individuals with communicable conditions. In the early part of this century, courts and legislatures adopted legal norms that imposed a duty to inform on physicians who knew that their patients could place family members or neighbors in danger because of infectious diseases. Failure to do so exposed them to civil liability (Hermann, 1986-1987).

With the decline of infectious diseases as a social threat by the mid-twentieth century, the "duty to inform" tradition had lost much of its significance. It was given new life, however, with the 1974 case of *Tarasoff* v. *Regents of the University of California* (17 C.3d 425, 131 Cal. Rptr. 14, 551 P.2d 334, 1976), which held that psychotherapists had a duty to exercise reasonable care to protect the identifiable potential victims of their patients' violent acts. Although some state courts have not accepted the *Tarasoff* doctrine, others have handed down rulings that limit the principle of the inviolability of physician-patient communications, holding that clinicians have either a duty to protect or warn identifiable individuals who might be harmed by their patients (Merton, 1982). It was that line of cases that set the stage for the debate over whether physicians could be held liable for failing to warn the partners of people infected with HIV who planned to act in a way that posed a risk of viral transmission.

The early and strict confidentiality rules surrounding HIV screening and medical records all but precluded physicians from performing *Tarasoff*-like duties in some states, most notably in New York and California. In recent years, however, confidentiality strictures have been modified in recognition that the limitations sometimes placed physicians in a position that violated professional ethical norms, the realization that some patients could pose a grave threat to unsuspecting partners, and the increasing importance of early therapeutic intervention. Such modifications were often opposed on grounds of the principle that physician-patient communications should never be violated (Kottow, 1986) and by those who argued that such breaches of confidentiality would have the counterproductive consequence of reducing patient candor, thus limiting the capacity of clinicians to counsel and persuade individuals who might harm their partners. Modifications in the standard of strict confidentiality have been given strong support in a number of state legislatures, and by the Public Health Service, the American Medical Association (1989), the Association of State and Territorial Health Officials (1988), and the American Bar Association (1989).

As of 1990, only two states had imposed on physicians a duty to warn unsuspecting partners, although federal authorities had imposed a duty of spousal notification on clinicians working at clinics of the National Institutes of Health when they believed that patients themselves would not undertake the task of notification. More important, about a dozen states had adopted legislation granting physicians a "privilege to warn or inform," thus freeing physicians from liability for either warning or not warning those at risk (Intergovernmental Health Policy Project, 1989). Reflecting profound concerns about the centrality of confidentiality to the struggle against AIDS, New York State's 1989 confidentiality statute (Public Health Law, Article 27-F) went further and, borrowing from the tradition of contact tracing, stipulated that the identity of the infected party not be revealed to those being warned. To those who believe that adequate warnings require, at least under some circumstances, that the identity of the infected party be revealed to the individuals placed at risk (e.g., the American Bar Association, 1990), such compromises represented an undue limitation imposed by a mistaken interpretation of the ethics of confidentiality.

QUARANTINE, ISOLATION, AND
CRIMINAL PROSECUTION

The question of how to respond to individuals whose behavior represents a threat to unknowing partners inevitably leads to a discussion of the public health tradition of imposing restrictions on liberty in the name of communal welfare. The issue of quarantine has haunted all such discussions—not because there was any serious consideration in the United States of the Cuban approach to AIDS (Bayer and Healton, 1989), which mandates the isolation of all persons infected with HIV—but because of fears that even a more limited recognition of the authority to isolate would lead to some intrusions on privacy and deprivations of freedom.

Use of Quarantine Statutes

Soon after he resigned as commissioner of health in New York City at the end of 1989, Stephen Joseph bluntly made the case for the careful exercise of the power of quarantine. He did so on the occasion of the continuing uproar surrounding the appointment of Woodrow Myers as his successor. Gay and civil liberties groups opposed Myers partly because he had supported quarantine legislation in Indiana and had reportedly exercised the authority then granted him under state law. They demanded that such policies never be pursued in New York. No such pledge could or should be made, stated Joseph in an editorial written for the *New York Times* (Joseph, 1990). Among his last formal acts had been the signing of a detention order for a woman with infectious tuberculosis because of her repeated unwillingness to take the medication that would render her noninfectious. In the editorial, Joseph (1990:A25) warned:

> It is virtually certain that at some point, a New York City Health Commissioner will be faced with an analogous situation concerning the transmission of the AIDS virus. When all lesser remedies have failed, can anyone doubt what would be the proper course of action for the Commissioner to take, faced with . . . an infected individual who knowingly and repeatedly sold his blood for transfusion.

When and if a treatment became available that would render HIV-infected people less infectious, "would there not then be a clear obligation to take all reasonable measures to ensure that the infected take their medication, thus protecting others?" (Joseph, 1990:A25). These statements represented the traditional claims of public health practice.

Although there was opposition to all efforts to bring AIDS within the scope of state quarantine statutes, more than a dozen states did so between 1987 and 1990.[3] Many of them used the occasion to modernize their disease control laws to reflect contemporary constitutional standards that detail procedural guarantees and to require that restrictions on freedom represent the "least restrictive alternative" available to achieve a "compelling state interest." In this regard, a return to traditional public health did in fact produce an important modification in central elements of the tradition, namely, an incorporation of more contemporary standards of civil rights.

Given both the new and old quarantine statutes, how frequently have states sought to impose public health restrictions on individuals because of their HIV-related behavior? Some notable instances have been reported in the media, but no systematic data have been published. A state-by-state survey conducted between June and November of 1990 by panel member Ronald Bayer found that more than 500 reports had been received by health departments regarding individuals whose behavior placed others at risk for HIV infection. Just over 350 formal investigations were undertaken to substantiate the accusations. The critical factor determining the level of reporting of "dangerous" AIDS-related behavior and the willingness to process such reports was the existence at the state level of formal mechanisms designed to respond. But in a number of states with a relatively large number of AIDS cases—California, New Jersey, and New York, for example—no such mechanism existed. Indeed, the vast majority of officially reported cases of "recalcitrant" behavior occurred in states with modest AIDS counts: Indiana, Minnesota, Missouri, Nevada, Oklahoma, and Washington. But even in those states that have sought to investigate reports about people whose behavior was thought to pose a social hazard, isolation was very rarely imposed, even for a brief period. More common was the decision to issue orders to "cease and desist" from actions that would lead to HIV transmission. In contrast, between 1981 and 1990, 400 people were institutionalized on a compulsory basis because of their failure to comply with tuberculosis control requirements.

Use of Criminal Statutes

After an initial hesitation to use existing public health statutes that attach criminal penalties to knowing transmission of venereal disease, and some confusion over their applicability, states began to enact new legislation that criminalized behaviors linked to the spread of AIDS. This legislative activity coincided with political receptivity to extend the authority of public health officials to control individuals whose behavior posed a risk of HIV transmission. Such use of the criminal law was broadly endorsed by the Presidential Commission on the HIV Epidemic (1988).

Between 1987 and 1989, 20 states enacted such statutes, almost all of which defined the proscribed acts as felonies, although older statutes usually treated knowing disease transmission as a misdemeanor. In addition, the Ryan White Comprehensive AIDS Resources Emergency Act of 1990 (P.L. 101-381) prohibited the Secretary of Health and Human Services from making a grant to a state unless it provides assurances that intentionally transmitting HIV is civilly and criminally actionable. This prohibition was put in the act in spite of a House committee report on the bill that acknowledged that virtually all states have available either AIDS-specific legislation that permits such prosecutions or broad statutory authority that would permit the prosecution of such individuals. In fact, aggressive prosecutors have relied on laws defining assaultive behavior and attempted murder to bring indictments even in the absence of AIDS-specific legislation.

Any effort to determine the extent to which prosecutions for HIV-related acts have occurred must confront the difficulty of monitoring the activity of local courts when there is neither a guilty verdict nor an appeal to a higher state tribunal. One survey, however, which relied on newspaper accounts as well as official court reports, estimated that between 50 and 100 prosecutions had been initiated involving acts as diverse as spitting, biting, blood splattering, blood donation, and sexual intercourse with an unsuspecting partner (Gostin, 1990).

Although small in number, criminal prosecutions have drawn great attention. In the vast majority of cases, there was either an acquittal or the prosecution was dropped, but in the small number of cases that produced guilty verdicts, some sentences were unusually harsh. In Nevada (where prostitution is legal and regulated), a woman was sentenced to 20 years imprisonment in 1989 under a statute that makes it a felony to solicit by anyone who tests positive for HIV (*State* v. *Kearns*, Nev. Dist. Ct., Clark Cty., No. 865848, March 9, 1989). In the same year, an Indiana appeals court upheld a conviction for attempted murder against a person who had splattered blood on emergency workers seeking to prevent him from committing suicide (*Indiana* v. *Haines*, 545 NE2d 834, Ind App 2d Dist 1989).

STATE AND LOCAL PUBLIC HEALTH PRACTICE

In addition to the effect of AIDS on some traditional public health practices, the HIV/AIDS epidemic has had an impact on state and local public health departments in established program areas and on the creation of new areas of work for those departments.

Infectious Disease Epidemiology

Before the advent of the HIV epidemic, it was widely thought that infectious diseases had peaked in the United States (and other developed countries). Indeed, the field of infectious disease epidemiology was nearly moribund, and epidemiology had turned its attention to the chronic diseases that are the major cause of death in developed countries (e.g., cardiovascular disease, cancer). In addition, the field of health promotion and disease prevention, although growing, was largely directed toward behaviors that contribute to chronic diseases: some attention was being paid to pregnancy and prevention of sexually transmitted diseases, but the emphasis had turned toward nutrition, weight control, smoking cessation, and other activities more closely linked to the major noninfectious killers. The HIV epidemic renewed interest in the epidemiology of infectious diseases (see "Recruiting and Training Providers" in Chapter 3). More important, perhaps, it lent a special urgency to issues of disease prevention and behavior modification.

The effect of the HIV epidemic on preventive public health has been in three main areas. First, it has heightened academic interest in, and awareness of, sexual activity as a vector for multiple diseases, including HIV and other sexually transmitted diseases. Thus, it has led to far more extensive study of the determinants of sexual behavior and variations by race, sex, geography, and educational status and to the determination of the effectiveness of different approaches changing individual behavior.

Second, the HIV epidemic has brought a new generation of practitioners with diverse backgrounds into the field of health promotion: community activists, academics, and even advertising executives with little previous background in public health have been recruited to apply their particular expertise to the area, resulting in an increased integration of their perspectives. The urgent nature of this task has also led to a rise in the attention paid to preventive issues in existing medical and public health journals and to the creation of organizations, journals, and other forums focused on health promotion generally and AIDS risk reduction in particular.

Third, the HIV epidemic has fostered and strengthened partnerships between departments of public health and community-based organizations. Such alliances were initially established because public health departments needed the assistance of groups that had the confidence of those hardest hit by HIV disease, particularly gay men. In the ensuing years, however, it has become clear that an additional reason for such alliances exists: the greater political acceptability of explicit sexual and drug education that is provided by independent organizations rather than by official agencies of government.

Clinical Services

Public health departments often serve as the "clinician of last resort" for people who lack adequate health insurance coverage. Clinics that are financed by or staffed and run by city, county, or state health departments have long provided treatment for gonorrhea, tuberculosis, and a variety of other usually communicable diseases, and, more recently, prenatal care for poor women. Such facilities can be categorical ones (e.g., tuberculosis, sexually transmitted disease, mental health, or prenatal care clinics) or more comprehensive (neighborhood health centers, primary care clinics, hospital-based clinics). HIV infection is medically relevant to many areas of clinical activity and thus has implications for services that must be provided.

Primary care is a responsibility of many local health departments, either directly or indirectly. Most city and county departments fund and manage neighborhood health centers or primary care clinics or both. Furthermore, public hospitals are important sites for the care of indigent people. Because the role of publicly funded clinics is to serve poor patients—who are increasingly represented in the HIV epidemic—such facilities are logically a major provider of HIV clinical services. Similarly, prenatal care for poor or uninsured women is often provided by publicly funded facilities. Because of the 25-35 percent probability that the child of an HIV-infected woman will also be infected, such facilities have also become major sites for HIV counseling and testing.

Sexually transmitted diseases (STDs) bear a special relationship to AIDS because people with such diseases may be biologically at higher risk to acquire or spread HIV infection and because, in an era of "safer sex," they give *prima facie* evidence of unsafe sexual behavior. STD clinics have become sites for intensified screening for HIV and referral for care. The epidemic has prompted efforts to provide a wider range of primary care services in these clinics and, increasingly, to initiate HIV-related research protocols there as well.

Tuberculosis is a major cause of clinical disease among HIV-infected individuals, particularly among drug users, minorities, and the poor. It is of special concern because, unlike HIV, it can be spread by ordinary, nonintimate contact and because of the emergence of strains that are resistant to treatment by currently available drugs (Altman, 1992). Screening for tuberculosis has thus become an important part of HIV care, and screening for HIV is a crucial part of evaluation of patients with tuberculosis. The presence of high rates of tuberculosis in the HIV-infected population has also been a recurring theme among those who call for quarantine or greater restriction of the liberty of HIV-infected people.

Methadone maintenance programs, formerly charged only with the dispensing of methadone to persons participating in drug treatment programs, are increasingly being urged to provide comprehensive primary care for their clients, largely because of the impact of HIV disease on the health of an otherwise generally healthy population.

In sum, the HIV epidemic has increased the range of clinical responsibilities of public health agencies and further strained already burdened resources. Furthermore, public health authorities are faced with a return to the ethical dilemmas of the pre-antibiotic era that arise from their dual function as providers of clinical services to individual patients and as protectors of the health of the public. In the former role, patient confidentiality and deferral to patient autonomy are generally accepted as the overriding consideration; in the latter role, disclosure to state agencies and the right of coercive restraint play a role. These roles are not easy to reconcile.

Expansion of the traditional responsibilities of categorical health programs is being contemplated on the basis of demonstrations of success in a few model programs. It remains to be seen whether successes in "leading-edge" programs can be used to transform more typical public health activities. In methadone maintenance, for instance, Montefiore Hospital in the Bronx has served as a model for the implementation of primary care, research, and other innovative programs. STD clinics in Baltimore are similarly a model for HIV testing and counseling, primary care, and clinical research in other STD clinics. But these programs received substantial benefits from their association with academic medical centers, subsidization of care through research grants, and other advantages that may be difficult to implement in other settings. It is not clear whether such efforts will be possible in an era of constrained public health resources.

The dramatic rise in AIDS expenditures at every level of government, at a time of increasing budgetary problems, constrains the resources that can be devoted to traditional areas of public health activity. In many cities, departments complain that care for STDs is underfunded because of the need to spend money on AIDS.

Planning and Financing Care

Public health departments have traditionally been responsible for planning and financing certain health care services for the indigent. Nowhere has the effect of AIDS on public health been more profound than in the energy consumed in this task, particularly at the state and federal levels. A large share of the cost of providing AIDS clinical care has been borne by Medicaid, and this proportion is increasing as the epidemic becomes more and more concentrated among the poor, who are less likely to have private medical insurance (Green and Arno, 1990). But the historic bias of private and public health insurance on inpatient care and curative (rather than preventive) therapy creates large gaps in medical coverage, particularly as medical intervention for HIV-infected individuals begins earlier in the course of the disease. While "presumptive eligibility" for Medicaid for people with full-blown AIDS has paid for inpatient care and other needs of patients in the latter stages of HIV disease, a growing number of infected persons need outpatient monitoring and drugs. They often find themselves unable to pay for their care and ineligible for Medicaid. Bills to expand Medicaid eligibility to all persons infected with HIV were proposed but defeated in Congress in 1990.

At the state level, public health departments are under considerable pressure to anticipate and plan for the specific health care needs of HIV-infected people, a task not traditionally carried out by these departments. Although most states have some form of "state health plan," they are not typically involved in detailed discussions of the types and amounts of clinical services required by people with specific diseases, such as lung cancer or diabetes. In the case of AIDS, however, most state health departments engaged community-based organizations, health care providers, academics, and others in discussions about such issues as the need for long-term or home care and the availability of physicians and dentists. One result of this involvement has been governmental sponsorship of professional education. The regional AIDS Education and Training Center program of the Health Resources and Services Administration (in the U.S. Department of Health and Human Services) is the major federal effort in this area, but many states also fund educational programs directed at professionals. Others have required documentation of HIV education as part of their general licensing and recertification processes.

Finally, the allocation of federal funds for AIDS clinical care may be a forerunner of new forms of control and allocation of health care funding. The 1990 Ryan White AIDS Resources Emergency Act dictates the creation of an innovative form of community consortium to allocate the funding the bill provides. The consortium must include local government, community-based agencies, and providers. Although analogous groups were once created for the distribution of funds for family planning, they have largely atrophied and were never as broad as those contemplated by the Ryan White legislation. With the growing debate over the reorganization of U.S. health care and various proposals for a more unified system of insurance and allocations, such consortia may provide a model for a more general reform.

CONCLUSIONS

𝒩In the first years of the AIDS epidemic, U.S. public health officials were stunned by the sudden emergence of an unexpected lethal threat. Under those circumstances, they had to negotiate the course of the public health strategy with representatives of a well-organized gay community and their allies in the medical and political establishments. Only such a collaborative relationship, it was believed, would prevent the surfacing of unproductive antagonisms. Only such a process would permit officials to gain access to communities with historically rooted antagonisms to government agencies. As a consequence, many of the traditional practices of public health that might have been brought to bear on the epidemic were rejected in favor of an exceptionalist approach.⟩

As the first decade of the epidemic drew to an end and as gay organizations increasingly shifted their organizational efforts toward issues involving access to therapeutic trials and treatment, public health officials began to reassert their professional dominance over the policy process. In doing so, they began to rediscover the relevance of their professional traditions to the control of the AIDS epidemic, although considerable questions remained about whether traditional measures would have any demonstrable impact on the epidemic's course. The return to more traditional public health approaches has been fostered by changing perceptions of the dimensions of the threat posed by AIDS. Early fears that HIV infection might spread broadly in the population have proven unfounded. As the focus of public health concern has shifted from gay men, among whom the incidence of new HIV infections has remained low for the past several years, to poor black and Hispanic drug users and their sexual partners, the influence of those who have spoken on behalf of the former has begun to wane. Black and Hispanic drug users, however, not only lack the capacity to influence policy in the way that gay men did, but those who speak on their behalf often lack the singular commitment to privacy and consent that so characterized the gay organizations. And as it has become clear that initial estimates of the level of infection first put forth several years ago were too high, the willingness to reconsider traditional policies has increased.

But most important in accounting for the changing course of public health policy has been the important advances in therapeutic prospects. The helplessness and fatalism of the early years has begun to wane, and a guarded optimism has begun to emerge. The prospects for better management of HIV-related opportunistic infections and the hopes of slowing the course of HIV progression itself through prophylaxis have increased the importance of early identification of those with HIV infection. That, in turn, has produced a willingness to consider traditional public health approaches to screening, reporting, and partner notification.

Although HIV disease may not continue to be treated as an exceptional disease, the new perspectives on public health prompted by its emergence will not disappear. The emphasis on mass behavioral change through education that had begun prior to the AIDS epidemic will continue to be of critical importance. Even the most ardent advocates of the relevance of traditional public health practice, the strongest opponents of HIV exceptionalism, recognize that mass educational campaigns will remain the single most important element in the public health strategy to contain HIV infection. And much was learned in the first decade of the AIDS epidemic about how to mobilize an effective public health education campaign—about the importance of engaging those who speak on behalf of those most at risk in the process of fashioning such efforts. These lessons could be applied profitably to the patterns of morbidity and mortality that represent so much of the contemporary threat to the public health.

In assessing the impact of AIDS on the practice of public health, it is important to remember that such practice entails not only education, surveillance, reporting, and other public health control measures, but also the delivery of primary health care services. State, county, and local public health programs have become, often by default, the providers of last resort for people with HIV disease who lack private insurance coverage. The inextricable link between HIV disease and other diseases and conditions prevalent in poor populations (e.g., drug addiction, tuberculosis, and sexually transmitted diseases) means that public health providers will face even greater challenges from the HIV epidemic in the 1990s. These challenges involve not only meeting the burden of growing caseloads, but also fashioning delivery systems that meet the many needs of people with HIV disease. The AIDS epidemic thus presents an opportunity and challenge for the revitalization of the practice of public health with regard to both infectious conditions and the chronic disorders that represent so much of the task of public health in the United States today (see Institute of Medicine, 1988b).

NOTES

1. Phenylketonuria is an inborn error of metabolism, detectable by genetic screening and treatable with a diet low in phenylalanine. The diet is extremely unpleasant and can be toxic in children who are misdiagnosed. Nevertheless, a change in diet for children with true PKU (as opposed to other benign forms of hyperphenylalaninemia) can prevent mental retardation. For a discussion of the lessons of PKU for mandatory screening programs, see Hardy (1991:82-83).

2. New York State's highest court refused to designate HIV infection a communicable and sexually transmitted disease, a move that would have "trigger[ed] statutory provisions relating to isolation and quarantine, reporting, mandatory testing and contact tracing" (slip op. at 6). The court concluded that "designating HIV infection as a communicable or sexually transmitted disease would be detrimental to the public health . . ." (slip op. at 11) (*New York State Society of Surgeons et al.* v. *David Alexrod*, 1991).

3. Based on a review of all AIDS-related legislation in the files of the George Washington University Intergovernmental Health Policy Project, Washington, D.C.

REFERENCES

Abraham, L. (1988) AIDS contact tracing, prison test stir debate. *American Medical News* July 8-15:4.

Altman, L.K. (1992) Top scientist warns tuberculosis could become major threat. *New York Times* February 11:B-6.

American Bar Association (1989) *Report from the House of Delegates, August 1989.* Chicago: American Bar Association.

American Bar Association (1990) *Policy on AIDS.* Chicago: American Bar Association.

American Medical Association (1989) Report X: AMA HIV policy update. In *AMA Proceedings of the House of Delegates.* December 3-6, 43rd interim meeting. Chicago: American Medical Association.

Andrus, J.K., D.W. Fleming, D.R. Harger, M.Y. Chin, D.V. Bennett, et al. (1990) Partner notification: can it control epidemic syphilis? *Annals of Internal Medicine* 112(7):539-543.

Arno, P.S., D. Shenson, N.F. Siegel, P. Franks, and P.R. Lee (1989) Economic and policy implications of early intervention in HIV disease. *Journal of the American Medical Association* 262:1493-1498.

Association of State and Territorial Health Officials, National Association of County Health Officials, U.S. Conference of Local Health Officers (1988) *Guide to Public Health Practice: HIV Partner Notification Strategies.* Washington, D.C.: Public Health Foundation.

Barnes, M. (1989) Toward ghastly death: the censorship of AIDS education. *Columbia Law Review* 89:698-724.

Barnes, M., N.A. Rango, G.R. Burke, and L.A. Chiarello (1991) The HIV-infected health care professional: employment policies and public health. *Law, Medicine & Health Care* 18:311-330.

Bayer, R. (1991a) *Private Acts, Social Consequences: AIDS and the Politics of Public Health.* New Brunswick, N.J.: Rutgers University Press.

Bayer, R. (1991b) Public health policy and the AIDS epidemic: an end to AIDS exceptionalism? *New England Journal of Medicine* 324:1500-1504.

Bayer, R., and C. Healton (1989) Controlling AIDS in Cuba. *New England Journal of Medicine* 320:1022-1024.

Burris, S. (1989) Rationality review and the politics of public health. *Villanova Law Review* 34:909-932.

Centers for Disease Control (CDC) (1988) Cooperative agreements for Acquired Immunodeficiency Syndrome (AIDS) prevention and surveillance projects program announcements and notice of availability of funds for fiscal year 1988. *Federal Register* February 5, 53(24):3554-3558.

Centers for Disease Control (CDC) (1990) Update: public health surveillance for HIV infection—United States, 1989 and 1990. *Morbidity and Mortality Weekly Report* 39:853, 859-861.

Centers for Disease Control (CDC) (1991) Guidelines for prophylaxis against *Pneumocystis carinii* pneumonia for children infected with human immunodeficiency virus. *Morbidity and Mortality Weekly Report* 40(RR-2):1-13.

Fox, D.M. (1986) From TB to AIDS: value conflicts in reporting disease. *Hastings Center Report* 16(6)(Suppl.):11-16.

Francis, D.P., R.E. Anderson, M.E. Gorman, M. Fenstersheib, N.S. Padian, et al. (1989) Targeting AIDS prevention and treatment toward HIV-1-infected persons. *Journal of the American Medical Association* 262:2572-2576.

Gostin, L.O. (1990) The AIDS litigation project: a national review of courts and human rights decisions. Part I: the social impact of AIDS. *Journal of the American Medical Association* 263:1461-1470.

Green, J., and P.S. Arno (1990) The medicalization of AIDS. Trends in the financing of HIV-related medical case. *Journal of the American Medical Association* 264:1261-1266.

Hardy, L.M., ed. (1991) *HIV Screening of Pregnant Women and Newborns.* Committee on Prenatal and Newborn Screening for HIV Infection, Institute of Medicine. Washington, D.C.: National Academy Press.

Hermann, D.H.J. (1986-1987) AIDS: malpractice and transmission liability. *University of Colorado Law Review* 58:63-107.

Institute of Medicine (1988a) *Confronting AIDS: Update 1988.* Washington, D.C.: National Academy Press.

Institute of Medicine (1988b) *The Future of Public Health.* Committee for the Study of the Future of Public Health. Washington, D.C.: National Academy Press.

Intergovernmental Health Policy Project (1989) HIV reporting in the states. *Intergovernmental AIDS Reports* 2(5):1-3.

Joseph, S.C. (1989) Remarks delivered at the Fifth International Conference on AIDS Plenary Program. Montreal, Canada.

Joseph, S.C. (1990) Quarantine: sometimes a duty. *New York Times* February 10:A25.

Kottow, M.H. (1986) Medical confidentiality: an intransigent and absolute obligation. *Journal of Medical Ethics* 12:117-122.

Lambert, B. (1989) In shift, gay men's health group endorses testing for AIDS virus. *New York Times* August 16:A1.

Lambert, B. (1990) AIDS policy dispute prompts a defense of a health official. *New York Times* January 12:28.

Lewis, C.E., and K. Montgomery (1990) The HIV testing policies of U.S. hospitals. *Journal of the American Medical Association* 264:2764-2767.

Merritt, D.J. (1986) Communicable disease and constitutional law: controlling AIDS. *New York University Law Review* 61:739-799.

Merton, V. (1982) Confidentiality and the "dangerous" patient: implications of *Tarasoff* for psychiatrists and lawyers. *Emory Law Journal* 31:263-343.

Moreno, J.D., and R. Bayer (1985) The limits of the ledger in public health promotion. *Hastings Center Report* 15:37-41.

New York Times (1991) New York widens plan to warn of AIDS exposure. *New York Times* March 17:A21.

Potterat, J.J., N.E. Spencer, D.E. Woodhouse, and J.B. Muth (1989) Partner notification in the control of human immunodeficiency virus infection. *American Journal of Public Health* 79:874-876.

Presidential Commission on the Human Immunodeficiency Virus Epidemic (1988) *Final Report*. Washington, D.C.: U.S. Government Printing Office.

Rhame, F.S., and D.G. Maki (1989) The case for wider use of testing for HIV infection. *New England Journal of Medicine* 320:1248-1254.

Toomey, K.E., and W. Cates, Jr. (1989) Partner notification for the prevention of HIV infection. *AIDS* 3(Suppl. 1):57-62.

U.S. Department of Health and Human Services (1991) *Healthy People 2000: National Health Promotion and Disease Prevention Objectives*. DHHS Pub. No. (PHS) 91-50212. Washington, D.C.: U.S. Government Printing Office.

3

Health Care Delivery and Financing

The U.S. health care system stands alone among advanced industrial countries in lacking a national program to ensure universal or nearly universal health insurance coverage. The various public and private insurance plans and delivery systems (such as the Veterans Administration health system) reflect what John Iglehart (1992:962) characterizes as "society's profound ambivalence about whether medical care for all is a social good, of which the costs should be borne by society, or a benefit that employers should purchase for employees and their dependents, with government insurance for people outside the work force." This ambivalence, and the resulting lack of any political consensus on how to finance and deliver health services, has resulted in an odd assortment of programs that does provide health insurance to about 85 percent of the population, but leaves some 36 million people uninsured. The uninsured are primarily full-time workers and their dependents who are employed in small firms at a low or the minimum wage. In addition, as health insurance premiums have escalated by 20 percent or more annually in recent years, employers have sought to contain costs by either reducing the value of the insurance coverage offered employees or by reducing the coverage provided for dependents. At the same time, insurance firms increasingly act unilaterally to avoid high (or "catastrophic") claims by dropping or limiting coverage for groups or individuals who are at high risk for serious illness. Thus, the security of health insurance even for the workers and their dependents who have coverage has deteriorated over the last decade.

Government spending on health services has increased continuously since the 1960s. The increases in spending have resulted primarily from inflation, technology changes, and increases in the volume of services that providers deliver; extensions of coverage to new population groups or improvements in benefits have accounted for a relatively minor proportion of the increase. In the last decade alone, federal health expenditures increased from 12 percent of the federal budget in 1980 to 15 percent in 1990. The increasing cost of Medicaid has resulted in severe problems for states and has occasioned difficult searches at the state level for means of containing (or shifting to the federal level) expenditures for health services.

The providers of health services—physicians, hospitals, other institutional and individual professions—are in a period of transition. The funds easily available for health care in the 1960s and 1970s, as Medicare, Medicaid, and private health insurance coverage paid charges as billed with few controls over services or rates, are now more constrained. Limits on Medicare and Medicaid reimbursement rates, the increasing reliance of private insurance plans on various types of managed care and administrative constraints on physician practice decisions, and new attention to areas such as medical devices and equipment are fundamentally changing the practice of medicine. Physicians are almost uniformly frustrated and angry over the loss of control they once exercised. The nation's 7,000 hospitals are similarly facing painful transitions, both as a result of Medicare rate limits and the explosion of new types of competitive delivery systems, such as ambulatory surgical centers and hospices. The growth in for-profit hospital chains in the 1970s and 1980s has deprived community hospitals of many privately insured, middle-class patients and further concentrated uninsured, multiproblem patients in public or inner-city voluntary hospitals.

The state of the U.S. health care system as it enters the 1990s has been described as a "paradox of excess and deprivation" (Enthoven and Kronick, 1989:29). As is discussed below and in the New York study (Chapter 9), the impact of the AIDS epidemic on the confederation of health care providers and insurers has been as varied as the system itself. Major portions of the financing and delivery systems have been largely untouched by the epidemic, others have made marginal changes, and those institutions that serve the populations at highest risk have been profoundly affected.

To simplify its task of describing the impact of the HIV/AIDS epidemic on the nation's health care system and the response of that system to the epidemic, the panel adopted four descriptive categories of the system: a provider of services, an employer of professional and other personnel, a marketplace for goods and services, and a major financial sector of the economy. Clearly, the health care system is far more complex and subtle than these gross categories suggest, but they provide a means of organizing and delimiting our analysis.

In each of its capacities, the health care system has been affected to a large or small extent by the HIV/AIDS epidemic. How lasting the impacts will be is not clear. For the health care system, as for any of the social areas and institutions discussed in this report, it is difficult to sort out the impact of HIV disease from a web of associated concerns. The connections between HIV disease and homosexuality, intravenous drug use, poverty, and racial or ethnic minority status contribute to this difficulty. For example, if physicians are disinclined to care for AIDS patients, is it because they fear AIDS? Or, even in the absence of HIV, would they be uncomfortable with patients who are gay or use intravenous drugs, daunted by the complexity of care or unwilling to render services in a context in which reimbursement may not even cover their costs? This chapter makes no claim to being exhaustive or even comprehensive on these issues; rather, it touches on a wide array of possible impacts on the health care in its functions as service provider, employer, economic market, and financing mechanism and suggests key aspects to be followed as the epidemic unfolds.

THE HEALTH CARE SYSTEM AS A SERVICE PROVIDER

Challenges for Traditional Health Care Delivery

AIDS presents a major challenge to hospitals, nursing homes, physicians, nurses, and other direct providers of health care services. The clinical characteristics of HIV/AIDS account for its difficulty in management. The disease is, first of all, a new one. Most medical knowledge is accumulated over decades, if not generations. Yet with HIV disease, the health care system is faced with the task of caring for approximately 1 million people in the United States who have a disease that has only been recognized for a few years and whose course, treated or untreated, is still only partly understood.

In total numbers, there are probably tens of thousands of persons with clinical manifestations of HIV disease; however, only a fraction of them require intensive medical care at any one time. The impact on the health care system must be measured by the volume of patients in particular locales and in light of the preexisting health care system. That large number of patients (combined with the crack cocaine epidemic, homelessness, and other problems) has resulted in a serious strain on an already high hospital occupancy rate. In other cities, the capacity of hospitals to absorb AIDS inpatients is not as pressing a concern as are the stigma and inadequate reimbursement associated with AIDS care.

Although more HIV-positive individuals will become ill in the next several years and most of them will require hospitalization, it is difficult to predict the magnitude of hospital-based and other services that will be required, largely because modes and standards of care change relatively quickly. Prediction of (and therefore planning for) specific quantities and types of clinical services and facilities can be extraordinarily difficult because of the rapidly changing nature of HIV clinical care.

One example of the evolution of HIV care is the changing need for inpatient hospital beds. Consider cryptococcal meningitis, a fungal infection of the central nervous system, which eventually attacks 10 to 15 percent of AIDS patients (non-HIV-infected people also occasionally contract the disease). Until recently, HIV-infected people with cryptococcal meningitis required several weeks of intravenous therapy with a relatively toxic drug, amphotericin B, followed by twice-weekly amphotericin B maintenance therapy for the rest of their lives. They constituted a substantial fraction of AIDS patients requiring hospital or nursing-home beds or intensive at-home therapy. Then, in the winter of 1990, a new oral antifungal drug, fluconazole, was licensed. It is equal to amphotericin B, at least for maintenance therapy; many patients who would formerly have required elaborate intravenous therapy (often in an institution) now take one pill a day at home.

Another challenge for the provision of direct services is the complexity of the disease. HIV disease attacks virtually every organ system of the body. The U.S. health care system has long been criticized for its failure to provide comprehensive, coordinated primary care and for too great a reliance on specialists and subspecialists. It is precisely such comprehensive, primary care that is necessary to cope with a disease that is chronic and disabling and that stubbornly refuses to be limited to any single organ system. In many ways, then, the calls for adequate ongoing medical care for HIV-infected persons reflect and reinforce other current demands for an overall reordering of staffing and reimbursement priorities in American health care.

The transmissibility of HIV poses another challenge to health care providers. Not only does the fear of acquiring HIV infection imperil recruitment and retention of health care professionals to work with HIV-infected patients, it also has the potential to drive a wedge between providers and their patients.

Organization of HIV/AIDS Care

A recurring question in the delivery of health care for people with HIV disease and AIDS involves how care ought to be organized and in what setting it might best be delivered. Various goals—increased survival, patient satisfaction, efficiency, economy, or quality care—may call for differing arrangements for delivering care. Optimal care for HIV disease may be difficult to accommodate within the extant organizational and reimbursement schemes of the health care delivery system. The newness, complexity, and transmissibility of AIDS, together with other problems associated with it, have tested traditional delivery mechanisms and forced the creation of new ones.

Hospital Care

The hospital is an essential source of care for people with AIDS, most of whom need to be hospitalized for diagnosis or treatment more than once as their disease progresses. The care of AIDS patients has been highly concentrated in inner-city public hospitals, which have also had to cope with inadequate reimbursements, staff shortages, lack of referral facilities, and the use of emergency rooms as sources of primary care (Andrulis, 1989).

Although the characteristics of the patient population with HIV disease and the resources to meet their needs vary from city to city, many health administrators and planners have looked to San Francisco's experience with the epidemic and its delivery of care as an exemplary model. The San Francisco model of care is distinguished by its reliance on extensive outpatient services and volunteer social support provided by a well-established gay community. Nevertheless, as Benjamin (1988:420) notes, "the fact remains that where life-threatening illness is concerned, for surprisingly large numbers of people in times of illness, be it ever so expensive there is no place like the hospital." Hence, even the San Francisco model includes a significant hospital component. San Francisco General Hospital, a municipal facility, created the nation's first dedicated inpatient hospital unit for AIDS care in 1983. Since then, care for patients with AIDS, the overwhelming majority of whom have been gay men, has been provided by multidisciplinary teams of physicians, nurses, psychologists, and social workers, supplemented by volunteers.

In cities in which the patient mix tends to include more intravenous drug users, AIDS-dedicated hospital wards have also been established. These wards have come to be accepted by physicians and patients alike, despite some initial misgivings that such centralization of care could further stigmatize patients, scare away health care workers, reinforce apprehensions about HIV transmission in a health care setting, and isolate the ward from the rest of the hospital. Disease-specific wards are not unprecedented. They are currently common in cancer treatment, and they have been prominent in treating diabetes, tuberculosis, and polio. Clinics dedicated to the care of HIV disease are also now common components of urban hospitals (Makadon, Delbanco, and Delbanco, 1990a; Turner, 1990).

The establishment of AIDS-specific hospitals was once contemplated in several cities, but it now seems unlikely. A New York City task force recommended against the creation of single-disease hospitals, in part because of the historical lessons provided by tuberculosis sanatariums and state mental hospitals. The task force concluded (Rothman, Tynan, and New York City Task Force on Single-Disease Hospitals, 1990:766) "[that] the creation of HIV-only hospitals would promote negative stereotyping . . . interfere with [patients'] freedom of choice [and] engender an unacceptably low quality of care." A proposal in San Francisco to create an AIDS-dedicated institution never came to fruition (Levine, 1990). The only AIDS-specific hospital actually established was in Houston. A joint venture of the University of Texas and American Medical International (the Institute for Immunological Disorders), the hospital was closed after losing $8 million in a little more than a year. Too few AIDS patients had enough private insurance coverage to support such a venture—two-thirds of the patients were indigent. In addition, some AIDS patients with insurance shunned the hospital, knowing that the name of the hospital merely appearing on their bills would alert their employers and insurers to the nature of their problem. The hospital may have also been a victim of its own success: it managed to provide treatment for many of its patients on a less costly and thus less lucrative outpatient basis.

The degree to which AIDS care should be rendered in centralized or specialized settings continues to be a matter of some debate. Hospitals that are experienced in providing AIDS care may be able to produce better outcomes. A study of 257 AIDS patients at 15 California hospitals, for example, found a significantly lower in-hospital mortality rate for *Pneumocystis carinii* pneumonia at the hospitals with more experience treating the disease (Bennett et al., 1989). The authors of the California study suggested three possible options: creating regional centers, promoting rapid but carefully monitored increases in the experience of low-volume hospitals, or providing focused educational efforts for facilities with little experience with AIDS. The implications of this study continue to be debated as the number of AIDS cases continues to grow and be geographically dispersed (Cotton, 1989; Greene, Leigh, and Passman, 1989).

Out-of-Hospital Care

AIDS has also had an impact on health care outside of hospitals. For example, AIDS has prompted a reexamination of the philosophy underlying hospice care. Hospice care, in the home and in specialized centers, emerged as an alternative to high-technology hospital care at the end of life. It involves palliative interventions and aggressive pain relief, and patients forgo any intrusive or curative procedures or experimental approaches. Hospice patients would rarely, for example, be readmitted to a hospital. They are typically cancer sufferers, whose disease has fairly well-defined stages and for whom the length of life remaining can be predicted with some certainty.

People with AIDS may not fit easily into the hospice scheme. The course of disease progression for AIDS is much less predictable than for many cancers. In the context of AIDS, hospice organizations have had to redefine palliative care to accommodate more therapeutic interventions for the continued use of zidovudine (AZT), the need for treatment of anemia (a frequent side effect of AZT), and the administration of intravenous therapies, such as gancyclovir, to treat cytomegalovirus retinitis, a sight-threatening condition. In addition, people with AIDS may wish to seek readmission to a hospital or undergo therapies (such as ventilator assistance) that are unavailable in traditional hospice settings.

One hospice administrator (quoted in Wallace, 1990:13) noted: "For the person with AIDS, hospice is less a gift from God and more the grim reaper . . . persons with AIDS, reacting to the prejudices against them can initially mistrust the motivations and altruism of hospice programs." In some cities, such as Boston, San Francisco, Seattle, and New York, hospices have been established exclusively for people with AIDS, which obviates some of the concerns about how traditional hospice services meet the needs of people with AIDS.

The hospice dilemma illustrates many of the tensions inherent in the shifting conceptualization of HIV disease from a terminal to a chronic illness. Other sources of tension arise in providing a context for decisions about forgoing life-sustaining care. In recent years, advocacy of "death with dignity" has increased with the growth of high-technology care. But advocating decisions about forgoing high-technology care may seem irrelevant to poor people who have tremendous difficulties in gaining access to any care at all.

Other out-of-hospital settings are also important to people with HIV disease, although traditional sources of long-term care have not always served them well. As people with HIV disease live longer, more are developing symptoms of dementia and neurological deficits, as well as the physical deterioration that requires supportive care. Many nursing homes have been reluctant to care for AIDS patients, citing the fears of other clients, inexperience with managing infectious disease, and lack of adequate reimbursement. Administrators of long-term care facilities have been reluctant to admit gay or intravenous-drug-using patients, who are typically younger than the rest of their patients. In skilled nursing facilities, the levels of intensity of services and the care available generally do not address the needs of people with HIV disease because of fluctuations between periods of acute illness and wellness (Benjamin, 1988).

HIV care has helped lead the way in the performance of lumbar punctures, transfusions, chemotherapy, and intravenous hydration in clinics rather than as formerly, during a hospital stay. Diminishing lengths of hospital stays for people with HIV disease are likely to be matched by increases in the acuity of illness among patients seen in clinics. A survey of 67 members of the National Association of Public Hospital with data on AIDS patients from 1985 to 1988 revealed a significant decrease in average length of stay. The average number of days per patient per year also declined, but that was offset by a slight increase in annual admissions per AIDS patients. In 1988 "the typical AIDS patient spent 29.1 days in the hospital but had 1.6 admissions" (Gage et al., 1991:42).

The advent of HIV disease has coincided with numerous initiatives to control the cost of health care. Because hospital care constitutes such a large percentage of total health care costs, many of the initiatives were designed to reduce inpatient stays: prospective payment, preadmission screening, and same-day surgery are the best-known examples. Thus, the fiscal environment and the desire of AIDS patients to remain outside the hospital have converged to favor greater use of nonhospital facilities.

Another beneficiary of more aggressive nonhospital care has been the growth of high-technology home care. Scores of small companies now provide equipment for intravenous, intramuscular, and aerosolized home therapies. Intravenous pumps, which once were complicated even for a nurse to operate, now work at the flip of a switch, allowing nurses to visit patients once a week at home rather than several times a day in the hospital (Manges, 1989; Podger, 1990). Industry analysts have predicted that home health care, which generates an estimated $15 billion of sales annually, will be the "fastest growing business segment from the mid-1990s until well into the next century" (Feder, 1991:C1). The AIDS market is a significant fraction of a fiercely competitive enterprise.

Many private insurers and government regulators are subjecting home health care bills to careful scrutiny because of the newness of administering complicated regimens in the home and the proliferation of equipment that can be used at home. Many start-up companies are facing difficulties in collecting bills; Selz (1990:B2) notes: "reimbursements [depend] heavily on compliance with numbingly complex and constantly changing government policy and procedure." As these difficulties are resolved, AIDS care may pave the way for the routine reimbursement of complex home-based treatments.

Connections with Community-Based Services

One striking development in the health care system is the close relationship that has evolved between medical providers and institutions, on one hand, and community-based agencies, on the other (see also Chapter 6). Some fields of medicine, such as oncology and diabetology, have long relied heavily on volunteers for services, ranging from hospice care to educational camps for juvenile diabetics. With HIV disease, however, the amount of community involvement in (and substitution for) medical services has been remarkable in both human and economic terms (Arno, 1986; Smith, 1989).

One activity of community-based agencies that has been widely advocated as a measure for containing the costs of HIV medical care and enhancing patient satisfaction and access to services is "case management" (Jellinek, 1988). Case-management programs tend to include at least the following elements: outreach, standardized eligibility screening, comprehensive assessment, initial care planning, service arrangements, ongoing monitoring, and periodic reassessments. To perform these wide-ranging tasks, a case manager may serve simultaneously as gatekeeper, advocate, educator, diagnostician, broker, and caregiver. First instituted in the United States in the 1940s through workmen's compensation and physical disability services, case management has more recently been refined in caring for elderly and mentally ill patients.

Case management has two major forms: a medical and a social service advocacy model. Under the medical model, case management is often hospital based and takes place primarily in the context of planning a patient's discharge. In the social service model, case management is oriented more toward providing social work and coordinating services to patient/clients. Under this model, the case manager may follow clients both in and out of hospitals. Traditionally, all case management programs try to centralize the responsibility for advocacy in one individual.

Although such systems have been widely encouraged because they are believed to improve the quality of care and reduce costs, evidence of their cost-effectiveness is lacking. In addition, experience with the advocacy model of case management among the elderly suggests that it may actually increase costs by increasing utilization of appropriate services by previously underserved clients (Benjamin, 1988).

A number of states now reimburse providers specifically for case-management services. Case management has been financed through enhanced service reimbursement and AIDS-specific waivers of standard rules for public financing (see below) or through special funding under Health Resources and Services Administration (HRSA) or private foundation grants. Most private insurers have some form of case management by which policy holders with high-cost illnesses are assigned to an individual (usually a nurse) who can investigate the patient's needs and authorize services that are cost-effective, even if they are not technically covered in the policy.

In the Ryan White Comprehensive AIDS Resources Emergency Act of 1990, case management was recognized as a primary service under Titles I and II and an optional service for early intervention under Title III. Even with this strong encouragement, the concept of case management remains somewhat unclear, and its benefits remain, in large part, unevaluated. In

1988 the Sierra Health Foundation of Northern California undertook a 3-year program of support for a regional case-management system. As this funding drew to a close, the foundation convened a group of national experts in case management to examine the concept and evaluate the efficacy of this service. While agreeing that case management seems to mean different things to different people, the conference participants reaffirmed the central concept of making available to clients assistance in maneuvering through the complex service system, advocating for patients, and enhancing preventive strategies. They suggested areas of research to clarify methods and outcomes. At the same time, they noted (Sierra Health Foundation, 1992:24): "case management is only as good as the services available for referral and that if services are not available for referral in the community, then case management can simply not access them."

THE HEALTH CARE SYSTEM AS EMPLOYER

Health care is the third largest industry in the United States. It employs 8 million people in a wide range of capacities. In many communities, the local hospital or medical school is one of the area's largest employers, particularly for highly paid professional staff and entry-level workers in clerical and janitorial positions.

Recruiting and Training Providers

Physicians

The term "AIDS physicians" refers to doctors who engage in a wide range of activities. In university facilities they are involved in basic, epidemiologic, and clinical research on the disease. In local communities they are the physicians who have seen a few patients with HIV disease and are willing to see more of them. Any physician identified as an AIDS care provider is likely to be involved not only in providing demanding patient care, but also in developing institutional policies, planning for care needs, and responding to media inquiries.

Among the challenges confronted in planning for the care of people with HIV disease is deciding what training is necessary to provide such care. There is no single subspeciality (with attendant prerequisites, board examinations, and certification) for AIDS care: no single medical discipline encompasses all the skills and training necessary to treat the wide spectrum of clinical manifestations of HIV disease (Bartlett, 1988; Cotton, 1988). The American Board of Internal Medicine entertained—and rejected—the notion of creating a new specialty for HIV care.

AIDS was originally thought to be a disease largely within the province of infectious disease experts. Indeed, a major impact of AIDS has been on the practice of infectious disease medicine. Infectious disease is a relatively new medical subspeciality and was for many years mainly hospital based; its practitioners provided consultation to other physicians and rendered relatively little ongoing primary care. The chronic nature of HIV disease has meant a radical change in the practice of many infectious disease specialists, who now often serve as primary care physicians for patients with HIV disease.

In the years just prior to the HIV epidemic, there were concerns about a projected oversupply of physicians in most medical specialties, including infectious disease.[1] In the late 1970s the president of the Infectious Disease Society of America said (Petersdorf, quoted in Bartlett, 1988:10): "Even with my great loyalty to infectious diseases, I cannot conceive of the need for 309 more infectious disease experts [the number taking the boards that year] unless they spend time culturing each other." By the end of the 1980s and after almost a decade of experience with AIDS, however, the situation had changed. In fact, according to a 1990 report in the *Annals of Internal Medicine*, infectious disease was the only medical specialty that needed more physicians.

General internists, family medicine specialists, and pediatricians are also potentially well suited to deliver primary care to people with HIV disease. They are dispersed geographically and experienced in primary care. A number of commentators (e.g., Northfelt, Hayward, and Shapiro, 1988; Smith, 1991) have proposed a range of AIDS-related services that primary caregivers might be expected to provide, including counseling about HIV transmission and prevention strategies, administering and integrating diagnostic tests, monitoring patient care during early HIV disease, and recognizing complications that require consultation or referral to a specialist.

AIDS arrived on the American health care scene when the preference of newly graduated physicians was shifting away from primary care specialties and toward such specialties as radiology, orthopedics, and otolaryngology. In particular, internal medicine, the specialty most likely to feel the impact of providing ongoing care for HIV-infected patients, had been undergoing a decline in interest for several years (McCarty, 1987). Some of the reasons for this trend include the technological focus of medical school training and the higher compensation in specialty fields. Specialties in which talking to and examining patients constitute the bulk of physicians' activities are not as highly remunerated as those involving diagnostic, therapeutic, and surgical procedures (although efforts are under way to redress these imbalances through changes in Medicare and other reimbursement schemes). Many physicians also begin medical practice encumbered by large educational debts, a further reason to avoid lower paying specialties.

Concern is growing that the burden of the epidemic may further dissuade young physicians from entering specialties such as internal medicine or from practicing in geographic locations where the burden or risk of caring for patients with HIV disease is perceived to be high (Ness et al., 1989). In some areas, AIDS remains an uncommon phenomenon; in others, it is prominent: "Today, a third-year medical student in New York City has more direct experience with [HIV] disease than a practicing internist in virtually any small town in the nation" (Cotton, 1988:520).

Surveys of physicians in training reflect concerns that AIDS will adversely affect training programs by skewing the mix of patients (Imperato et al., 1988). Such concerns tend to overlook the wide spectrum of diseases represented by AIDS and the historical fact that physicians have always been trained by studying the most prevalent disease at the time, such as tuberculosis or syphilis.[2] Moreover, physicians in training at sites where AIDS is prevalent tend to overestimate significantly the proportion of patients with AIDS under their care, perhaps because of anxiety or stress associated with HIV disease or the exigencies of caring for patients with such great needs (Cooke and Sande, 1989; Hayward and Shapiro, 1991).

No firm evidence is yet available to determine whether HIV disease is contributing to the continuing decline in popularity of primary care specialties and causing young physicians to shun areas with a high prevalence of AIDS when making career choices. As with topics treated in other chapters of this report, confounding factors make it difficult to sort out the particular impact of HIV disease. Some cities where AIDS is prevalent have also suffered declines in the quality of life that make them less attractive to young professionals. But many urban hospitals with high proportions of AIDS patients are also prestigious teaching centers, and a few of the specialties in which occupational risk has been particularly feared, such as orthopedic surgery, are particularly well paid. Thus, there are incentives that might draw graduate physicians toward AIDS care.

A recent survey of internal medicine and family practice residents in ten geographically representative states showed that 77 percent rated their ambulatory care of AIDS patients an excellent educational experience. Yet 23 percent of the residents stated that, given the choice, they would not take care of *any* patients with AIDS (Hayward and Shapiro, 1991).

Nurses

Assessing the impact of AIDS on the supply of nurses is somewhat more problematic, although hospitals, nursing homes, and other institutional health care providers are currently experiencing staffing problems, and the National Commission on AIDS (1990) identified a shortage of nurses as an obstacle to improved care of AIDS patients.

Nurses and their professional associations have not figured prominently in debates about AIDS care. Nurses have a different perspective on the debate about professional obligations toward HIV-infected individuals than physicians. The decision about whether to treat a particular patient is seldom within a nurse's purview. As hospital employees, nurses have little, if any, freedom in choosing which patients to serve (nor do patients have much say in choosing their nurses). But nurses are the most constant providers of round-the-clock care for persons with AIDS, whose physical and emotional needs are great.

Fox, Aiken, and Messikomer (1991:249) have speculated about the impact of AIDS on the nursing profession:

> [Because of the lack of a cure for AIDS, it is] the caring of precisely the sort that nurses are uniquely trained to perform, that makes a difference. [As a result of AIDS] nurses are gaining recognition from physicians, as well as from patients and their families, for their caring attitudes and competence. . . . [One specific impact of AIDS has been to help] loosen the tight association of nursing care with 'women's work' through the conspicuous number of male nurses who are engaged in the clinical care of AIDS patients.

At San Francisco General Hospital and in other AIDS-dedicated units where multidisciplinary models of care have been developed to integrate physical and psychosocial care both in and out of the hospital, nurses have played a key role. In fact, AIDS service programs have been a vehicle for introducing organizational reforms that have long been sought by the nursing community and urged by expert advisory panels. It remains to be seen whether organizational changes made in response to AIDS will affect hospitals more broadly.

Confronting Occupational Risks

A singular and profound impact of AIDS has been a renewed appreciation for the risk of disease transmission in providing health care. Despite the well-known presence of many occupational risks (including infectious hazards, such as hepatitis B[3]), infection control in hospitals received very little attention until the dramatic increase in public and professional concern stimulated by the potential risk of HIV transmission. AIDS has prompted not only extensive assessments of risk in health care settings, but also searching examinations of how conscience, codes of ethics, moral obligations, and legal duties define the extent of the duty to treat (see "Defining the Scope of Professional Obligations," below).

Taking care of patients has always been a risky enterprise. In the 1800s and much of the 1900s, physicians and other health care workers faced fearsome epidemics of cholera, yellow fever, and influenza (Fox, 1988). The polio epidemic of the 1950s is within the memory of some who practice medicine today. Physicians' historical willingness to risk personal danger to care for their patients during epidemics has been important in forging a positive public attitude toward medicine and its practitioners (Kim and Perfect, 1988).

Many current practitioners, however, entered medicine at a time when risks of personal danger were not a major concern. Risks previously thought acceptable or commonplace may be viewed differently, however, in an era of high-tech medicine characterized by rapid advances in virology, immunology, and epidemiology. As Arras (1988:17) comments:

> Prior to the development of antibiotics, antisepsis, and vaccines, the entire world might be said to have constituted a 'high risk group' for early death from pestilence and other killer diseases. . . . Present day physicians . . . no longer believe that anyone, especially themselves, should die from infectious disease.

Health professionals are at risk of occupational HIV infection largely through exposure by accidental cuts or punctures incurred while caring for HIV-infected patients.[4] Once HIV was identified as the cause of AIDS and serologic tests for determining HIV antibody status were made available in 1985, prospective studies were undertaken to identify the extent of HIV infection acquired in hospital and clinic settings. A growing body of literature has emerged to quantify the frequency of needlestick injuries, the risk of seroconversion following a single needlestick from an infected patient, and the cumulative risks of practice over the course of a career in particular subspecialities or geographic locations (see Gerberding et al., 1990; Henderson et al., 1990).[5]

In May 1987 a report by the Centers for Disease Control (1987b) documented HIV infection in three health care workers who were exposed to HIV-infected blood through abrasions in the skin or splashes to mucous membranes. The anxiety prompted among health care workers by this report of seroconversions without needlestick exposures was quickly evident. It gave rise to a series of recommendations from the CDC and to a new regulation from the Occupational Safety and Health Administration (OSHA) for infection control measures ("Bloodborne Pathogens Standard," 29 CFR 1910.1030, 1991). Generally known as "universal precautions," the measures are designed to avoid exposure to blood and body fluids regardless of whether patients or health care workers are believed to be infected (Centers for Disease Control 1987a, 1988; U.S. Department of Labor, 1987). More recent recommendations have suggested a protocol for prophylaxis with AZT following needlestick exposure from infected patients (Centers for Disease Control, 1990), although there is doubt as to the efficacy of even immediate treatment (Lange et al., 1990).

The risks are not the same in all settings or in all health care specialties. A survey of 26 sentinel hospitals by the CDC revealed that an average of

1.3 percent of patients tested in these hospitals were HIV positive. The highest rate was at the University of Medicine and Dentistry in Newark, New Jersey, where 7.8 percent of patients tested HIV positive (St. Louis et al., 1990). Other studies of urban hospital emergency rooms have revealed disturbing rates of HIV infection (e.g., Kelen et al., 1989).

Attempts are being made to monitor health care workers' attitudes toward infection control and to define sources of risk (Gerberding and Schecter, 1991). The techniques and behaviors in health care settings that must be modified to reduce HIV transmission risks, however, may be as difficult to change as risky sexual behavior and drug-use habits. Health care procedures are learned behaviors and habits of many years' duration. More needs to be known about how to change infection-control practices and how psychological factors contribute to assessing and reducing risks. The spectrum of possible responses is wide: some health care workers may deny their risks and take few or no precautions; others may exaggerate risks and refuse to care for patients they believe to be HIV positive (Cotton, 1988; Rosenthal, 1990).

Concerns about HIV-infection risks have two sound bases: even remote risks are real, and with HIV the risk is of a lethal disease. The health care workers at greatest risk, such as surgeons, often voice skepticism about the scientific advice on risk reduction. Scientific information by itself about the nature of risk can only partly mitigate the fear of contracting a potentially fatal disease. Health care professionals who come in frequent contact with the blood and body fluids of patients who are likely to be HIV infected remain deeply concerned, even while appreciating the statistical information about the remoteness of risks.

Health care workers' concerns about becoming sick and dying following occupational exposure to HIV may be exacerbated by worries about breach of confidentiality, loss of employment and employee benefits, and possible economic ruin (Aoun, 1989; Cadman, 1990). Proof-and-causation problems may make it difficult to recover damages for workplace injuries in tort suits against hospitals or manufacturers. A health care worker who contracted HIV would have to prove that the HIV transmission occurred in the hospital and that the hospital was negligent—events that, because of the lengthy incubation period of the virus, may have occurred years previously. Meanwhile, the insurer and hospital might try to uncover the worker's sexual and drug-use history to ensure that other risk factors are not present.

Workers' compensation is a way to compensate for workplace injuries without a showing of fault. Although it is available to health care workers who are hospital employees, workers' compensation is better suited to dealing with traumatic injury than long-term disability. Workers' compensation has serious limitations in the context of HIV injury. For example, benefit levels are tied to the salary at the time of injury or death, which may be unfair for interns and residents or student nurses, all of whom could anticipate greater salaries later in their careers (Brennan, 1987; Cooke and Sande, 1989; Hauptman and Feinberg, 1990).

HIV-Infected Practitioners and Risks to Patients

It is not just caregivers who are worried about HIV transmission in health care settings. HIV-positive health care workers can transmit the virus to patients in the course of rendering care. Even remote or theoretical possibilities of caregiver-to-patient transmission can spark a great deal of concern. A Texas pediatrician was forced to close his practice within days after it became known through local news stories that he was HIV positive (Appelbome, 1987).

The death of Dr. Rudolph Almarez, a breast cancer surgeon who had operated on as many as 2,000 patients before he died from AIDS, generated considerable concern in Baltimore. Soon after his case was made public in 1990, a Baltimore law firm began to solicit clients to seek legal advice whether they were infected or even knew their serostatus. Clients were advised that emotional distress might be grounds for recovery against the hospital where Dr. Almarez practiced, and lawsuits were filed. In two separate cases, however, a Baltimore judge dismissed complaints based on fear of exposure to AIDS. The judge noted that there were no allegations that Dr. Almarez had not followed recommended infection control procedures or that any accident had occurred during surgery. The plaintiffs did not allege Dr. Almarez had infected them. A "look-back" study failed to uncover any HIV-positive patients (*Rossi* v. *Almarez, Faya* v. *Almarez*, Baltimore City Cir. Ct. Nos. 90344028 CL123396; 90345011 CL12345g, May 23, 1991).

Of the 202,843 cases of AIDS reported as of 1990, less than 5 percent are known to have been among health care workers. This is a slightly smaller fraction than is proportional to their number in the population at large. The attention to occupational risk for health care providers has overshadowed the fact that many more health care workers have become infected off the job, through unprotected sex or intravenous drug use. Health care workers with AIDS have included 679 physicians, 42 surgeons, 156 dentists and dental hygienists, and 1,199 nurses (Barnes et al., 1990). Many of the infected workers are HIV positive but have yet to develop AIDS. A number of look-back studies have been conducted of patients of infected health care workers to develop approximations of patient risk, but they are expensive to conduct and fraught with methodologic difficulties (Danila et al., 1991). The only alternative to developing estimates of risk of transmission is the development of theoretical models (Office of Technology Assessment, 1991).

Despite the theoretical risk to patients of HIV transmission in health care settings, there was little discussion in the late 1980s among professional associations and government officials about actions to be taken should a case of practitioner-to-patient transmission occur.[6] Nor were there guidelines as to what kind of procedures HIV-infected health care workers should be permitted to perform or who among colleagues, employers, or patients should be apprised of their HIV status. In the absence of clear policy guidelines, cases were handled on an ad hoc basis. An HIV-positive dental student from Washington University St. Louis was dismissed; a Chicago neurologist obtained a consent decree from a federal court that allowed him to practice but limited his involvement in certain invasive procedures; a director of anesthesiology was denied contact with patients and then disciplined when he personally assisted a patient who had vomited and was in immediate danger of aspirating; a gynecologist was forced to abandon a lucrative medical partnership despite his offer to do no work requiring physical contact with patients (Gostin, 1990:2091).

It became apparent that risks to patients in health care settings, if exceedingly remote, was more than theoretical when the CDC reported the possible transmission of HIV to Kimberly Bergalis, a patient in the Florida dental practice of David J. Acer, who died of AIDS. In 1991 the CDC announced that five patients had likely become infected in the course of treatment by Dr. Acer.[7] Ms. Bergalis's case sparked a firestorm of controversy and intense public policy debate concerning HIV testing in health care settings and possible strictures on practicing by HIV-positive health care workers. Ms. Bergalis, who died from AIDS in December 1991, blamed her illness on public health officials in a highly publicized letter published in *Newsweek* (Kantrowitz, 1991). In media appearances and in congressional testimony, the Bergalis family launched a campaign calling for mandatory testing of health care workers and disclosure of test results.

The issue of disclosure of caregivers' HIV status to patients is a critical policy concern. In a Gallup poll conducted among 1,014 adults in May 1991, 87 percent of the general public believed that doctors and dentists should be tested for AIDS, and 84 percent believed that nurses should be tested. In another study, more than one-half of patients surveyed said they would seek care elsewhere if they found out their physicians were caring for people with HIV disease (Gerbert et al., 1989).

In July 1991, largely as a result of the Bergalis case, the CDC published new guidelines reiterating the need for strict adherence to universal precautions and infection control procedures (Centers for Disease Control, 1991). The guidelines also stated that health care workers who perform "exposure-prone invasive procedures" should know their HIV status. Infected health care workers were directed not to perform such procedures unless they sought counsel from an expert panel as to the circumstances, "if any," under which it would be appropriate to do so. A few days before the guidelines were issued, an additional clause was added at the behest of Senator Orrin Hatch (R-Utah) and Health and Human Services Secretary Louis Sullivan (Gautier, 1991): the "informed consent" provision in the CDC guidelines requires that HIV-infected health care workers disclose their seropositivity to prospective patients undergoing exposure-prone, invasive procedures.[8]

On August 16, 1991, the CDC had announced the initiation of a process to develop a list of exposure-prone, invasive procedures to serve as a guide for local review bodies. Although the CDC anticipated completing the development of such a list by November 15, 1991, in order to clarify what it wanted states to do, a November 4 meeting revealed widespread discontent among the medical and public health community with CDC's approach (Altman, 1991). Virtually all medical and professional associations except the American Medical Association refused to cooperate in the list-making endeavor because they were not convinced that there existed sufficient scientific evidence on which to base such a list. In October 1991 Congress passed an appropriations bill that included an amendment requiring states to institute the CDC guidelines or their "equivalent" or risk the loss of Public Health Service funds (Treasury, Postal Service, and General Government Appropriations Act, 1992, P.L. 102-141 Sec. 633 (1991)). However, on July 30, 1992, the National Commission on AIDS recommended against both mandatory testing for doctors and mandatory notification of patients because the risks of infection are so remote and disclosure so detrimental to a provider's career (National Commission on AIDS, 1992; Leary, 1992).

Many questions remain to be answered as professional associations, state and local policy makers, and hospital administrators and risk managers sort out federal directives and make policy. The ethical arguments on both sides of the issue are complex (Gostin, 1989; Daniels, 1992). Perhaps the overarching question, in the words of former New York State Health Commissioner David Axelrod, is the extent to which "highly unusual circumstances" should "dictate broad policy questions" (Altman, 1990). As has been apparent in other settings, such as schools, workplaces, and prisons, sober appraisals of risk can easily be overwhelmed by fear, prejudice, misunderstandings, and the impact of highly publicized individual cases.

The Burden of Caring for AIDS Patients

Because of its clinical complexities, its dire nature, and the stigma that surrounds it, AIDS poses considerable challenges for caregivers. The range of opportunistic infections involved means that virtually any organ system, and often many at the same time, can be subject to rare and potentially life-threatening infections or malignancies. In addition to complex medical needs, complex psychosocial needs that are evident in other chronic and terminal illnesses may have special urgency in AIDS patients. Whether because of medical problems, discrimination, or both, people with HIV disease may lose jobs, housing, and the support of families and friends.

The reasons that physicians might choose to limit their involvement with HIV disease are varied (Volberding, 1989:748):

> Many may feel intimidated by the rapidly growing medical complexity of AIDS-associated illnesses and by the numerous diagnostic and therapeutic approaches available. Some may be afraid of becoming infected with HIV in the course of treating patients. Others, like so many in our society, may fear the sex- and drug-related behavior that accounts for much of HIV transmission (a fear that contributes to discrimination against patients with AIDS). Finally, physicians may feel unable to cope with the severe psychological stress of caring for the young, dying, disfigured, and isolated patient—the patient that is so typical in this epidemic.

Patients with AIDS are younger, on average, than others with life-threatening or chronic illnesses. They often are contemporaries of their physicians in age, social class, and education. Many health care providers who have taken on large numbers of patients with HIV disease are themselves gay and may share a special fear of the virus with their patients. The psychological toll of losing tens or hundreds of previously healthy patients can be enormous. Grief, hopelessness, and frustration about the limitations in treatment for HIV make caring for persons with AIDS a challenge.

The Influence of Prejudice

A cornerstone of a physician's ethic has been objectivity in the care of patients. Physicians try to put aside personal feelings about the life-styles, values, and morals of their patients (Groves, 1978). Yet such objectivity may be difficult to maintain. Physicians may occasionally express overt dislike and frank prejudice for patients whose life-styles they find disagreeable. Physicians may be uncomfortable in treating gay patients or discussing sexuality (Kelly et al., 1987a,b; Lewis, Freeman, and Corey, 1987). Conversely, patients may be unwilling to share information about their life-styles that may be relevant to their health care (Dardick and Grady, 1980). Prejudice may be expressed in subtle devaluations of stigmatized patients in ways that providers may not even realize.

Some observers have wondered whether "submerged prejudices enhance the apprehension of danger" of HIV transmission (Jonsen, 1990:158) and find some evidence for this in the contrasting attitudes about HIV and hepatitis B. Many health care workers have seemed to overlook the danger of hepatitis, while expressing serious concerns about HIV.

Reluctance to treat patients with HIV disease has been documented, at least to a certain extent, in a number of surveys:

A survey of 258 New York City interns and residents in hospitals with a large AIDS patient census revealed that roughly 50% were "mildly, moderately, or extremely" resentful of having to take care of AIDS patients. If given a choice, 25% said they would stop taking care of AIDS patients; 24% believed that refusing to care for AIDS patients would not be unethical (Link et al., 1988).

A 1987 survey of second-year medical students revealed that 7% thought they should be allowed to decline taking a history from a patient with AIDS; 14% thought they should be allowed to refuse to examine such a patient; and 32% felt they should be able to decline to draw blood (Imperato et al., 1988).

Answers to hypothetical questions on surveys do not necessarily reflect what health care workers actually do when put to the test. As an example, a 1986 survey of 325 orthopedic surgeons in the United States revealed that nearly 50 percent agreed that a surgeon was ethically obligated to operate on HIV-positive patients whenever surgery was medically indicated; yet only 4 percent of the respondents had themselves declined to operate on HIV-positive patients (Arnow et al., 1989).

Refusal to care for people with AIDS or HIV disease, or those at risk, may result in a broad range of harm. Refusal to treat can lead to systematic denial of access and substandard care. People who are refused care may ultimately never find it, or they may be harmed by delays if their condition worsens as a result of a refusal. Being refused care stigmatizes patients and adds to the considerable psychological burdens of living with HIV disease. Such refusals can also exacerbate the risk for health care professionals who remain steadfast in their willingness to treat and, hence, assume a disproportionate burden of caring for HIV disease. In addition, providers who care for people with AIDS have themselves experienced stigma and discrimination.

Defining the Scope of Professional Obligation

One impact of AIDS has been the revival of interest in the history of physicians' response to occupational risk (Friedlander, 1990; Kim and Perfect, 1988). Bosk and Frader (1991:268) note: "AIDS as a total social phenomenon has become the lens for focusing on the obligations of the members of the medical profession." However, history provides an imprecise guide to physicians' individual or collective duties to care for patients with contagious diseases. As revealed in the recent spate of histories occasioned by the HIV epidemic, physicians as esteemed as Galen and Sydenham fled from patients with contagious diseases. Others stayed behind, caring for patients at considerable personal risk (Zuger and Miles, 1987). In European cities during the intermittent plagues that persisted from the fourteenth to eighteenth centuries, some localities passed laws forbidding physicians to leave during times of plague. More commonly, however, local governments contracted with "plague doctors"—younger, relatively inexperienced physicians, often from the countryside, who were willing to risk the dangers in exchange for salaries, citizenship, and entry into restrictive physicians' guilds (Fox, 1988).

In the United States, the duty to assume risks in caring for contagious patients, first articulated as a personal religious obligation by colonial physician Benjamin Rush, was codified as a professional duty by the American Medical Association (AMA) in 1847: "And when pestilence prevails, it is their [physicians'] duty to face the danger and to continue their labors for the alleviation of suffering, even at the jeopardy of their own lives." The duty remained part of the AMA's code of ethics until 1957, when it was jettisoned during the exuberance of the first years of the antibiotic era.[9]

The obligation to care for patients with contagious diseases stands alongside a tradition of freedom of choice in American medicine. "The right to refuse to care for a particular patient, either by not accepting that person as a patient or by discharging oneself from responsibility in a recognized way, is deeply embedded in the ethos of American medicine" (Jonsen, 1990:159). Self-employed physicians have no legal obligations to provide particular services to individual patients, unless some relationship already exists. Medical ethicists have sought to establish the source of collective and individual professional obligations to treat people with HIV disease (Pellegrino, 1987; Daniels, 1991). Some have argued that an obligation derives from distinctive characteristics of medicine as a learned profession or a vocation to which one is called (Emanuel, 1988). Others have argued for a "virtue-based ethic" that mandates physicians to commit themselves to obligations beyond what is narrowly required by law or by contract, recognizing the moral nature of medical practice (Zuger and Miles, 1987).

The situation is different for institutions and their employees. Nurses, for example, as hospital employees, seldom have any freedom in choosing which patients to serve (nor do patients have much to say in choosing their nurses). Hospitals with emergency rooms must offer services to all patients with emergencies. Federal laws provide stiff fines for "dumping" unstable patients on other facilities. Although anti-dumping laws may help ensure safe patient transfer, they do not guarantee that patients with HIV disease will receive the services of any particular institution. Private hospitals are likely to continue to refer patients with HIV disease to public or charity hospitals, along with other patients whose care is complex and for whom there are inadequate reimbursements (Andrulis, 1989; Gage et al., 1991).

THE HEALTH CARE SYSTEM AS A MARKET

Another social impact of AIDS on the health care system is economic. Any epidemic as extensive as that of HIV/AIDS is bound to create markets for new products and services. Although the size and permanence of these markets are difficult to estimate, the following are likely to be the major ones:

- pharmaceuticals
- medical devices
- health care services (other than those of physicians)
  — home care
  — institutional care (e.g., nursing homes)
- educational services
- management and other consultative services

The World Health Organization (1992) estimates the number of HIV-infected people worldwide at 8 to 10 million. Nevertheless, the main marketing focus for therapeutic products of pharmaceutical companies has been the United States and other developed countries because of the expense of the newly developed drugs. AZT, for example, costs patients in the United States $2,000-$3,000 per year, and the potential market for AZT in North America, Europe, and Japan is quite large. The Pharmaceutical Manufacturers Association estimated that some 90 compounds were in some phase of clinical testing as of early 1990. In what is perhaps a first, pharmaceutical companies have been under attack from AIDS activists for the prices charged for drugs. Such attacks have led to challenges to the patent rights of Burroughs-Wellcome to AZT and attempts to revise the federal Orphan Drug Act (National Commission on AIDS, 1991).

Vaccine production is another potentially profitable area for pharmaceutical companies—virtually everyone in the world is a candidate for an effective HIV vaccine, if one can be developed and distributed at a reasonable cost. Aside from the formidable technical challenges in creating an HIV vaccine, there are substantial financial and social barriers. Many of the difficulties revolve around the issue of liability for damages arising from injuries, which are almost inevitable in any vaccination program as broad as that contemplated for HIV (Keystone Center, 1990).

Another market exists for medical devices. Increased costs are associated with the barrier protections adopted by hospitals as a means of minimizing health care workers' contact with blood and body fluids. The items involved include latex and vinyl gloves, protective gowns, face masks, protective eye wear, and containers for disposing of needles and other sharp instruments. The HIV epidemic has spurred the development of needles and syringes that can be disposed of with minimal risk of needlesticks.

Attention in this area has been given to technique (e.g., avoiding "recapping" needles) and technologies (redesigning syringes, needles, and other sharp instruments) (Gerberding and Schecter, 1991).

Few studies have been made of the actual costs of implementing universal precautions. In their study of a 900-bed teaching hospital, Doebbeling and Wenzel (1990) estimated an increase of $350,900 annually for barrier protections against HIV infection. They extrapolated from their data to arrive at an estimated cost nationwide of $336 million for universal precautions in 1989.

Home health care is now a $15 billion a year business (Feder, 1991). The technical capacity of the industry and its acceptance by medical providers have been spurred by the HIV epidemic. This development is the result of a "push"—the desire of payers and hospitals to find lower cost ways of administering intravenous therapy—and a "pull"—the preference of many AIDS patients to be at home rather than in a hospital. Some companies, however, have come under criticism for their high prices, a reflection of the consumer activism that exists in other areas of the system (Green and DeStefano, 1991).

The need for institutions, professionals, and managers to deal with the epidemic has also led to the creation of an AIDS consulting and educational "industry." Pamphlets, audio- and videotapes, lectures, presentations, seminars, and conferences abound on topics ranging from HIV prevention among minority adolescents to surrogate screening techniques that help to identify and avoid underwriting insurance for HIV-infected individuals.

Two states (Washington and Kentucky) have passed laws requiring documentation of HIV education as a condition of licensure of certain health professionals. The effectiveness of such provisions is unclear, as is the potential precedent for the requirement of other disease-specific knowledge.

HEALTH CARE FINANCING

A study of the first 10,000 patients with AIDS showed the average direct medical costs from diagnosis to death to be approximately $147,000 (Hardy et al., 1986). This figure, announced at a press conference in 1985, took on a life of its own in the early years of the epidemic (Oppenheimer and Padgug, 1991). Combined with widespread uncertainty about the extent of HIV infection in the population and its clinical course, the estimate prompted serious concerns about the ability of the health care system to meet the challenge of paying for the necessary care. The $147,000 figure was based on data from hospital charges that were skewed in favor of New York City municipal hospitals, but the AIDS caseloads of those hospitals comprised primarily intravenous drug users, who often suffered from a number of concomitant illnesses and required more hospitalization than gay men with AIDS. Since 1985, data from other studies have yielded a more complete picture of the direct and indirect costs of AIDS and have shifted the focus of concern.

First, the per-patient costs for AIDS-related medical care have been dropping. Most estimates now place direct lifetime medical costs between $40,000 and $50,000.[10] The reduction is attributable to several developments: greater medical familiarity with the disease; more aggressive outpatient management of traditionally inpatient procedures, such as transfusions and lumbar punctures; effective outpatient regimens for such diseases as *Pneumocystis carinii* pneumonia and cryptococcal meningitis; and the availability of largely volunteer-based social service supports that allow management of sick patients at home and in less costly institutions than hospitals (Arno, 1986; see also Chapter 6).

The direct medical cost of caring for persons with AIDS consumes only a small fraction of national health expenditures—less than 2 percent. For this reason, AIDS has been described as a financing rather than a cost problem. It is rapidly becoming a burden for local governments in cities with a high prevalence of HIV disease (National Commission on AIDS, 1991).

AIDS care is also increasingly the province of public health care financing mechanisms; the burden is shifting more to Medicaid (Green and Arno, 1990). This is true in large part because the epidemic is increasingly manifested among intravenous drug users and poor people, who are unlikely to have private insurance. In addition, patients who may initially have had private insurance through the workplace lose their coverage after they become unable to work (Yelin et al., 1991) and turn to Medicaid and other public programs for indigent care. Furthermore, since a record of a positive HIV test renders someone virtually ineligible for individually underwritten private insurance—or may be considered a "preexisting condition," precluding claims for non-HIV illnesses—there are an unknown number of people whose employment or economic situation would ordinarily be sufficient to obtain insurance, but who now cannot do so.

Although the overall effect of AIDS on Medicaid expenditures is not overwhelming, its impact is considerable in those states with large numbers of cases. The AIDS epidemic also arose when Medicaid was becoming the fastest-growing segment of many state budgets—roughly 15 percent of expenditures in 1992, compared with 7 percent 10 years ago. Medicaid is thus facing cutbacks in many states, and the increasing demand for AIDS care competes with the need to provide other health services.

In the world of private insurance, AIDS has mainly had the effect of adding another screening test to the 15 percent of the insurance market that is medically underwritten: that is, individual medical exams are required as proof of "insurability." (Most insurance is provided though the workplace and does not require individual health assessments.) Several states, including California and Massachusetts and the District of Columbia, initially banned the use of HIV antibody testing for private insurance purposes. All have now, amidst considerable controversy, reversed that stand (Intergovernmental Health Policy Project, 1990).

Despite the considerable per-patient cost of direct medical care of HIV disease, especially to the public sector, there have been few major structural changes in the health care financing system in response. Indeed, the response to AIDS has been described as "incrementalist." Adjustments have been made here and there in existing financing mechanisms, but no large-scale changes have been made. Providers, including hospitals, nursing homes, and physicians, have claimed that AIDS patients are more costly than others. Regulators and rate setters have thus been forced to examine the structure of their reimbursement systems to incorporate this "exception." In New Jersey, for example, this examination has contributed to a major effort to provide more flexibility in determining rates for all diseases.

Various proposals have been put forward for HIV-specific funding of care. Among them are the inclusion of HIV as a categorical disease covered by Medicare, similar to end-stage renal disease (ESRD) (Makadon et al., 1990b) and designation of HIV disease as a Medicaid-eligible condition, at least for outpatient care and prescription drugs. Such structural reforms have generally been rejected by the executive and legislative branches of state governments on two major grounds: concerns over the equity of HIV-specific funding streams (Roper and Winkenwerder, 1988) and the potentially large impact on already strained entitlement programs, much as the Medicare ESRD program has grown far larger than was expected at its inception.

One federal development has been the creation of the Public Health Service's AIDS Drug Reimbursement Program, a pool of money earmarked for assisting patients who are neither insured nor affluent enough to pay for expensive HIV-related drugs, now including AZT, pentamidine, and gancyclovir. This fund, initiated soon after the licensing of AZT, was created from funds already earmarked for AIDS research and care in agencies of the Public Health Service (P.L. 100-71; P.L. 100-471; P.L. 100-116; S. 2240; Merlis, 1990).

What structural financing innovations have been initiated have largely been at the state level. They have included enhanced Medicaid reimbursement for AIDS care, in New Jersey and New York (Rango et al., 1990); creation of AIDS centers with core funding in New Jersey, New York, and California (Williams et al., 1990); and regional centers for people with HIV disease in Maryland and Massachusetts (Smith et al., 1990); and, a number of states have obtained waivers of Medicaid regulations from the Health Care Financing Administration, allowing them to provide medical and other services not usually covered by Medicaid.

The current costs for care of AIDS patients has thus a noticeable, but not overwhelming impact on health care financing, except in those places where a heavy caseload must be supported by an already stressed system. However, it might be asked what the impact will be over the next decade, as those who are infected but not yet symptomatic begin to require more extensive health care. This question cannot be readily answered. It is extraordinarily difficult to project beyond a year or two the costs of AIDS care or the needs for health personnel, because of rapidly changing standards of care. The past few years have seen some developments that have lowered costs and others that have increased them. In the diagnosis of *Pneumocystis carinii* pneumonia, for instance, a new technique to induce sputum for laboratory analysis has lowered the number of costly bronchoscopies. Introduction of that technique has also required readjustments of the projections of pulmonary specialists needed to perform those bronchoscopies. Similarly, future development in drug therapy, success in orally administered outpatient treatment for conditions that currently require hospitalization, and therapeutic and preventative advances make accurate predictions of future costs and personnel virtually impossible.

CONCLUSIONS

The impact of AIDS on the health care system, with all its complexities, is not easily summarized. In part this is because of the greatly disparate geographic impact of the epidemic and differences in preexisting local configurations of health care. In some areas, such as New York City, growing numbers of HIV and AIDS patients have put severe strains on already beleaguered public and university teaching hospitals. Other local health care systems, with fewer cases and smaller inpatient hospital censuses, have been better able to absorb the influx of people with HIV disease or AIDS. Although many more people will be diagnosed with AIDS in coming years, prediction and planning for specific quantities and types of health care services are made difficult by the rapidly changing nature of HIV-related clinical care.

AIDS does seem to be having an impact on certain ways in which health care is delivered. The HIV epidemic may have increased the trend to deliver care beyond the inpatient hospital setting, either in clinics or in patients' homes. Many procedures for people with AIDS that formerly required hospitalization (e.g., transfusions, chemotherapy, and intravenous hydration) are now being done in clinics, and intravenous, intramuscular, and aerosolized therapies are increasingly being delivered at home. And AIDS is helping pave the way for the routine reimbursement of quite complex treatments that are critical not only for HIV-related care, but also for other chronic and terminal illnesses.

The trend toward out-of-hospital care, whether in clinics, hospices, or patients' homes, is being driven by cost concerns and the desire of many ill people to remain in comfortable and familiar surroundings with loved ones. With the AIDS epidemic, these trends are also accompanied by concerns about how to ensure continuity of care and bring rationality to a fragmented health care system.

Although many people with HIV disease face daunting problems in gaining access to and being able to pay for needed care—problems that are only likely to increase as the epidemic becomes more widespread among intravenous drug users and their sexual partners and poor residents of inner cities—AIDS has not been a catalyst for large-scale reform of health care financing. The chorus of voices calling for reform of the health care system has been growing louder in the early 1990s, but it seems to have less to do with AIDS and more to do with the realization that many of the working poor and middle class (nearly 40 million Americans) find private health insurance beyond their reach and public programs inadequate.

Early concerns about the ability of the private health care system to pay for AIDS care now seem somewhat alarmist. The direct medical costs of caring for persons with AIDS consumes 2 percent or less of national health expenditures. As noted above, AIDS has thus been described as a financing rather than a cost problem. This characterization, however, should not detract from the realization of the tremendous burden HIV disease poses for those who are afflicted with it, as well as for providers and governments in areas with high prevalences of HIV disease. The multifaceted impact of AIDS has meant that any financing reforms in response to the epidemic have tended to be of a piecemeal, tinkering-around-the-edges nature, rather than wholesale or systemic.

The HIV epidemic may also be having an impact on the training and recruitment of physicians and other health care workers, but the number of confounding variables makes it difficult to sort out the impact of HIV disease on the attitudes and behaviors of health care professionals. Some caregivers may be attracted by the challenges AIDS care poses; others may find the same challenges daunting. Some physicians may be wary of establishing practices among certain populations or in certain areas hard hit by AIDS, although in many instances those areas are where the most prestigious medical institutions and teaching centers are located. Further study will be necessary to determine the impact of HIV on the decisions of physicians and other caregivers about specialties and practice locations.

Perhaps the most profound impact of AIDS on health care has been a renewed appreciation of, and heightened attention to, the risk of blood-borne pathogens. These include, but are not limited to, HIV. Many health care workers who were trained in an era of scientific derring-do and medical hubris are coming to realize that medicine has always posed dangers for practitioners. AIDS is prompting an extensive reassessment, not only of the scientific and technical aspects of those risks and how to quantify them, but of how conscience, codes of ethics, moral obligations, and legal duties affect practitioners' duties to treat patients who pose risks of potentially lethal infections.

NOTES

1. The Graduate Medical Education National Advisory Committee report (U.S. Department of Health and Human Services, 1981) predicted a physician oversupply of 70,000 by 1990.

2. Sir William Osler's (1906) injunction to "know syphilis in all its manifestations and relations and all other things clinical will be added unto you" could be recast for the modern practitioner. To "know AIDS" implies knowledge of the toll HIV disease takes on a variety of organ systems, as well as associated illnesses, such as tuberculosis, and other sexually transmitted diseases, including syphilis (Nunn et al., 1990; Quinn et al., 1990).

3. Hepatitis B, a blood-borne infection transmitted by the same routes as HIV, is transmitted in occupational settings to as many as 5,900-7,400 health care workers each year—as many as 200 to 300 of whom will eventually die from hepatitis-related complications (U.S. Department of Labor, 1991).

4. The CDC has documented 37 cases of health care workers with no other apparent risk factors who have seroconverted following occupational exposure to HIV; virtually all of the cases involved needlesticks or other deep punctures with instruments contaminated with HIV-infected blood. Health care workers have voiced considerable skepticism about whether the CDC-reported cases represent the full extent of occupationally acquired HIV infection (Rosenthal, 1990).

5. The most commonly cited figure for risk of seroconversion following a single needlestick exposure is 1:250. This is an "average" estimate. A more accurate assessment of the probability involved in a particular case would depend on the clinical stage of HIV infection of the source patient and the quantity of the inoculate, which in turn is related to needle type and size, the depth of penetration, and the type of gloves worn.

6. A substantial fraction of medical students, interns, and even practicing physicians are not vaccinated for highly infectious diseases that might pose a threat to patients. A 1990 survey of medical schools found that one-third do not require their medical students to be vaccinated. Up to 20 percent of medical students have not been immunized against measles and rubella, and anywhere from 40 to 90 percent have not been immunized against hepatitis B or influenza (Nazario, 1990; Poland and Nichol, 1990).

7. Investigators have been unable to determine exactly how Dr. Acer's patients were infected; it was established that he and his staff followed standard sterilization procedures (Palca, 1992).

8. Congress held hearings on the issue of HIV in health care settings, and in July 1991 the Senate voted 80-18 for an amendment that would have mandated prison terms of not less than 10 years or fines of up to $10,000 or both for HIV-infected health care workers who knew they were seropositive but failed to notify prospective patients before performing invasive procedures (Gautier, 1991). The amendment was ultimately rejected by a congressional conference committee, but its passage in the Senate by such a wide margin reflected the immediate impact of Kimberly Bergalis and the cluster of cases in Dr. Acer's dental office. It should be noted, however, that those cases are the only known cases involving HIV transmission to patients in a health care setting.

9. The 1957 revised code reads: "A physician, shall, in the provision of appropriate

patient care, except in emergencies, be free to choose whom to serve." When AIDS appeared on the scene, the AMA's Judicial Council reaffirmed physicians' duties: "A physician may not ethically refuse to treat a patient whose condition is within the physician's current realm of competence solely because the patient is seropositive. . . . Neither those who have the disease [AIDS] nor those who have been infected with the virus should be subjected to discrimination based on fear or prejudice, least of all by members of the health care community" (American Medical Association, 1987:1360). Freedman (1988) has critiqued contemporary codes of professional ethics as they relate to obligations to care for HIV disease.

10.   There are other many prevalent chronic illnesses with high average costs per patient, such as end-stage renal disease.

REFERENCES

Altman, L.K. (1990) AIDS testing of doctors is crux of thorny debate. *New York Times* December 27:A1.

Altman, L.K. (1991) Unexpected defiance greets AIDS guidelines. *New York Times* October 15:C-1.

American Medical Association, Council on Ethical and Judicial Affairs (1987) Ethical issues involved in the growing AIDS crisis. *Journal of the American Medical Association* 259(9):1360-1361.

Andrulis, D.P. (1989) *Crisis at the Front Line: The Effects of AIDS on Public Hospitals.* New York: Priority Press.

Aoun, H. (1989) When a house officer gets AIDS. *New England Journal of Medicine* 321:693-696.

Applebome, P. (1987) Doctor in Texas with AIDS virus closes his practice amid a furor. *New York Times* October 1:A16.

Arno, P.S. (1986) The non-profit sector's response to the AIDS epidemic: community-based services in San Francisco. *American Journal of Public Health* 76:1325-1330.

Arnow, P.M., L.A. Pottenger, C.B. Stocking, M. Siegler, and H.W. DeLeeuw (1989) Orthopedic surgeons' attitudes and practices concerning treatment of patients with HIV infection. *Public Health Reports* 104:121-129.

Arras, J.D. (1988) The fragile web of responsibility: AIDS and the duty to treat. *Hastings Center Report* 18(Suppl.):10-20.

Barnes, M., N.A. Rango, G.R. Burke, and L. Chiarello (1990) The HIV-infected health care professional: employment policies and public health. *Law, Medicine & Health Care* 18:311-330.

Bartlett, J.G. (1988) Who will take care of patients with AIDS? *Washington Post* April 5(Health Suppl.):10-11.

Benjamin, A.E. (1988) Long-term care and AIDS: perspectives from experience with the elderly. *Milbank Quarterly* 66:415-443.

Bennett, C.L., J.B. Garfinkle, S. Greenfield, D. Draper, W. Rogers, et al. (1989) The relation between hospital experience and in-hospital mortality for patients with AIDS-related PCP. *Journal of the American Medical Association* 261:2975-2979.

Bosk, C.L., and J.E. Frader (1991) AIDS and its impact on medical work: the culture and politics of the shop floor. In D. Nelkin, D.P. Willis, and S.V. Parris, eds., *A Disease of Society: Cultural and Institutional Responses to AIDS.* New York: Cambridge University Press.

Brennan, T.A. (1987) The acquired immunodeficiency syndrome (AIDS) as an occupational disease. *Annals of Internal Medicine* 107:581-583.

Cadman, E.C. (1990) Physicians in training and HIV (letter). *New England Journal of Medicine* 322:1392-1393.

Centers for Disease Control (CDC) (1987a) Recommendations for prevention of HIV transmission in health-care settings. *Morbidity and Mortality Weekly Report* 36:3S-18S.

Centers for Disease Control (CDC) (1987b) Update: human immunodeficiency virus infection in health-care workers exposed to blood of infected patients. *Morbidity and Mortality Weekly* 36:285-289.

Centers for Disease Control (CDC) (1988) Update: acquired immunodeficiency syndrome and human immunodeficiency virus infection among health-care workers. *Morbidity and Mortality Weekly Report* 37:229-234, 239.

Centers for Disease Control (CDC) (1990) Public Health Service statement on management of occupational exposure to human immunodeficiency virus, including considerations regarding zidovudine postexposure use. *Morbidity and Mortality Weekly Report* 39(RR-1):1-14.

Centers for Disease Control (CDC) (1991) Recommendations for preventing transmission of human immunodeficiency virus and hepatitis B virus to patients during exposure-prone invasive procedures. *Morbidity and Mortality Weekly Report* 40(RR-8):1-9.

Cooke, M., and J.A. Sande (1989) The HIV epidemic and training in internal medicine: challenges and recommendations. *New England Journal of Medicine* 321:1334-1338.

Cotton, D.J. (1988) The impact of AIDS on the medical care system. *Journal of the American Medical Association* 260:519-523.

Cotton, D.J. (1989) Improving survival in acquired immunodeficiency syndrome: is experience everything? *Journal of the American Medical Association* 261:3016-3017.

Daniels, N. (1991) Duty to treat or right to refuse. *Hastings Center Report* 21(2):36-46.

Daniels, N. (1992) HIV infected health care professionals: public threat or public sacrifice? *Milbank Quarterly* 70(1):3-42.

Danila, R.N., K.L. MacDonald, F.S. Rhame, M.E. Moen, D.O. Reier, et al. (1991) A lookback investigation of patients of an HIV-infected physician: public health implications. *New England Journal of Medicine* 325:1406-1411.

Dardick, L., and K.E. Grady (1980) Openness between gay persons and health professionals. *Annals of Internal Medicine* 93:115-119.

Doebbeling, B.N., and R.P. Wenzel (1990) The direct costs of universal precautions in a teaching hospital. *Journal of the American Medical Association* 264:2038-2087.

Emanuel, E.J. (1988) Do physicians have an obligation to treat patients with AIDS? *New England Journal of Medicine* 318:1686-1690.

Enthoven, A., and R. Kronick (1989) A consumer choice health plan for the 1990s: universal health insurance in a system designed to promote quality and economy. *New England Journal of Medicine* 320:29-37.

Feder, B.J. (1991) Where the boom is in health care. *New York Times* December 26:C-1.

Fox, D.M. (1988) The politics of physicians' responsibility in epidemics: a note on history. *Hastings Center Report* 18(Suppl.):5-10.

Fox, R.C., L.H. Aiken, and C.M. Messikomer (1991) The culture of caring: AIDS and the nursing profession. In D. Nelkin, D.P. Willis, and S.V. Parris, eds., *A Disease of Society: Cultural and Institutional Responses to AIDS.* New York: Cambridge University Press.

Freedman, B. (1988) Health professions, codes, and the right to refuse to treat HIV-infectious patients. *Hastings Center Report* 18(Suppl.):20-25.

Friedlander, W.J. (1990) On the obligation of physicians to treat AIDS: is there a historical basis? *Reviews of Infectious Diseases* 12:191-203.

Gage, L.S., V.B. Weslowski, D.P. Andrulis, E. Hintz, and A.B. Camper (1991) *America's Safety Net Hospitals: The Foundation of Our Nation's Health System.* Washington, D.C.: National Association of Public Hospitals.

Gautier, E. (1991) Hysteria v. reason: health care workers and HIV transmission. *The Exchange* 16:1-9.

Gerberding, J.L., and W.P. Schecter (1991) Surgery and AIDS: reducing the risk (editorial). *Journal of the American Medical Association* 265:1572-1573.

Gerberding, J.L., C. Littell, A. Tarkington, A. Brown, and W.P. Schecter (1990) Risk of exposure of surgical personnel to patients' blood during surgery at San Francisco General Hospital. *New England Journal of Medicine* 322:1788-1793.

Gerbert, B., B.T. Maguire, S.B. Hulley, and T.J. Coates (1989) Physicians and acquired immunodeficiency syndrome: what patients think about human immunodeficiency virus in medical practice. *Journal of the American Medical Association* 262:1969-1972.

Gostin, L.O. (1989) Hospitals, health care professionals, and AIDS: the "right to know" the health status of professionals and patients. *Maryland Law Review* 48:12-54.

Gostin, L.O. (1990) The AIDS litigation project: a national review of court and human rights commission decisions, Part II: Discrimination. *Journal of the American Medical Association* 263:2086-2093.

Green, J., and P.S. Arno (1990) The "Medicaidization" of AIDS: trends in the financing of HIV-related medical care. *Journal of the American Medical Association* 264:1261-1266.

Green, M., and G. DeStefano (1991) *Making a Killing on AIDS: Home Health Care and Pentamadine*. New York: City of New York Department of Consumer Affairs.

Greene, J., M.R. Leigh, and L.J. Passman (1989) AIDS treatment center: is the concept premature? (letter). *Journal of the American Medical Association* 262:2537-2538.

Groves, J.E. (1978) Taking care of the hateful patient. *New England Journal of Medicine* 298:883-887.

Hardy, A.M., K. Rauch, and D. Echenberg, et al. (1986) The economic impact of the first 10,000 cases of acquired immunodeficiency syndrome in the United States. *Journal of the American Medical Association* 255:209-211.

Hauptman, P.J., and M.B. Feinberg (1990) Occupational exposure to HIV among house staff (letter). *New England Journal of Medicine* 323:1356.

Hayward, R.A., and M.F. Shapiro (1991) A national study of AIDS and residency training: experiences, concerns, and consequences. *Annals of Internal Medicine* 114:23-32.

Henderson, D.K., B.J. Fahey, M. Willy, J.M. Schmitt, K. Carey, et al. (1990) Risk for occupational transmission of human immunodeficiency virus type 1 (HIV-1) associated with clinical exposures: a prospective evaluation. *Annals of Internal Medicine* 113:740-746.

Imperato, P.J., J.G. Feldman, K. Nayeri, and J.A. DeHovitz (1988) Medical students' attitudes towards caring for patients with AIDS in a high incidence area. *New York State Journal of Medicine* 88:223-228.

Inglehart, J.K. (1992) The American health care system. *New England Journal of Medicine* 326(14):962-967.

Intergovernmental Health Policy Project (1990) State financing for AIDS: options and trends. *Intergovernmental AIDS Report* 3:1-8, 12.

Jellinek, P.S. (1988) Case managing AIDS. *Issues in Science and Technology* 4(Summer):59-63.

Jonsen, A.R. (1990) The duty to treat patients with AIDS and HIV infection. In L.O. Gostin, ed., *AIDS and the Health Care System*. New Haven, Conn.: Yale University Press.

Kantrowitz, B. (1991) Doctors and AIDS: should patients and doctors have the right to know each other's HIV status? A pair of new cases in Minneapolis reignites the debate while the first victim of doctor-to-patient transmission lies dying. *Newsweek* July 1:48.

Kelen, G.D., T. DiGiovanna, L. Bisson, D. Kalainov, K.T. Sivertson, et al. (1989) Human immunodeficiency virus infection in emergency department patients: epidemiology, clinical presentations, and risk to health care workers: The Johns Hopkins experience. *Journal of the American Medical Association* 262:516-522.

Kelly, J.A., J.S. St. Lawrence, S. Smith, Jr., H.V. Hood, and D.J. Cook (1987a) Medical students' attitudes toward AIDS and homosexual patients. *Journal of Medical Education* 62:549-556.

Kelly, J.A., J.S. St. Lawrence, S. Smith, Jr., H.V. Hood, and D.J. Cook (1987b) Stigmatization of AIDS patients by physicians. *American Journal of Public Health* 77:789-791.

Keystone Center (1990) *Keystone AIDS Vaccine Liability Project.* Keystone, Colo.: The Keystone Center.

Kim, J.H., and J.R. Perfect (1988) To help the sick: an historical and ethical essay concerning the refusal to care for patients with AIDS. *The American Journal of Medicine* 84:135-138.

Lange, J.M., C.A. Boucher, C.E. Hollak, E.H. Wiltink, P. Reiss, et al. (1990) Failure of zidovudine prophylaxis after accidental exposure to HIV-1. *New England Journal of Medicine* 322:1375-1377.

Leary, W. (1992) Mandatory AIDS test for doctors opposed. *New York Times* July 31:A11.

Levine, C. (1990) In and out of the hospital. In L.O. Gostin, ed., *AIDS and the Health Care System.* New Haven, Conn.: Yale University Press.

Lewis, C.E., H.E. Freeman, and C.R. Corey (1987) AIDS-related competence of California's primary care physicians. *American Journal of Public Health* 77:795-799.

Link, R.N., A.R. Feingold, M.H. Charap, K. Freeman, and S.P. Shelov (1988) Concerns of medical and pediatric officers about acquiring AIDS from their patients. *American Journal of Public Health* 78:455-459.

Makadon, H.J., S.F. Delbanco, and T.L. Delbanco (1990a) Caring for people with AIDS and HIV infection in hospital-based primary care practice. *Journal of General Internal Medicine* 5:446-450.

Makadon, H.J., G.R. Seage, III, K.E. Thorpe, and H.V. Fineberg (1990b) Paying the medical cost of the HIV epidemic: a review of policy options. *Journal of Acquired Immune Deficiency Syndromes* 3:123-133.

Manges, M. (1989) Do-it-yourself: innovations make it possible for more patients to stay at home and still be cared for. *Wall Street Journal* November 13:B14.

McCarty, D.J. (1987) Why are today's medical students choosing high-technology specialties over internal medicine? *New England Journal of Medicine* 317:567-569.

Merlis, M. (1990) Acquired immune deficiency syndrome (AIDS): health care financing and services. Issue Brief No. IB 87219. U.S. Library of Congress/Congressional Research Service, Washington, D.C.

National Commission on AIDS (1990) *Research, the Workforce, and the HIV Epidemic in Rural America.* Washington, D.C.: National Commission on AIDS.

National Commission on AIDS (1991) *America Living with AIDS: Transforming Anger, Fear, and Indifference into Action.* Washington, D.C.: National Commission on AIDS.

National Commission on AIDS (1992) *Preventing HIV Transmission in Health Care Settings.* Washington, D.C.: National Commission on AIDS.

Nazario, S.L. (1990) Non-vaccinated health workers spread disease. *Wall Street Journal* November 23:B1.

Ness, R., C.D. Killian, D.E. Ness, J.B. Frost, and D. McMahon (1989) Likelihood of contact with AIDS patients as a factor in medical students residency selections. *Academic Medicine* 64:588-594.

Northfelt, D.W., R.A. Hayward, and M.F. Shapiro (1988) The acquired immunodeficiency syndrome is a primary care disease. *Annals of Internal Medicine* 109:773-775.

Nunn, P., D. Kibuga, A. Elliott, and S. Gathua (1990) Impact of human immunodeficiency virus on transmission and severity of tuberculosis. *Transactions of the Royal Society of Tropical Medicine and Hygiene* 84(Suppl. 1):9-13.

Office of Technology Assessment (OTA) (1991) *HIV in the Health Care Workplace.* Washington, D.C.: Office of Technology Assessment.

Oppenheimer, G.M., and R.A. Padgug (1991) AIDS and the crisis of health insurance. In F. Reamer, ed., *AIDS and Ethics.* New York: Columbia University Press.

Osler, W. (1906) *Aequanimitas With Other Addresses*. London, England: HK Lewis & Co. Ltd.

Palca, J. (1992) CDC closes the case of the Florida dentist. *Science* 256:1130-1131.

Pellegrino, E.D. (1987) Altruism, self-interest and medical ethics. *Journal of the American Medical Association* 258:1939-1940.

Podger, P.J. (1990) Home intravenous care catches on rapidly. *Wall Street Journal* July 18:B1.

Poland, G.A., and K.L. Nichol (1990) Medical schools and immunization policies: missed opportunities for disease prevention. *Annals of Internal Medicine* 113:628-631.

Quinn, T.C., R.O. Cannon, D. Glasser, S.L. Groseclose, W.S. Brathwaite, et al. (1990) The association of syphilis with risk of human immunodeficiency virus infection in patients attending sexually transmitted disease clinics. *Archives of Internal Medicine* 150:1297-1302.

Rango, N., I. Feldman, G. Burke, E. Anderson, and S. Anderman (1990) Enhanced Medicaid rates for the treatment of HIV. Paper presented at the Sixth International Conference on AIDS, San Francisco.

Roper, W.L., and W. Winkenwerder (1988) Making fair decisions about financing care for persons with AIDS. *Public Health Reports* 103:305-308.

Rosenthal, E. (1990) Practice of medicine is changing under specter of the AIDS virus. *New York Times* November 11:A-1.

Rothman, D.J., E.A. Tynan, and the New York City Task Force on Single-Disease Hospitals (1990) Advantages and disadvantages of special hospitals for patients with HIV infection: a report by the New York City Task Force on Single-Disease Hospitals. *New England Journal of Medicine* 323:764-768.

Selz, M. (1990) Home health-care companies learn painful lesson: insurers' slow payment can stunt growth even in a booming industry. *Wall Street Journal* March 26:B-2.

Sierra Health Foundation (1992) Report of the National Symposium on Case Management and HIV/AIDS. Sierra Health Foundation, Sacramento, Calif.

St. Louis, M.E., K.J. Rauch, L.R. Petersen, J.E. Anderson, C.A. Schable, et al. (1990) Seroprevalence rates of human immunodeficiency virus infection at sentinel hospitals in the United States. *New England Journal of Medicine* 323:213-218.

Smith, M.D. (1989) The role of community-based organizations in containing the costs of the AIDS epidemic. Paper presented at the Fifth International Conference on AIDS, Montreal.

Smith, M.D. (1991) Primary care and HIV disease. *Journal of General Internal Medicine* 6(Suppl. 1):S56-S62.

Smith, M.D., R.B. Murray, S. McAvinue, M. Suldan, and R.E. Chaisson (1990) Cost-effectiveness of aerosolized pentamidine (AP) prophylaxis against *Pneumocystis carinii* pneumonia. Paper presented at the Sixth International Conference on AIDS, San Francisco.

Turner, B. (1990) Models of ambulatory care: opportunities for SGIM. *Society for General Internal Medicine News* 13:2,4-5.

U.S. Department of Health and Human Services (1981) *Summary Report of the Graduate Medical Education National Advisory Committee*, Vol. 1. DHHS Publ. No. (HRA) 81-651. Washington, D.C.: U.S. Department of Health and Human Services.

U.S. Department of Labor, Department of Health and Human Services (1987) Guidelines on AIDS and hepatitis B. *Federal Register* (52):41818-41824, October 30.

U.S. Department of Labor, Occupational Safety and Health Administration (1991) Occupational exposure to bloodborne pathogens. Final rule. *Federal Register* (56):64004-64182, December 8.

Volberding, P. (1989) Supporting the health care team in caring for patients with AIDS. *Journal of the American Medical Association* 261:747-748.

Wallace, W.E. (1990) Hospice and AIDS: clinical issues which affect care. *American Journal of Hospice & Palliative Care* 7:13-16.

Williams, N., A. Lin-Greenberg, F.K. Goldschmidt, and D. Ngumezi (1990) Individual and institutional measures of efficacy in an early HIV therapeutic intervention program. Paper presented at the Sixth International Conference on AIDS, San Francisco.

World Health Organization (WHO) (1992) *WHO Global Programme on AIDS: Current and Future Dimensions of the HIV/AIDS Pandemic.* Geneva: World Health Organization.

Yelin, E.H., R.M. Greenblatt, H. Hollander, and J.R. McMaster (1991) The impact of HIV-related illness on employment. *American Journal of Public Health* 81:79-84.

Zuger, A., and S.H. Miles (1987) Physicians, AIDS and occupational risk: historic traditions and ethical obligations. *Journal of the American Medical Association* 258:1924-1928.

4

Clinical Research and Drug Regulation

In perhaps no other area has the impact of AIDS been more clear than in the identification, clinical testing, and regulation of new drugs. The effects have been so extensive and the pace of change so rapid that it is difficult to describe all the important events within the confines of a single chapter. Yet it is still too soon to identify changes that are merely transient phenomena versus those that will endure (Henninger, 1990). Although there are early indications that the changes witnessed in AIDS research may be affecting pharmaceutical development for other diseases, it remains unclear whether AIDS will appreciably alter the development of drugs in general, especially for conditions that are less lethal or less common.

Perhaps the most profound change wrought by AIDS in the area of drug development is simply the dramatic increase in public awareness, especially regarding the very existence, as well as the structure and purpose, of clinical trials. Terms such as "randomized," "placebo," and "double-blind," although perhaps not household words, are nonetheless regularly used in the mass media. Debate about the ethics and scientific validity of clinical trials occurs not only among physicians, statisticians, and ethicists, but also among patients, activists, and politicians. AIDS has opened the arena of clinical investigation—the organization, ethics, and politics of research—to media and public scrutiny.

The impact of the HIV/AIDS epidemic on clinical research poses a series of important questions with broad implications for the practice of science and medicine. For example, to what extent have changes been driven by scientific, ethical, economic, or political considerations? Has AIDS merely accelerated changes that were already occurring in cancer research, or do they represent a clear departure from the practices of the last two decades? When changes have occurred, have they been defined narrowly for AIDS or more broadly constructed? How can change be monitored in the future, and can the likely long-term critical impact of such change be predicted?

This chapter begins with a brief historical perspective on clinical research and drug development prior to the advent of the HIV/AIDS epidemic. It is important that the interplay of politics, science, and ethics in this area be recognized as an ongoing dynamic during the twentieth century; it has been shaped by AIDS but it was not created by it. The chapter then describes drug development from 1981 through late 1991—the age of AIDS—and analyzes the impact of social institutions and events on the process and, conversely, the impact of the process on such institutions as the Food and Drug Administration and the National Institutes of Health. The development of social and political activism is examined as a major force for generating change. Finally, the chapter summarizes how key areas in clinical investigation and drug regulation have been shaped by the HIV/AIDS epidemic.

HISTORICAL PERSPECTIVE[1]

Several developments of the post-World War II era establish a baseline for evaluating changes driven by the HIV/AIDS epidemic. Those developments relate to four major historical shifts: (1) the development of randomized clinical trials as orthodox research methodology, (2) changes in federal drug regulation, (3) the evolution of protections for human research subjects and the growing recognition of ethical dilemmas inherent in research, and (4) the rise of patient advocacy and the changing dynamics of patient-physician relationships. In the postwar era, and especially since 1960, considerable change has taken place in each of these areas. The AIDS epidemic has had powerful effects on clinical research and the culture of science.

Randomized Clinical Trials

Although experimental approaches to clinical medicine date to antiquity, it was only in the 1940s and 1950s that contemporary approaches to the evaluation of medical treatments and technologies were fully articulated and began to be put into practice. Randomized clinical trials—experiments in which human subjects are randomly assigned to experimental and nonexperimental (control) groups for purposes of comparison—offer researchers considerable advantages in evaluating new drugs and other medical technologies. First, variability among subjects will, on average, be equally distributed, thereby reducing the potential for selection bias. Second, because such studies are generally conducted on a double-blind basis (i.e., neither the researcher nor subject knows which group a given subject is in), randomized clinical trials offer a mechanism for reducing investigator bias (W.A. Silverman, 1985). Third, randomized clinical trials permit the use of sophisticated statistical tests of significance in the comparison of treatments. According to their proponents, prospective, double-blind trials offer the potential to place clinical medicine, at long last, on a truly scientific base (Marks, 1990). As biostatisticians have recognized, the development of randomized clinical trials was perhaps the most important methodologic advance associated with the scientific basis of therapeutics (Zelen, 1990).

Despite these advantages, randomized clinical trials did not immediately become the basic rule of clinical investigation. Such studies were expensive to conduct, administratively complex, and required new skills that many investigators lacked. Furthermore, investigators expressed a critical awareness of the difficult ethical dilemmas posed by randomized trials. As statistician A. Bradford Hill (1951:279) explained:

> The first step in such a trial is to decide precisely what it hopes to prove, and secondly to consider whether these aims can be ethically fulfilled. It need hardly be said that the latter consideration is paramount and must never, on any scientific grounds whatsoever, be lost sight of. If a treatment cannot ethically be withheld then clearly no controlled trial can be instituted.

Researchers, attuned to this question, attempted to specify those conditions under which a particular treatment could be withheld for the purposes of a randomized trial (Chalmers, Block, and Lee, 1972). According to most researchers, randomization could be justified only in instances in which there was genuine ignorance concerning the advantages and disadvantages of an experimental drug; only then could a researcher claim "therapeutic indifference" (Hill, 1963:1047):

> It must be possible ethically to give *every* patient admitted to a trial any of the treatments involved. The doctor accepts, in other words, that he really has no knowledge at all that one treatment will be better or worse, safer or more dangerous, than another. . . . If the doctor does not believe that, if he thinks even in the absence of any evidence that for the patient's benefit he ought to give one treatment rather than another, then that patient should not be admitted to the trial. Only if, in his state of ignorance, he believes the treatment given to be a matter of indifference can he accept a random distribution of patients to the different groups. . . . By certain omissions from a trial we may limit the generality of the answer given by it, but on

ethical grounds that, in my experience, must be accepted [emphasis in original].

In order to retain this state of ignorance as the process of collecting data began, trials were designed to isolate researchers from findings. This was accomplished by establishing an advisory panel, usually including expert biostatisticians, to monitor the data as they accrued. Such panels were empowered to halt a trial at the earliest time that a scientific conclusion, usually defined as statistically significant, could be reached. In practice, despite this mechanism, such determinations about when a trial should be ended proved to be complex (Chalmers, Block, and Lee, 1972).

In addition to the justification of therapeutic indifference, proponents of randomized trials also cited the fact that experimental preparations were sometimes scarce and that randomization offered a means of allocating drugs in a socially constructive manner (Rutstein, 1970). Such was the case with the Medical Research Council's streptomycin trials of 1946 (Hill, 1963:1043):

> When, in 1946, the Medical Research Council's Streptomycin in Tuberculosis Trials Committee set out to investigate the effect of that drug in pulmonary tuberculosis it was faced with no serious ethical problem. The antibiotic had been discovered two years previously . . . the published clinical results were distinctly encouraging though not conclusive. Yet overriding all this evidence in favour of the drug was the fact that at that time exceedingly little of it was available in Great Britain. . . . Except for that situation it would certainly on ethical grounds have been impossible to withhold the drug from desperately ill patients. *With* that situation, however, it would, the Committee believed, have been unethical *not* to have seized the opportunity to design a strictly controlled trial [emphasis in original].

Despite these early attempts to define clear ethical criteria for randomization, withholding unproven but potentially beneficial treatments has remained controversial. So-called treatment indifference is far more simple to establish in theory than in practice (Johnson, Lilford, and Brazier, 1991). Drugs are subjected to controlled trials because there is already some evidence that they *may* be effective. This hope, which may or may not be borne out through further investigation, nevertheless shapes the research environment, especially in instances in which there is little to offer patients with serious, life-threatening disease. Jonas Salk, for example, opposed double-blind trials of the vaccine he developed against polio. In Salk's mind, the research he had already conducted demonstrated the effectiveness of the vaccine; to conduct a full-fledged randomized trial, he concluded, would be merely a "fetish of orthodoxy" and would lead to more new and unnecessary cases of paralytic polio among the group receiving the placebo. Other researchers countered that without a full randomized clinical trial the effectiveness and safety of the vaccine would never have scientific and medical credibility, a requirement if doctors, parents, and children were to accept immunization (Carter, 1966; Brandt, 1978a). In this respect, it was argued that only through rigorous trials would it be possible to avoid "therapeutic anarchy," in which clinicians, based on experience and anecdote, would do as they saw fit. Randomized trials would add scientific evidence and legitimacy to clinical judgment (Feinstein, 1967). Proponents also pointed out that only randomization could adequately identify not only the beneficial impacts of experimental drugs but also their significant dangers and side effects (Chalmers, Block, and Lee, 1972).

The difficult ethical considerations that attend randomized clinical trials remain a critical part of the debate concerning "therapeutic research," a term used to denote research conducted on subjects who, it is hoped, will benefit from the experimental preparation. When are randomized trials justified? How should they be organized? Is it ethical, in effect, to toss a coin to assign patients to a particular treatment? How can the conflicts between the desire to further scientific knowledge and the commitment to act in the interest of individual patients be resolved? Does the very act of randomization violate basic norms of the doctor-patient relationship (Fried, 1974; Schaefer, 1982)?

In randomized clinical trials, conflicts inevitably arise between the group and the individual, between the desire for scientific advancement and an individual patient's welfare. Attempts have been made to moderate such conflicts, but they can never be absolutely and categorically resolved. All these issues were debated prior to the AIDS epidemic, but the epidemic gave them a new immediacy. What would be the nature of clinical research in the midst of the epidemic (Eckholm, 1986)? With the onset of the epidemic and the establishment of a research program, the techniques of drug evaluation and experimentation and the ethics of randomized clinical trials came under intense scrutiny.

The Food and Drug Administration and
the Politics of Drug Regulation

Since the early twentieth century, federal regulation of food and drugs had been largely reactive to scandals and tragedies in which consumers of unsafe products were harmed. Upton Sinclair's *The Jungle* (1906) helped to spur Congress to pass the first major piece of protective legislation in 1906, which prohibited false and deceptive labeling of food products and medications (Pure Food and Drug Act, P.L. 59-384). Prior to that time, a vigorous market had existed for nostrums and patent medicines, many of which made sweeping claims for miracle cures. Nevertheless, the act had no provisions requiring evidence that a drug be safe or effective. The impact of the act was undermined by a Supreme Court ruling in 1912 requiring the Food and Drug Administration (FDA) to demonstrate not only that a particular claim was false, but also that it had been made with the intent to deceive. Promotional claims for useless and dangerous products, not surprisingly, continued to flourish (Quirk, 1980; Okun, 1986; Young, 1990).

In 1938 Congress again took action, this time enacting the Food, Drug, and Cosmetic Act (P.L. 75-717), which required that drugs be established as safe through "adequate tests" prior to marketing. Unfortunately, a tragedy helped to break the legislative deadlock that preceded passage of this act. Elixir sulfanilamide, a new sulfa drug marketed for children, was suspended in a solvent that could lead to immediate death; by the time the drug was withdrawn, more than 100 deaths had occurred. With the new legislation, the FDA was mandated to review safety data on drugs and remove dangerous products from the market.

Despite growing methodologic sophistication and rigor in the design and execution of drug trials during the 1950s and 1960s, it soon became clear that the public was still not always protected from pharmaceuticals that were either inadequately tested or produced. As late as the early 1960s, randomized clinical trials continued to be the exception rather than the rule in testing new therapeutic interventions.

Spurred by another series of scandals, Congress in 1962 enacted the Kefauver-Harris amendments to the Food, Drug, and Cosmetic Act of 1938 (Harris, 1964; Quirk, 1980). The notorious "Cutter incident" of 1956, in which 11 children died as a result of being inoculated with improperly produced Salk polio vaccine, was a powerful indicator of the need for better governmental regulation of biologic and pharmaceutical products. This tragedy was soon followed by the thalidomide disaster; children born to mothers who had taken this sedative had severe congenital malformations (Insight Team, 1979). Although thalidomide had not been marketed in the United States, it had been made available in loosely conducted premarketing studies. Both incidents pointed to weaknesses in the federal regulatory process. The Kefauver-Harris amendments to the Food, Drug, and Cosmetic Act required for the first time that before FDA approval was granted, a company had to categorically demonstrate through animal and human studies that a drug was safe and efficacious. (Prior to 1962 federal law had required that drugs be safe, but no specification regarding efficacy was mandated.) The amendments were a major impetus for the conduct of randomized clinical trials, which soon became the only accepted criterion for evaluating new drugs.

By 1970, with the growth in influence of the National Institutes of Health and the rise of biostatistics as a distinct discipline (Marks, 1990), the nature and methods of drug evaluation had achieved a form of scientific and bureaucratic orthodoxy. Moreover, as medical costs rose precipitously during these years, interest in comparing treatments, not just on the basis of efficacy, but also on the basis of costs, was heightened and spurred more trials. A report by the Office of Technology Assessment (1983) concluded that randomized clinical trials offered a particularly effective methodology for evaluating a full range of medical interventions and technologies. Furthermore, the report concluded, such trials should become the basis for evaluating standards of medical practice, as well as for public policy.

The regulatory ethos established in the wake of the Kefauver-Harris amendments emphasized caution. The repercussions of approving a dangerous drug were typically perceived as being greater than those that would attend restricting the marketing of a potentially beneficial drug. Although some critics have recently called this view of regulation "paternalistic" (Delaney, 1989a,b), it reflected a growing recognition that the evaluation of pharmaceuticals was a complex scientific, political, and economic process. Individual patients and individual physicians, it was argued, could not make decisions about safety and effectiveness in a clear or objective manner. Any substantive evaluation required the aggregation and evaluation of large data sets. Thus, the government should mediate by establishing clear criteria, mandating trials, and evaluating industry claims before allowing drugs to be marketed. Rather than being seen as paternalistic, this approach was more often viewed as a significant role of the government in a consumer-oriented, government-regulated economy. In addition, as skepticism about medical technologies and interventions grew during the 1970s and 1980s, the FDA was often criticized for not being aggressive enough in its regulatory mission (Mintz, 1967; Silverman and Lee, 1974; Wolfe and Coley, 1980; U.S. Department of Health and Human Services, Advisory Committee on the FDA, 1991).

The Kefauver-Harris amendments shifted the regulatory burden from premarket *notification* of a new drug to premarket *approval*. The legislation required "substantial evidence" of efficacy, including "adequate and well-controlled investigations, by experts qualified by scientific training and experience to evaluate the effectiveness of the drug involved." This change obviously required the development of detailed criteria and bureaucratic mechanisms to evaluate the safety and efficacy of drugs. Under the regulations established to meet the requirements of the amendments, companies or other researchers seeking to have a product approved must first submit an investigational new drug application. The application had to show that initial screening and animal testing for toxicity had been completed and offer a thorough justification and plan for testing human subjects.

Generally, randomized clinical trials are divided into three phases: phase I trials typically assess data on safety; phase II trials evaluate efficacy; and phase III trials compare the prospective drug with standard therapy, usually on a randomized, double-blind basis. This process can take considerable time, and a variety of approaches to streamlining the procedures have been proposed. In the view of the pharmaceutical industry, which typically bears the costs of clinical trials, the Kefauver-Harris amendments raised the cost of researching, developing, and marketing new products.

In the face of the AIDS epidemic, FDA's policies of cautious protection came under fire. Given attempts to modify regulatory practices, it will be critical in the future to monitor the potential effects of changes on new drug development, both for HIV and other diseases. How, in the context of the AIDS epidemic, has the FDA balanced its duties to ensure safe and effective drugs against its duty to make potentially beneficial agents available on a timely basis? (Edgar and Rothman, 1991). And how are changes in the regulatory environment likely to affect research and development in the pharmaceutical industry?

Protecting Human Research Subjects

Just as changes in the regulation of new drugs were spurred by a series of scandals, so, too, were attempts to protect human subjects driven by reports of serious abuses. Efforts to improve the regulatory capacities of the FDA were followed by a heightened public concern about the ethics of human subject research. Widespread reports of experiments in which research subjects were unaware of their involvement led to calls for more vigorous protections (Gray, 1975; Barber, 1976; Katz, 1984). Henry Beecher's (1966) review of unethical experimental protocols in the *New England Journal of Medicine* (see also Rothman, 1987b) was soon followed by exposes of the Public Health Service's Tuskegee syphilis experiment, in which some 400 African American sharecroppers were denied treatment in a study of the natural history of the disease (Brandt, 1978b; Jones, 1981; Thomas and Quinn, 1991).

As a result of these reports, Congress in 1974 established the National Commission for the Protection of Human Subjects (Rothman, 1991; Jonsen, 1984). The commission devised general ethical principles for the conduct of human experimentation, which it issued in its 1978 "Belmont report" (National Commission for the Protection of Human Subjects, 1978). Three principles were to form the basis for the evaluation of experimental protocols and provide a guide for obtaining informed consent, establishing favorable risk-benefit ratios, and equitably selecting test subjects: respect for persons, beneficence, and justice. A central tenet of the Belmont report was the need to be rigorous in differentiating experimentation from therapy. The commission argued that therapeutic research had the potential of subjecting patients to risky and dangerous experimentation offered in the hope of therapeutic benefits. The heavy emphasis implicit in the work of the commission, as well as its formal title, was the need to *protect* individuals from potentially dangerous research—that is, that government must set limits on researchers and their prospective subjects. In this context, taking part in an experiment was typically viewed as a sacrifice that citizens, in the name of the public good, might periodically be called on to perform. Most commentators emphasized, however, that all too often the burden of medical progress fell inadequately on vulnerable populations—the uneducated and minorities (Katz and Capron, 1975). The commission reiterated its support for clinical investigation and scientific research, but it sought to establish clear principles on which to evaluate research on human subjects and specific mechanisms to protect human subjects *from* possible harm.

The findings of the commission were supported by the federal government in the subsequent requirements for institutional review boards to evaluate research protocols in advance of their implementation. Any institution that received federal funds was required by law to establish such a board to review all proposed research on human subjects and to assess the procedures for obtaining each subject's informed consent. In fact, most research institutes, regardless of funding sources, did establish institutional review boards. The effect of the boards was to create a somewhat more restrictive environment for clinical investigation by establishing clear requirements for consultation and oversight. The era of autonomous research had come to an end.

The HIV/AIDS epidemic suddenly and dramatically fractured the risk-aversive ethic of human experimentation, raising again fundamental questions regarding the nature of clinical investigation and research ethics (Levine, 1988). The epidemic created a constituency that would find the protections of the past too restrictive. It created a constituency of individuals eager to take risks with unproven therapies. In the midst of the AIDS epidemic, when access *to* clinical trials has become a bitterly contested question, it is worth remembering that only a short time ago the focus of discussion was the protection of research subjects *from* potentially dangerous experimental protocols. What the regulatory process had failed to recognize was that in certain specific situations individuals might be eager to have access to experimental drugs even if their safety and efficacy had yet to be proven by scientific criteria. The AIDS epidemic made clear that risk can only be defined in a very specific personal and social context. In this respect, an appropriate margin of safety for any set of clinical trials cannot be uniformly set.

Patient Advocacy and Activism

The critiques of medical experimentation articulated in the 1970s were not new, but they were being expressed with considerable vigor. Efforts to protect human research subjects were part of a larger social movement that reflected a shift in the medical balance of power. Many have called AIDS activism unique—and certainly in some ways it has been unprecedented—but it can be understood in the context of changes in medical relationships and authority that have characterized American medicine since the late 1960s (Jonsen, 1991; Rothman, 1991).

Although there is no adequate history of the patient-doctor relationship, it is widely recognized that fundamental cultural changes in the nature of this relationship have occurred since the mid-1960s. Since that time, there have been several changes that reflect, if not characterize, a shift away from "medical paternalism": a growing skepticism by patients of medical and scientific authority; a deeper commitment to disclosure and consent by physicians; the legal codification of informed consent, as well as clearer promulgation of patients' "rights"; and the establishment of institutional mechanisms, such as internal review boards to protect human subjects. All these developments reflected significant change in the general practice of medicine and the nature of clinical investigation (Katz, 1984; Faden and Beauchamp, 1986).

The rise of AIDS activism can be understood only in the context of the critical shifts in the medical culture just noted and the gay rights movement of the 1970s and 1980s (D'Emilio, 1983). The development of organized activist groups provided an institutional vehicle for articulating critiques of traditional research approaches and federal regulatory mechanisms (see Chapter 6). Those critiques reflected the powerful conflicts in values and priorities revealed by the epidemic, as well as a more general erosion of medical and scientific authority. This social process, as noted, was already under way before the onset of the epidemic; the sacrosanct world of scientific and medical investigation had been opened to public scrutiny, regulation, and criticism. Research, in this new context, would fundamentally require active participation and negotiation between researchers and subjects.

The AIDS epidemic would severely strain virtually every assumption of what had come—over a 20-year period—to be the guiding, orthodox assumptions regarding clinical research and the regulation of new drugs. Every aspect of the process by which new pharmacologic agents were identified, evaluated, regulated, and allocated would be tested by the exigencies of epidemic disease. Questions basic to the epistemologic foundations of biomedicine—questions of verifiability, reproductibility, proof, variability, safety, and efficacy—would all be subject to debate and reevaluation. In this respect, the epidemic has already had a profound social impact on science and medicine.

THE FIRST DECADE OF AIDS

The recognition of the first case of AIDS in the summer of 1981 was an abrupt event, but a basic understanding of its cause, epidemiology, and natural history evolved over a period of 5 years. During that time, despite great limitations of knowledge, many treatments were pursued and some therapeutic successes claimed.

Kaposi's sarcoma and *Pneumocystis carinii* pneumonia (PCP) were the two diseases that heralded the arrival of the epidemic. Both diseases had been seen before (in elderly and cancer patients, respectively), and drugs already licensed were commonly used to treat the disorders, generally with good results. Indeed, it was the sudden marked increase in requests for a drug long used to treat PCP, pentamidine, that provided one of the first pieces of evidence that AIDS was an epidemic disease.

Frustration that PCP and other complications in AIDS patients were not amenable to conventional therapies led to a host of alternative approaches, including vitamins, holistic therapies, and imported, non-FDA-approved drugs. At the same time, the failures led scientists to consider the infectious and neoplastic aftermath of AIDS's destruction of the immune system as essentially insurmountable and to concentrate on the central immune defect underlying the disease as the proper focus for drug research. Heroic interventions, such as bone marrow transplants in twins (one infected with HIV and one not) and aggressive chemotherapy for Kaposi's sarcoma, were attempted. As patients continued to die despite these measures, AIDS increasingly came to be viewed as an untreatable disease, and medical and lay literature emphasized the need to respect the rights and needs of individuals with a fatal disease of short duration, including their right to refuse intubation and resuscitation, their need for companionship and personal assistance, and the need to create low-cost, compassionate, out-of-hospital care.

The year 1985 was a landmark year in the epidemic. First, it was revealed that movie star Rock Hudson had AIDS and that he had traveled to France to obtain HPA-23, an antiviral agent that French researchers had hailed at a press conference as curing several patients with the disease. Patients in the United States, desperate for therapy, questioned why a potentially useful drug could not be brought into this country. Affected individuals became increasingly aware of the often painfully slow process of drug evaluation and licensing regulated by the FDA. When additional experience with HPA-23 did not confirm early promising results, however, the wisdom of traditional methods of drug testing seemed to be substantiated.

Second, suramin, an agent that had been licensed for over 50 years and that had been used worldwide to treat sleeping sickness, was identified as having strong *in vivo* anti-HIV activity and was quickly put into a small, phase I trial in several institutions. Surprisingly, the drug produced severe and apparently new side effects in many recipients and led to at least two deaths. The experience with suramin again appeared to validate the preeminence of orthodox clinical trials.

The Emergence of AZT

In the winter of 1985-1986, preliminary studies of a previously discarded anticancer agent, zidovudine (AZT), were begun by Drs. Samuel Broder and Robert Yarchoan at the National Cancer Institute (Wastila and Lasagna, 1990). The work of Broder and Yarchoan was carried out under the drug development program initiated by the National Cancer Institute (NCI) under the authority provided by the 1971 National Cancer Act. AZT appeared to increase patient well-being and possibly to slow progression of the disease, although it was not obviously curative. Because of acceptable toxicity, a phase II clinical trial was mounted by Burroughs-Wellcome, Ltd., in the late winter of 1986. Originally planned to last for 27 weeks of observation per patient, the trial was halted prematurely in September 1986 because of significantly greater survival rates in those receiving AZT in comparison with those receiving a placebo. At the time the trial was ended, most patients had been observed for only a short period of time. With this dramatic finding, the world of clinical research was turned upside down.

Virtually overnight, AIDS patients and others demanded that AZT be made immediately available. Burroughs-Wellcome established a compassionate-plea mechanism for drug distribution, modeled on the compassionate, investigational new drug (IND) mechanisms developed by NCI in the early years of its drug development program (see below). Physicians were required to document that patients had AIDS as evidenced by PCP or advanced AIDS-related complex (ARC), the characteristics of the trial participants. Generally used only for small numbers of patients with life-threatening conditions, the compassionate IND mechanism was a cumbersome, ad hoc process requiring active participation by individual physicians to obtain a drug and document its use. It had never before been applied in the wide manner an epidemic required. Although immediate problems of access were thus solved, it was clear that this mechanism would be quickly overwhelmed. Faced with urgent demands, the FDA hastened AZT through the regulatory process by easing requirements for animal and preclinical data. On January 16, 1987, the FDA convened a meeting of its Anti-Infective Advisory Committee to consider FDA approval. The advisory committee voted 10 to 1 for licensing AZT despite the expedited procedures (Nussbaum, 1990).

Dissent in the research community regarding this decision was muted but real. Concerns were raised that despite specific labeling that identified the drug as useful only in patients who had AIDS as evidenced by PCP or severe ARC, even asymptomatic patients might demand and physicians acquiesce to treatment with AZT, thereby risking major adverse effects in patients who might expect at least several healthy years if untreated. In contrast, others believed that all patients with AIDS, not only those who had PCP, were equally in danger of death and should receive the drug and that the labeling was thus too narrow. In an unprecedented program, Burroughs-Wellcome announced plans to collect postlicensing data on 20,000 patients receiving AZT to lessen the possible danger of widespread use of a drug on the basis of minimal data on toxicity and efficacy.

The Rise of Advocacy

As AZT quickly made its way from test tube to pharmacy in 1987, two other major developments occurred: AIDS activists, most notably represented by the AIDS Coalition to Unleash Power (ACT-UP), became increasingly visible, and the primary federal mechanism for the conduct of clinical trials, the AIDS Clinical Trials Group of the National Institute of Allergy and Infectious Diseases, expanded rapidly. Advocacy by grassroots organizations in the gay community had been strong almost from the beginning of the epidemic. Initially focusing on issues of discrimination and access to health care, such groups became increasingly involved with issues of experimental treatments.

Advocacy groups made the FDA their prime focus, and from 1987 to 1989 they steadily and forcefully challenged the FDA to widen and speed the availability of drugs for AIDS. In addition, the Reagan administration, with its general philosophy of deregulation, became a sympathetic (if ironic) partner in the push toward greater consumer choice in AIDS drugs. Together, patient activism, a political climate favoring deregulation, and the exigency of an epidemic disease drove the most dramatic changes in drug regulation since the Kefauver-Harris legislation of 1962.

Initially, the changes were largely modifications of existing programs. As noted above, prior to 1987 physicians treating patients with life-threatening disease for which they had exhausted all licensed therapeutic options, could (on a case-by-case basis) obtain therapeutic agents that were still under investigation. Several variations on the basic process evolved, but terminology and procedures were ambiguous, and use of the various processes was sporadic and not well known in the medical community. Several attempts had been made to codify the "compassionate use of drugs," but regulation by the FDA only occurred in 1987 under pressure from AIDS activists.

The 1987 IND regulations require that the disease for which the drug is to be used be "severe or immediately life-threatening," although specific diseases meeting this criterion are not specified. They also require that there is no licensed therapeutic option for the disease, that clinical trials or studies be ongoing or completed, and that the sponsor is in fact seeking marketing approval. In most instances, companies can charge for the drug. The intent of the 1987 regulations was to retain close control of treatment IND use but to enable it to be granted in a uniform way and earlier in the drug-approval process, as early as the completion of promising phase I studies.

Another landmark event occurred in 1988 when the Presidential Committee on Regulatory Relief, chaired by (then) Vice President George Bush, approved importation of limited supplies of foreign drugs for personal use. The FDA also developed the "expedited review procedure for drugs to treat life-threatening and severely debilitating diseases," through which drug sponsors could trade early involvement of the FDA in the drug development process for the promise of more efficient approval later. The FDA also demonstrated increasing willingness to provide treatment IND distribution. The 1987 regulations were viewed by the FDA as variously defined for only a few drugs and unlikely to be highly attractive to drug sponsors because of the cost of early FDA involvement. Others have noted that the regulations seemed to change the definition of "severe" in such a way that a relatively large number of drugs might in fact be included.

Despite these changes, which permitted patients a greater degree of personal choice in deciding which drugs to take, activists charged that the FDA interpreted the 1987 regulations too conservatively, only approving drugs for which phase II trials were completed or nearly completed, as a bridge between trials and FDA approval. Activists pushed for the creation of a novel mechanism to widen patient access, a concept that came to be called the "parallel track."

The parallel track concept was loosely modeled on an approach to clinical trials common in Europe to obtain definitive information about treatment efficacy. As ultimately implemented in the United States, however, the parallel track became primarily a drug distribution mechanism that foreshortens phase II and virtually eliminates phase III of clinical trials. Such an approach is scientifically valid only if joined to intensive postmarketing surveillance. Although the parallel track was described as an alternative phase II model, permitting it to fit within the regulatory framework of the standard FDA procedures, it was in reality an ad hoc concession to public pressure that demanded wide distribution of clinically unproven new drugs. By contrast, the compassionate IND offered limited availability of drugs that had demonstrated clinical efficacy, but were not yet fully approved. AIDS activists argued that as soon as drugs had been shown to be safe and at all effective in phase I trials, they should be made available to persons who could not enter phase II trials because of ineligibility or geographic barriers. The parallel track, then, would be a large-scale release of an unapproved drug in lieu of the physician-initiated, case-by-case treatment IND request. It was designed to broaden dramatically the availability of experimental drugs at the earliest possible time. New York's ACT-UP, which had become increasingly knowledgeable and sophisticated about drug approval, did the most to popularize this concept.

The first public discussion of the parallel track concept occurred in April 1988 under the leadership of the AIDS Clinical Trials Group. Dr. Anthony Fauci, associate director of the National Institute of Allergy and Infectious Diseases and AIDS coordinator for NIH, ultimately became a defender of the process, which he argued could be accomplished without sacrificing the integrity of concurrent formal clinical trials. Others, including the FDA's then Chief of Antiviral Drug Products, Dr. Ellen Cooper, contended that the 1987 treatment IND regulations were themselves sufficiently flexible to permit very early access and that no new mechanism was needed.

As the parallel track concept became widely discussed in the summer of 1989, enthusiasm was mounting for dideoxyinosine (ddI), a drug similar in composition and mechanism of action to AZT. Dideoxyinosine had shown dramatic *in vitro* inhibition of HIV replication and, in phase I studies, acceptable toxicity and some evidence of possible efficacy. Phase II trials of the drug were being quickly designed by the sponsor, Bristol-Myers Squibb, and activists pushed for wide access to the drug for those who were ineligible for trials and for concurrent formal trials. Thus, before the parallel track was fully developed as a concept, the White House decided to authorize its implementation, without the usual normal consultation with the scientific community. Because the decision to implement a parallel track circumvented normal procedures, both within the federal government and the larger scientific community, it emerged without the essential component of postmarketing scientific review. Indeed, it is questionable that such a review could be either designed or implemented for the HIV/AIDS patient group due to problems such as compliance with treatment protocols and extensive self-medication. A program was set up by the FDA that, for all intents and purposes, represented a parallel track. Perhaps because it was not officially viewed as such, or because of the great pressure to begin, no evaluation component was included in the program. Moreover, the formal clinical trial of the drug had, in retrospect, especially stringent criteria for entry: a large percentage of people with severe HIV disease were excluded and thus had no alternative for getting ddI other than enrolling in the expanded access program. Finally, initiation of expanded access actually preceded the beginning of the phase II trials, which resulted in a situation in which, within months, thousands of patients had enrolled in an expanded access program, but the number of participants in the formal trial was significantly less than initial projections.

Many observers have cautioned that the ddI experience may be unique and cannot be used to determine the likely success of the parallel track mechanism. Indeed, debate continues as to what the exact purpose of the parallel track should be. Some argue that through such an approach valuable data could be obtained concerning safety and efficacy, data of sufficient quality even for the purposes of drug licensing. Others have argued that such data would be flawed and that expending the resources required to collect and analyze the data would be counterproductive to the central goal of increasing access.

Although the intention of the parallel track concept was that drugs would be supplied free to participants, no consideration was given to how the costs of laboratory monitoring and physician visits would be handled. Thus, those costs, traditionally covered by sponsors of research in formal clinical trials, have fallen on the patients themselves and, in some cases, third-party payers. This situation has led to the virtual exclusion of poor people from the expanded access program, despite the fact that one of the goals of the parallel track concept was to increase access. Lack of access for poor people has played an important part in recent demands by activists groups for very early licensing of drugs—immediately after phase I trials if any efficacy is demonstrated.

In July 1991, an advisory committee of the FDA recommended the approval of ddI (Kolata, 1991), and the FDA commissioner completed the final steps for approval. Thus, in the space of a very few years, radical changes in drug regulation have occurred, and for the first time, they have been due not to public reaction to a fatal drug toxicity, but to strong consumer activism by a group of affected patients and their advocates.

The Integration of Activists in the Clinical Trials Process

As activists achieved success in altering the regulation of drugs from 1987 to 1989, they began to turn their attention to the actual design and conduct of clinical trials, criticizing what they perceived as the failure of the AIDS Clinical Trials Group to test and deliver effective therapies rapidly. Although the group did not control many of the clinical trials being conducted in the United States, it had a critical mass of investigators, and its budget had grown considerably. Thus, it offered an identifiable and powerful target against which activists could organize their efforts to reform clinical trials. Over the next 3 years, activism exerted an unprecedented influence over the clinical trials process. The fifth annual International AIDS Conference, which met in Montreal in June 1989, proved to be pivotal in this regard. At the time, most activism was still being directed at the FDA and the regulatory process, but activists were also openly critical of the AIDS Clinical Trials Group, which they accused of having produced no tangible results despite an investment of hundreds of millions of dollars. In Montreal, ACT-UP New York circulated a highly specific critique of the group's programs and protocols and called for sweeping changes in trial design (ACT-UP, 1989).

Investigators and statisticians initially offered predictable defenses of the traditional clinical trials process, but shortly after the Montreal meeting, as attention was focused on the surprising adoption of the parallel track concept by Dr. Anthony Fauci, an equally surprising event occurred. Dr. Susan Ellenberg, chief of the Biostatistics Branch of National Institute of Allergy and Infectious Diseases (NIAID) told activists and others that she found real merit in proposals for alternative designs (Green et al., 1990). She organized an NIH-FDA conference on clinical trial design in November 1989 and subsequently formed a statistical working group within the AIDS Clinical Trials Group as a forum in which novel trial designs could be debated and developed by statisticians, clinical investigators, activists, and persons with AIDS. This working group, which continues to meet, provided the first inroad for activists into the mainstream process of the AIDS Clinical Trials Group.

In September 1989, NIAID had awarded a large contract for statistical support to the Statistical and Data Analysis Center at the Harvard School of Public Health. This group, which had been providing limited statistical consultation to NIAID during 1989, began to provide increasing expertise in the design and analysis of trials. Senior statisticians at the center brought their significant experience in clinical trials in cancer to AIDS and formed a community advisory board to keep local community groups aware of their activities and to explain statistical issues in trials (Valdiserri, Tama, and Ho, 1988).

Later, the NIAID Division of AIDS and the leadership of the AIDS Clinical Trials Group (at least as a group) also became more amenable to inclusion of activists after several came uninvited to a meeting of the group in November 1989. Whether this cooperation represented the activists' banging down the door or clinical researchers' opening it is unclear. (To date, few of the principal individuals involved have written about or publicly discussed their recollection of these events.) Several individual trial sites (called AIDS clinical trial units) formed local community advisory boards to provide two-way communication of issues and concerns. Increasing interaction occurred among members of the AIDS Division staff and activists. A series of discussions and planning meetings ensued, and by July of 1990 Dr. Anthony Fauci announced that activists would have representation on all committees and in all activities of the AIDS Clinical Trials

Group (ACTG). The Community Constituency Group (CCG) was established as a formal committee of the ACTG.

After several years of growth, the CCG now consists of 24 members with diverse representation from the AIDS community. The CCG has come to play an active role in the ACTG: two positions on the ACTG Executive Committee are allotted to the CCG, and CCG members serve on each of the core committees. The CCG also works closely with the individual AIDS Clinical Trials Units (ACTUs), each of which is required to establish a local Community Advisory Board (CAB). Communication between the staff at the ACTU, CCG, and CAB has ensured broader input and enables the trial sites to effectively address patients' concerns, and other pertinent issues, such as recruitment, compliance, and retention.

It is perhaps too early to evaluate the full impact of these developments on the conduct of clinical trials. The process has certainly changed, but it is still unclear how decisions concerning which trials to mount and how to conduct and interpret them will be made. Clearly, the entire process will be open and highly visible. It is likely that studies will take longer to design because of the number of people who are providing input, but it is also more likely that the final trial designs will be more agreeable to patients and activists, which might lead to faster identification of participants and improved retention of them in studies (Arras, 1990).

Activists are also turning their attention back to the FDA. As discussed above, activists argue that expanded access, no matter how designed, will never achieve widespread distribution of drugs because of the cost of patient monitoring. Thus, they argue that the earliest possible licensing should be the goal. To that end, San Francisco's Community Consortium of Bay Area HIV Care Providers used a little-known legal mechanism of a citizen petition of the FDA to seek the release of ddI (and ddC) on the basis of short-term effects on laboratory markers (Kolata, 1990).

CURRENT ISSUES AND PRACTICES

Drugs and Alternative Therapies

Drugs used in the treatment of AIDS and related disorders have come from a variety of sources. Encouraged by the efficacy of AZT, the National Cancer Institute launched an ambitious program of *in vivo* drug screening in 1986, as part of which it has evaluated hundreds of drugs through the same simple assay that first identified AZT as a candidate for treatment. Antiviral drugs, such as ddI and ddC, have resulted from this process. As more became known about the early pathogenesis of HIV disease and its effects on the immune system, the first of the so-called designer AIDS drugs, soluble CD4, was put into trial.

The relatively large number of antiviral agents that have been shown to have activity in the test tube was not anticipated even a few years ago, and their existence has raised new issues regarding priorities in drug testing. At present, simultaneous trials of several agents are ongoing. Whether it is most efficient to test drugs in this manner or whether it would be better to rank drugs and test them in sequence (i.e., starting a new trial only when a previous one has enough subjects) is a matter of ongoing but ill-defined debate. Arguments on the basis of personal choice, which have been predominant in the epidemic (Delaney, 1989a,b), would seem to support the current system of multiple trials. Some have argued that federally sponsored trials might be conducted sequentially, but not the myriad of trials sponsored by pharmaceutical companies and others whose research and development information is proprietary. For a brief time, the AIDS Clinical Trials Group considered requiring that pharmaceutical companies virtually hand over promising drugs they wanted put into the group's trials, but in 1990 the pendulum seemed to swing back to individual companies' dictating many of the details of drug design and monitoring. Thus, it is likely that multiple experimental studies will continue to be conducted concurrently.

Even more interesting is the issue of how resources should be divided between testing candidate antiviral drugs and evaluating drugs used to treat the myriad of complications associated with HIV disease. Critics of the use of resources for the investigation of such supportive therapies have drawn an analogy with the polio epidemic of the 1950s, likening testing of drugs for opportunistic infections to investing large resources in the development of a better iron lung. They argue that the emphasis should be on the underlying cause of AIDS. This viewpoint has been criticized by some clinical investigators, who point out that prophylaxis of PCP has been perhaps more influential in extending survival than the use of AZT. The argument in favor of focusing on causes has also been heavily criticized by activist groups, who interpret the approach as "writing off" the hundreds of thousands of patients with severely impaired immune systems who are perhaps unlikely to benefit from antiviral therapy, however effective it may be, but who still might benefit at least modestly from more effective therapies for opportunistic infections and tumors. Debate on this issue became so intense that congressional hearings were held on the subject, and budgets for opportunistic infection therapies were increased (U.S. Congress, 1991).

Although the debate has often been deemed a political one—between scientists with conflicting research agendas or between future patients and current ones—there remains fundamental scientific uncertainty about the most efficient approach to prolonging the life of AIDS patients. It is likely that interest and resources will continue to shift between the antiviral approach and the supportive (opportunistic infections) approach as new information is obtained concerning the pathogenesis of the disease and as new drugs are identified.

Along with numerous antivirals that emerge from the National Cancer Institute, there have been agents whose proponents, often patients or their advocates, cite dramatic if anecdotal case histories to support their claims of efficacy. So-called alternative therapies include not only drugs identified in the laboratory, but also traditional (folk) remedies used by ethnic minorities and nonmedicinal therapies, such as acupuncture, visualization, meditation, and special diets (Hand, 1989).

The use of alternative therapies is widespread among persons with HIV infection, especially gay men; less is known about the therapeutic choices of ethnic minorities. Alternative therapies were initially prohibited for patients in federal trials, but it quickly became clear that many patients continued to use them without reporting such use (Arras, 1990). Concerned that the possible effects of such unknown therapies might adversely affect interpretation of the trial design and aware that some patients were refusing to enter or stay in trials because of these prohibitions, clinical researchers gradually came to tolerate their use.

Nonmedicinal healing regimens and approaches in which empowerment of patients is encouraged ("survivors" rather than "victims"), already used by cancer patients prior to the AIDS epidemic, have increased in popularity during the AIDS epidemic for all life-threatening diseases. Although the degree of activism that has arisen in response to AIDS has yet to be seen for cancer, there are indications that it may occur for breast cancer, a disease that, like AIDS, can be associated with a long period of clinical well-being after initial diagnosis. Breast cancer patients are beginning to move beyond individual empowerment to group empowerment as a means of fighting the disease. Breast cancer advocates are demanding increased research funding, better dissemination of information concerning treatment options, and a more patient-centered approach to decision making (Gross, 1991). Although it did not rise directly from AIDS activism, it is probable that some of the inspiration for the new activist approach to breast cancer came from media coverage of AIDS activism, as well as from the feminist and natural childbirth movements.

Who Performs Clinical Trials

Clinical trials have been traditionally performed almost exclusively in tertiary care (specialized teaching or research) hospitals and clinics by academic physicians. Virtually all federally sponsored research and most of the research sponsored by the pharmaceutical industry has been conducted in this way. The advantages of such a centralized approach have included the interest and expertise of physicians at these sites, many of whom are conducting basic research in the disease; the ability to develop dedicated facilities that are highly efficient for the conduct of such research (clinical research centers); the availability of specialized laboratory testing and nursing personnel trained in the requirements of research; and the availability of people to constitute an institutional review board to provide approval and oversight of the study and ensure proper protection of subjects.

The first significant changes in the traditional approach to clinical trials resulted from the large expansion in clinical research funded through the National Cancer Institute. The increasing numbers of young oncologists trained in the cancer research centers saturated the positions available in cancer centers and resulted in significant numbers of fully trained clinical oncologists establishing practices in smaller cities and towns, distant from cancer research centers. In response to this development, NCI established the Community Clinical Oncology Program (CCOP), which enabled community-based oncologists to be tethered to cancer centers and to use state-of-the-art cancer drugs in research protocols that were fully integrated into center-based clinical trials. CCOP has been extremely successful, but critical to that success are the well-established links with cancer centers and the available pool of oncologists fully trained in clinical research methods.

AIDS has strained the traditional system for clinical trials in several ways. First, unlike the situation for other fatal diseases, in which primary care physicians did not feel competent to treat unusual and severe diseases (like cancer), many community physicians with practices comprising mostly gay men acquired extensive experience in the management of HIV disease. Those physicians were often unwilling to transfer even part of the primary care of their patients to clinical investigators. Patients, too, wanted to remain with their physicians, many of whom were more tolerant than the medical establishment of alternative therapies. In addition, many gay patients had a deep distrust of a medical system that they saw at best as unwelcoming and often openly condemning of their life-styles.

As previously noted, access to investigational therapy has increasingly been viewed as a right rather than a burden (Annas, 1988; Bayer, 1990). Even a large and multicentered system may be "unfair"—in not meeting the needs of infected persons if there are geographical and financial barriers to access. Thus, many AIDS patients and their advocates have argued that studies could be done more efficiently and equitably and with increased patient compliance if community physicians and their offices participated in the conduct of clinical trials (Merton, 1990). An early example of such a community network was the Community Consortium of Bay Area HIV Care Providers, headed by Donald Abrams, a San Francisco physician. This group performed a study of the efficacy of three different doses of aerosolized pentamidine in the prevention of PCP, a trial that ultimately provided the basis for the licensing of aerosolized pentamidine for this purpose by the FDA (Abrams, 1990).

Both the American Foundation for AIDS Research and the National Institute of Allergy and Infectious Diseases have established a formal network of community-based trials (and some sites receive funding from both sources). In addition to sponsorship of clinical trials, the network's program will include establishment of an observational database to collect information gathered during the routine care of patients by their primary physicians. It is hoped that the database will provide information that will be useful in studying the natural history of HIV disease, in assessing the use of particular therapies by people with HIV disease, and perhaps, in projecting those patients' resource needs. Such databases have been developed to a lesser extent for other diseases and have been suggested as a means of creating an accurate historical group and thereby lessening the need for randomized trials.

It will be important to monitor the types of community studies done and their success in improving patient participation and retention and to delineate any drawbacks to the approach, such as decreased ability to monitor or respond to drug toxicities. It will also be important to determine whether a national system can retain the flexibility of a more grass-roots structure while providing the capability to mount large trials.

Almost from the beginning of the AIDS epidemic, patient advocacy groups took on the role of medical advisers through the creation of patient information newsletters (Steinbrook and Lo, 1990; Bishop, 1991). In San Francisco, *AIDS Treatment News* began appearing in May 1986 and grew from a biweekly column in a local gay newspaper to a newsletter with a circulation of about 5,000 (James, 1989). Also in 1986 in New York City, the Gay Men's Health Crisis began to publish *Treatment Issues*, an update on research in progress, complete with extensive references to the medical literature. The American Foundation for AIDS Research publishes the *AIDS/HIV Experimental Treatment Directory*. Buyers' clubs were also formed to import and distribute drugs that were not approved for use in the United States or approved drugs that were available more cheaply in other countries. Such groups were instrumental in educating patients about therapeutic options and creating in many areas a climate of debate on AIDS care and research. These developments reflected a new "consultant" ethos among potential and actual research subjects.

Such advocacy took on a whole new dimension, however, when one such group, San Francisco's Project Inform, under the direction of Martin Delaney, carried on its own study of compound Q, a cucumber derivative that had been used as an abortifacient in China and was reported to have significant *in vitro* activity against HIV. This study was conducted without oversight by FDA or an institutional review board, which sparked criticism from a number of lawyers and bioethicists. Project Inform argued that this was an ethical trial because patients were already taking the drug on their own, and the trial afforded at least some oversight by a participating physician. When it was learned that two patients in the study had become comatose and died shortly after taking the drug, the FDA stepped in and halted the trial. Interestingly, Delaney was later permitted to reinstitute the trial after filing a treatment IND application and forming an institutional review board for oversight. This decision was especially noteworthy in light of the heavy hand of the FDA in past dealings with even minor clinical trial infractions: "wrongdoing" investigators were often barred for life from conducting further drug trials. It remains to be seen whether the creation of community research consortiums will decrease the interest of advocacy groups in mounting their own trials and increase the level of cooperation and compliance among patients/subjects.

Activists have also become researchers in other less dramatic ways. As noted above, activist representatives now sit on many major scientific committees, including the Executive Committee of the AIDS Clinical Trials Group and several AIDS clinical trial units have community advisory boards. The mission of the latter is currently evolving, but they will likely at least informally review studies to be done at each site. Activists also routinely publish articles on AIDS therapies and have suggested novel approaches to trial design. Indeed, they have been more visible in strategic planning concerning trial design and conduct than the AIDS Clinical Trials Group or other academically based organizations.

The Design of Clinical Trials and Access to Them

AIDS has deepened and broadened critiques of clinical trials as the "gold standard" approach to the testing of new drugs. Such criticism certainly predated AIDS, but it focused largely on the ethics of trials (Beecher, 1966; Rothman, 1987a,b); criticism of AIDS-related trial design also includes methodologic issues.

Traditionally, clinical trials have been designed to ensure that answers are arrived at as quickly as possible and with no associated uncertainties as to whether the drug itself or confounding factors produced the observed effect. Thus, subjects in trials have no serious diseases other than the one under investigation and are not taking other medications. Definitive events are chosen for measurement of drug effect, such as survival, objective clinical improvement (such as disappearance or shrinkage of tumors), or in some cases, the return of an abnormal laboratory or clinical measurement to normal (Weiss and Mazade, 1990). When such laboratory measurements are chosen, they must have been previously shown to correlate to survival or clinical outcomes. For example, since it has been shown that lowering of blood pressure by drugs leads to a decrease in strokes and deaths, new drugs are licensed if they can be shown to lower blood pressure; it is not required that subjects be followed until the occurrence of stroke or death.

The smallest number of patients necessary to detect a predetermined effect of a drug are studied because, it is argued, it would be unethical to subject more people to experimental therapies than those needed to demonstrate an effect. To detect possible side effects of drugs, physical examinations and laboratory testing are generally performed frequently and thoroughly.

AIDS, however, is a complex disease. Its very name, acquired immune deficiency syndrome, reveals a key feature that makes traditional trial design problematic: HIV's destruction of the immune system manifests itself clinically through a host of secondary diseases, such as PCP, cerebral toxoplasmosis, atypical mycobacterial disease, and unusual tumors. Over 30 such diseases have been identified, and the majority of patients develop three or more of them during their lifetimes. Thus, it is not possible to find a population of HIV-infected patients in the late stages of disease who could be considered free of other serious disease. Patients entering a trial typically have several opportunistic infections, each of which may be treated by one or more drugs, each drug with its own side effects and interactions with other drugs. It is not uncommon for patients with AIDS to take ten or more such medications. Monitoring of toxicity due to an experimental drug is therefore difficult because observed side effects may be due to medications other than the experimental agent or because of interactions with that agent.

The use of definitive outcomes in AIDS research to determine drug efficacy is becoming increasingly problematic. AIDS is a chronic disease: using survival as an outcome, especially in trials of asymptomatic persons, would entail many years of treatment and observation before the value of a therapy could be ascertained. Choosing the development of CDC-defined AIDS as the outcome shortens the duration of a trial somewhat, but that outcome may be delayed by the simultaneous use of prophylactic drugs for opportunistic infections. For this reason, some people have proposed using surrogate markers, that is, laboratory indicators of disease progression that could give early evidence of drug effect. Of the markers proposed, the measurement of the absolute number of CD4 cells is currently considered the most promising. Indeed, at this time, many AIDS investigators favor basing trials and early drug licensing on CD4 counts in lieu of clinical outcomes. However, other researchers have pointed out that even in diseases for which some drugs have been shown to have the same effect on surrogate markers and clinical outcomes, other drugs may have a beneficial effect on markers but not show clinical benefit, or may even cause clinical harm. Conversely, some drugs may have clinical benefit without having any effect on surrogate markers. Two recent trials not involving AIDS illustrate this issue. In one study, interferon was of dramatic benefit in the treatment of chronic granulomatous disease (CGD), an inherited disorder leading to life-threatening infections. However, all laboratory tests of neutrophil function (the affected cell in CGD) failed to show any improvement. In contrast, a recent large clinical trial (Cardiac Arrhythmia Suppression Trial) looking at prevention of sudden death due to cardiac arrhythmias after myocardial infarction (heart attack) was stopped when two agents (ecainide and flecanide) were found to suppress cardiac arrhythmias, but paradoxically, to lead to sudden death (Ruskin, 1989).

In addition to emphasizing the need to include in trials people whose clinical status is representative of all those with the disease, AIDS trials have also raised the issue of access to trials for groups that historically have been excluded (passively or actively) from participation, such as intravenous drug users, minorities, and women of childbearing age. Initially, AIDS trials almost exclusively enrolled white, middle-class gay men. These participants were, in general, better educated than average, usually well informed about treatment options, and able to enter and remain in trials. As AIDS increased among intravenous drug users and their sexual partners, advocacy groups began to argue not only for increased enrollment of these groups in trials, but also for the provision of social support services to enable participation, such as translators, transportation vouchers, and child care services. Advocates have argued that inclusion of a demographically representative group of patients is warranted not only for reasons of fairness (recognizing that for a disease with few options for licensed drug treatment, experimental trials are themselves rare), but also because drugs may have different efficacy or toxicity on demographically different patient groups.

Thus, arguments of justice and science have been put forth to support increased access. Trial sponsors and community leaders now publicly support this approach, but there is as yet little indication that groups other than gay men are entering trials in appreciable numbers. Indeed, the pragmatic obstacles to such participation are considerable. In a recent report, the National Commission on AIDS (1991:104) noted:

> the difficulties in deciding who pays for health care associated with research vividly reveals the discontinuity in federal health programs. NIH-based researchers claim no jurisdiction over health care provision, and the federal agencies responsible for the reimbursement and delivery of health care, HCFA and HRSA, are not designing program strategies that would take these research-related issues in account.

NIH, charged with conducting drug trials, has no mandate or funding support to provide health care services.

There has been little research to explore the desire or capabilities of underrepresented groups to participate in trials. Some have argued that at least among African Americans, distrust of the medical system is so high and the collective memory of clinical trial abuses (as in the Tuskegee syphilis study) so strong that many people are actively opposed to participation

(Brandt, 1978a; Thomas and Quinn, 1991). Particular questions have been raised about children and women.

Children

The ethical issues inherent in including children in trials, long debated for other diseases, are even more complex in relation to HIV disease. In general, candidate AIDS drugs are moving into trials on the basis of relatively less preclinical and toxicologic data, which increases traditional concerns over possible adverse outcomes for children in trials. Most children with HIV disease have mothers who themselves have the disease, many of whom are unable to care for their children. For this reason, and in some cases because of ongoing maternal drug use, many HIV-infected children are in foster care (see Chapter 8). It has proven difficult to obtain consent for enrolling such children in trials (Martin and Sacks, 1990). Yet the natural history of HIV disease in children differs appreciably from that in adults, which is an argument for earlier and fuller trials involving children. Lacking such trials, therapy for children has lagged behind that for adults, and guidelines for translating the results of trials to clinical practice have been limited to adults, leaving practicing pediatricians uncertain as to how to treat children.

In the case of AZT, use in symptomatic children was not approved until April 1990—fully 3 years after the drug was licensed for adult use. Moreover, licensing was granted by virtue of a regulatory waiver because the limited trials conducted among children did not satisfy minimal FDA requirements. As a result of that experience, pediatric trials of ddI were started very soon after adult trials were initiated and were designed to satisfy FDA licensing requirements. In addition, it has recently been suggested that because opportunistic infections occur in children too infrequently to warrant separate pediatric trials, children should instead be included in adult trials, with appropriate modification of dosage (Nolan, 1990). Thus, it is likely that, at least for AIDS, and possibly for other life-threatening diseases, there will be a shift toward earlier, larger trials among affected children.

Women

The issue of inclusion of women of childbearing age in trials, especially pregnant women, has been the subject of much debate (Levine, 1990). Early trials often explicitly excluded pregnant women. At a minimum, all trials have required a negative pregnancy test at entry and have stipulated that birth control must be practiced. Whether because of these restrictions or because women are less aware of trials and more likely to face numerous barriers to participation, as of the end of 1991 fewer than 7 percent of participants in the AIDS Clinical Trials Group trials were women.

AIDS trials are not unique in having few women participants (Cotton, 1990a,b). Indeed, the norm in clinical trials for a wide variety of illnesses has been explicitly to exclude women. Despite NIH guidelines requiring that any research protocol not including women offer a justification for the exclusion, a study released by the U.S. General Accounting Office (1990) demonstrated that few federally sponsored studies complied with those guidelines. That report, widely covered by the media, resulted in congressional inquiry into the lack of inclusion of women in trials and the creation of a new post of assistant director of the NIH for women's research. Recent NIH directives require, not merely encourage, the participation of women (and minorities) in federally funded research (National Institutes of Health, 1990; Dresser, 1992). AIDS was not the cause of the debate concerning this issue, but it certainly sharpened that debate because AIDS is now a leading cause of death in women of childbearing age.

Inclusion of pregnant women in AIDS trials has created an arena for debate concerning larger social issues. Because most cases of pediatric AIDS are a result of transmission of the virus from mother to fetus, proposals for treatment of the mother in an attempt to prevent such transmission have been offered. At the time of this writing, a study designed to treat pregnant women with AZT to prevent such transmission has recently begun. The protocol for this study (the so-called AIDS Clinical Trials Group protocol 076) has been the subject of more debate and controversy than that for any other AIDS trial; that 2-year debate illustrates the changing climate regarding treating pregnant women with experimental therapies.

The trial was originally designed to treat newborn infants with either AZT or a placebo (chosen at random) for 6 weeks in an attempt to prevent or ameliorate HIV infection, because, at that time, most investigators were unwilling to treat pregnant women with AZT. Although some of this reluctance stemmed from concerns over maternal side effects (the drug causes anemia when given at high doses), even greater reservations were related to fetal toxicity, especially the possibility of inducing birth defects. Unfortunately, key information needed to assess the risk-benefit of treatment during pregnancy for mother and fetus was, and to a large degree still is, unavailable. Estimates of the overall risk of transmission from mother to fetus have decreased steadily from approximately 50 percent to 25-35 percent (Hardy, 1991), and preliminary data and extrapolation from other diseases have raised the possibility that the virus might be transmitted during the birth process itself. A registry of over 40 cases in which pregnant women had received AZT during at least part of their pregnancy revealed no cases of teratogenicity likely due to AZT. Armed with these admittedly limited data, the investigators for protocol 076 proposed including women in the third trimester of pregnancy, on a randomized basis, to receive either AZT or a placebo until the birth of the child. The newborn would then receive the same medication as the mother for an additional 6 weeks after birth. This design was chosen to decrease the risk of fetal malformation by starting therapy well after organ development was complete. Study organizers believed that the risk of giving AZT to an uninfected fetus was acceptable because of the inability to identify such fetuses and the relatively high likelihood of transmission. Thus, the pediatricians who designed the trial believed the study to be timely and ethical.

Criticism of the design, however, was immediate and severe. Advocates of women with HIV disease and some AIDS Clinical Trials Group investigators argued that the focus of the protocol, including any risk-benefit analysis, should be the pregnant woman, not the fetus. Previously expressed concerns that women were considered of importance in the epidemic only in relation to their role as "vectors" of disease to their unborn children or as sexual partners seemed to them to be borne out by the design of protocol 076 (Mitchell, 1988). Critics also pointed out that AZT had been demonstrated to prolong life in patients with AIDS and to delay progression to AIDS in asymptomatic HIV-infected individuals with CD4 counts below 500. They argued that by randomizing pregnant women to receive AZT or a placebo, the design would deny some women essential therapy in order to determine the effects of the drug on preventing fetal transmission. To meet concerns that in this protocol, and others, decisions regarding the treatment of women were not being addressed by those qualified to make them, a working group composed of obstetrician-gynecologists, internists, and pediatricians was established within the AIDS Clinical Trials Group. The working group has since been raised to the level of a full scientific committee and presumably will be consulted regarding all studies in which pregnant women will be enrolled.

Ultimately, the FDA asked its Anti-Viral Advisory Committee to review protocol 076. That review, in September 1990, resulted in recommendations to radically redesign the study. In general, the recommendations supported the view that women should be the focus of the trial. Thus, the committee recommended that women with AIDS or severe immune dysfunction be excluded and given AZT. Women with moderate immune dysfunction, although eligible, would be told that if they were not pregnant, AZT would often be recommended, although the risk of delaying therapy for 6 months was believed to be small. Randomization much earlier, just after the first trimester, was recommended to maximize the possible benefit in preventing fetal transmission.

Advocates have recently voiced new doubts about the ethical propriety of the protocol. They point out that the carcinogenic effects of AZT in women are unknown because studies of AZT have included very few women.

(Female rodents given a high dose of AZT for prolonged periods have developed cervical dysplasia.) Advocates argue that the prime group to be recruited for this study (HIV-positive women with more than 500 CD4 cells) receive no known benefit from AZT and face a possible hazard in its use, genital carcinogenesis. Again, they argue that the protocol subsumes the interests of the mother to those of the fetus.

However this debate evolves and whatever final shape protocol 076 takes, it is clear that this experience has altered how pregnant women are viewed as trial subjects, and it has highlighted the lack of information on gender-specific treatment effects in women. Whether it will have far-reaching effects on how decisions are made regarding the use of experimental or standard therapies with pregnant women with other diseases is unclear, but given that the entire area of research in women's health is undergoing dramatic evolution, it is likely that developments regarding AIDS will be scrutinized and considered as possible models.

Dissemination of Information

Peer-Reviewed Reporting of Clinical Research

Dissemination of information regarding research results has traditionally occurred first through peer-reviewed scientific and medical publications. This process begins with an author's writing and rewriting of a manuscript and submitting it to a journal, initial editorial consideration, and, usually, referral to outside reviewers. Editors then compile and compare reviews and make a final decision regarding publication. Papers may be accepted outright, accepted under the condition that changes are made, returned to the author for possible resubmission, or rejected outright. Rejected manuscripts are almost always submitted to other journals, beginning the time-consuming review process again. Once a paper is accepted for publication, considerable time usually occurs before it is actually published, often 6 months to 1 year. After publication, months to years may elapse before the results of the research make their way into clinical practice or are widely accepted and taught by the scientific community. Codification of results into textbooks and removal of outdated or even disproved information from textbooks may take longer.

Although cumbersome, this process has on the whole been viewed as appropriate. Outside peer review—in theory and usually in practice—provides an objective assessment of the accuracy and relevance of research findings by experts in the same field. It has benefits for authors, who are often given advice by reviewers that strengthens or extends their work, and society benefits from the prevention of dissemination of information that is not sound. These advantages have been considered to outweigh the inherent disadvantage of delay. However, many people have questioned whether in the case of clinical research that appears to show a significant therapeutic benefit for serious diseases or that demonstrates a previously unknown toxicity of accepted therapy the slow and orderly process of peer review and publication is in fact appropriate.

Studies pertaining to AIDS have not been the only ones in which disclosure before publication has been championed or actually occurred. Repeatedly in the past decade, authors, journalists, physicians, and public health officials have protested specific instances in which promising results were delayed from public announcement for months prior to journal publication. In response to these criticisms, some journals have adopted various "fast track" approaches to manuscript review and publication, in essence identifying some manuscripts as high priority and hastening them through the process. In addition, several government agencies have themselves asked for permission from journal editors to release information to the lay press and medical practicing communities before manuscript publication and in some cases, even before manuscript review. For example, in May 1988, the National Cancer Institute sent out a "Clinical Alert" informing the public that adding chemotherapy to initial surgery for women with node-negative breast cancer increased survival. Publication of the findings in the *New England Journal of Medicine*, which had agreed to the "Clinical Alert," did not occur until 9 months later. Similar announcements in the past 5 years have included information concerning a protective effect of corticosteroids for spinal cord injury, a news conference to announce an unexpected mortality from two widely used antiarrhythmic drugs in a large clinical trial, and announcements of termination of a clinical trial of AZT versus a placebo in delaying the progression to AIDS among HIV-positive asymptomatic subjects.

Such announcements have been criticized, however, as not providing sufficient information to permit physicians and patients to proceed with clinical care, for which they would want to have detailed information, such as drug dosage, drug side effects and interactions, and any caveats concerning the applicability of the results to types of patients other than those included in the trial. In addition, although most promising studies that have been announced in this way had some level of review by such groups as independent data-safety monitoring boards, early release of their results came with the risk that the information would be found to be inaccurate, which would lead to the need for rapid retraction and, perhaps, to morbidity and mortality.

The issue of whether a more pragmatic approach to traditional peer review is needed is just beginning to be fully considered. Some people have suggested that guidelines should define studies that are of sufficient importance and whose inherent design and internal review mechanism are of sufficient rigor that they should be singled out for rapid, intensive review and early disclosure of relevant results. It is likely that continued refinements, large and small, will be proposed that will alter the process of research review and dissemination. Because of the large number of AIDS-related clinical studies, including clinical trials, and the urgency of AIDS research, it is likely that much of the debate and change will take place in the context of the epidemic.

Non-Peer-Reviewed Publications

The dissemination of AIDS research information through AIDS-specific, nontraditional means has been explosive. Among the most interesting of these are patient-oriented publications, which started out very modestly but have grown in sophistication and influence as well as circulation. *AIDS Treatment News* (mentioned above), which is produced in San Francisco by John S. James (a former computer programmer), has a circulation of about 5,000. Another influential newsletter is San Francisco Project Inform's *PI Perspective*. Supported by a staff of 11 and numerous volunteers, it has a circulation of 50,000. Project Inform also operates an AIDS treatment hotline (Bishop, 1991).

Many mainstream AIDS researchers and clinicians are subscribers to AIDS treatment newsletters, and a few even contribute to such publications. Often, these publications provide editorial comment on many aspects of the epidemic, such as regulation and access to drugs, HIV antibody testing among various groups at risk, and immigration and travel restrictions for HIV-positive individuals. Compilation and updating of information regarding all known AIDS drugs has been done for several years by the American Foundation for AIDS Research through its *AIDS/HIV Treatment Directory*. The Public Health Service operates a toll-free hotline (1-800 TRIALS-A) that provides information on federally sponsored clinical trials and industry-sponsored efficacy trials.

From the beginning of the epidemic, the problem of teaching busy practitioners about a new disease of rapidly growing prevalence and importance was appreciated. A variety of newsletters for primary care practitioners were established to meet this need, such as *AIDS Alert*, *AIDS News*, and *AIDS Clinical Care* (published by the Massachusetts Medical Society, publishers of the *New England Journal of Medicine*). These publications are uniquely suited to providing up-to-date information on AIDS through a mixed format of in-depth clinical reviews, annotated summaries of articles in leading peer-reviewed journals, and reporting of late-breaking stories of interest. They fill a gap between mass media reporting and traditional peer-reviewed journals and as such are uniquely suited to the exigencies of the epidemic.

Science and Health Reporting in the Mass Media

During the 1980s medical and scientific reporting in the mass media became increasingly well supported and sophisticated, changing from simple repetition of the abstracts and press releases that accompanied publication of articles in medical journals to careful and then highly critical commentary. Major newspapers often employ several full-time science and medical reporters, and local and network television shows regularly air health segments. As science and medicine have become big business, they have become big stories. Because of the dramatic nature of the HIV/AIDS epidemic, the changes it has generated in all aspects of science and medicine, and its extraordinary social ramifications, AIDS has become the biggest of those stories and as such has driven many of the media changes that have occurred (Kinsella, 1989).

Ironically, there was almost total avoidance of AIDS by the media early in the epidemic. The turning point came in the mid-1980s, and it is often tied to the coverage given to Rock Hudson when it was learned that he had AIDS. Now, virtually all AIDS stories of importance and most minor ones are covered by the daily print media. Indeed, many AIDS researchers rely first and foremost on several key newspapers to keep themselves abreast of AIDS research news. The number of public service announcements, local and national "AIDS specials," and AIDS segments on major television news shows has been remarkable. Indeed, the Public Broadcasting System had for some time a regular feature, "AIDS Quarterly," hosted by anchor Peter Jennings; it has continued but is now the "Health Quarterly."

CONCLUSIONS

It is impossible at this juncture in the HIV/AIDS epidemic to reach any definitive conclusions about its long-term impact on clinical research and the regulation of new drugs. It is apparent that patient activism, a political climate favoring deregulation, and the exigencies of the AIDS epidemic have generated the most significant reevaluation of the research and regulation processes to occur since World War II. As this chapter shows, the AIDS epidemic has had profound effects on the conduct and nature of clinical research and on the regulation of drugs.

First, not since randomized clinical trials became the orthodox mode of clinical investigation had the most basic approaches and assumptions regarding research methodologies been open to searching critique in the context of an epidemic disease. AIDS has led to a fundamental reconsideration of basic methodologies for establishing the efficacy and safety of pharmaceuticals. New approaches to experimentation—to shorten the time required, as well as to alter the criteria for assessment—are actively being explored. Moreover, the very legitimacy of randomization has been called into question as the ethics of withholding treatments has loomed large in the context of the epidemic. At this time it seems clear that randomized clinical trials will continue to have a significant role in clinical investigation, but that they will be designed in new ways in order to answer a revised set of questions. Moreover, it seems likely that the new methodologic approaches will not be limited to AIDS investigations, but, rather, will be diffused to other research fields. Although randomized clinical trials continue to offer significant scientific advantages for the evaluation of new drugs, it seems likely that in the context of AIDS, alternative approaches to clinical investigation will be proposed and evaluated in the years ahead.

Second, there has been a dramatic shift in the face of the epidemic from a restrictive ethos for regulating new drugs to a new, less restrictive environment. Nevertheless, the balance between protection and access is likely to be the focal point of intense debate in the future. The evolution of the parallel track, expanded compassionate drug allocations, and the general trend to expedite trials—all are clear indicators of the impact that the HIV/AIDS epidemic has had on drug regulation. Although the epidemic has spurred these changes, it now seems likely that in certain instances attempts will be made to expedite the regulatory process for drugs for other diseases, especially those for life-threatening or previously untreatable conditions. Reports of toxicity, morbidity, or, especially, drug-related mortality, however, could lead to new restrictions in the future.

Third, changes in clinical trials and the regulation of new drugs are obviously having a related impact on the pharmaceutical industry. Although the issue of the relationship between federal research and private industry has been most vocally raised in the instance of AZT, fundamental questions of public-private cooperation in research and development have been posed by the epidemic. To date, many of these complex issues have been resolved essentially on an ad hoc basis, but that public-private relationship, which is outside the scope of this chapter, merits much more attention. Moreover, the incentives and disincentives for the development of new drugs in a new regulatory environment also needs much more scrutiny.

Fourth, to a degree that few could have anticipated, AIDS has influenced the nature and meaning of the ethics of human investigation. AIDS has forced clinical medicine to consider the variable of time in a new way: added to the normative care and precision of clinical investigation has been the new demand of urgency. The epidemic will not pause for the traditional modes of science; AIDS has forced the acceleration of the procedures and processes of clinical investigation, as well as the mechanisms of regulation. The scientific community has accepted the acceleration of clinical trial phases in the context of AIDS, recognizing the urgency of early access and allocation of new drugs for a disease that is fatal and principally strikes young people. Similar pressures were building prior to AIDS for early access to new cancer drugs. However, there is also serious concern in the research community that an effective research tool may be compromised and that the implications for both safety and efficacy of new therapeutic agents have not been fully assessed. Thus, the long-term impact of these changes is not known. Although, in the past, the very term "therapeutic research" was held in disrepute, the lines between experimentation and therapy have now been blurred. Activists have chanted, "a drug trial is health care, too." The basic concept of human experimentation has been radically altered—from protecting individuals from research to attempting to ensure individuals access to research. These changes can be fully understood only in the context of the powerful and effective social and political activism that the HIV/AIDS epidemic has generated.

NOTE

1. This section is based in part on a paper prepared for the panel by Harry M. Marks of the Institute for the History of Medicine at the Johns Hopkins University, "Historical Perspectives on Clinical Trials" (August 1990).

REFERENCES

Abrams, D.I. (1990) Alternative therapies in HIV infection. *AIDS* 4:1179-1187.
AIDS Coalition to Unleash Power (ACT-UP) (1989) A National AIDS Treatment Research Agenda. Paper distributed at the Fifth Annual International Conference on AIDS, Montreal, June 4-9.
Annas, G.J. (1988) AIDS, judges and the right to medical care. *Hastings Center Report* 18(4):20-22.
Arras, J.D. (1990) Noncompliance in AIDS research. *Hastings Center Report* 20:24-32.
Barber, B. (1976) The ethics of experimentation with human subjects. *Scientific American* 234:25-31.
Bayer, R. (1990) Beyond the burdens of protection: AIDS and the ethics of research. *Evaluation Review* 14:443-446.
Beecher, H.E. (1966) Ethics and clinical research. *New England Journal of Medicine* 274:1354-1360.
Bishop, K. (1991) Underground press leads way on AIDS advice. *New York Times* December 16:A-10.
Bozette, S.A., F.R. Sattler, J. Chiu, A.W. Wu, D. Gluckstein, et al. (1990) A controlled trial of early adjunctive treatment with corticosteroids for *Pneumocystis carinii* pneumonia in the acquired immunodeficiency syndrome. *New England Journal of Medicine* 321:1451-1457.
Brandt, A.M. (1978a) Polio, politics, publicity, and duplicity: ethical aspects in the development of the Salk vaccine. *International Journal of Health Services* 8:257-270.
Brandt, A.M. (1978b) Racism and research: the case of the Tuskegee syphilis study. *Hastings Center Report* 8:26-27.
Carter, R. (1966) *Breakthrough: The Saga of Jonas Salk*. New York: Trident.

Chalmers, T., J. Block, and S. Lee (1972) Controlled studies in clinical cancer research. *New England Journal of Medicine* 287:75-78.

Cotton, P. (1990a) Examples abound of gaps in medical knowledge because of groups excluded from scientific study. *Journal of the American Medical Association* 263:1051, 1055.

Cotton, P. (1990b) Is there still too much extrapolation from data on middle-aged white men? *Journal of the American Medical Association* 263:1049-1050.

Delaney, M. (1989a) The case for patient access to experimental therapy. *Journal of Infectious Diseases* 159:416-419.

Delaney, M. (1989b) Patient access to experimental therapy. *Journal of the American Medical Association* 261:2444-2447.

D'Emilio, J. (1983) *Sexual Politics, Sexual Communities: The Making of a Homosexual Minority in the United States, 1940-1970.* Chicago: University of Chicago Press.

Dresser, R. (1992) Wanted: single, white male for medical research. *Hastings Center Report* 22(1):24-29.

Eckholm, E. (1986) Should the rules be bent in an epidemic? *New York Times* July 13:E30.

Edgar, H., and D.J. Rothman (1991) New rules for new drugs: the challenge of AIDS to the regulatory process. In D. Nelkin, D.P. Willis, and S.V. Parris, eds., *A Disease of Society: Cultural and Institutional Responses to AIDS.* New York: Cambridge University Press.

Faden, R.R., and T.L. Beauchamp (1986) *A History and Theory of Informed Consent.* New York: Oxford University Press.

Feinstein, A. (1967) *Clinical Judgment.* Baltimore, Md.: Williams and Wilkins.

Fried, C. (1974) *Medical Experimentation: Personal Integrity and Social Policy.* New York: American Elsevier.

Gray, B. (1975) *Human Subjects in Medical Research: A Sociological Study of the Conduct and Regulation of Clinical Research.* New York: John Wiley and Sons.

Green, S.B., S.S. Ellenberg, D. Finkelstein, A.B. Forsythe, L.S. Freedman, et al. (1990) Issues in the design of drug trials for AIDS. *Controlled Clinical Trials* 11:80-87.

Gross, J. (1991) Turning disease into a cause: breast cancer follows AIDS. *New York Times* January 7:A1.

Hand, R. (1989) Alternative therapies used by patients with AIDS (letter). *New England Journal of Medicine* 320:672-673.

Hardy, L.M., ed. (1991) *HIV Screening of Pregnant Women and Newborns.* Committee on Prenatal and Newborn Screening for HIV Infection, Institute of Medicine. Washington, D.C.: National Academy Press.

Harris, R. (1964) *A Real Voice.* New York: Macmillan.

Henninger, D. (1990) Will the FDA revert to type? *Wall Street Journal* December 12:A16.

Hill, A.B. (1951) The clinical trial. *British Medical Bulletin* 7:278-282.

Hill, A.B. (1963) Medical ethics and controlled trials. *British Medical Journal* 1:1043-1049.

Insight Team (of the *Sunday Times* of London) (1979) *Suffer the Children: The Story of Thalidomide.* New York: Viking Press.

James, J.S. (1989) *AIDS Treatment News.* Berkeley, Calif: Celestial Arts.

Johnson, N., R.J. Lilford, and W. Brazier (1991) At what level of collective equipoise does a clinical trial become ethical? *Journal of Medical Ethics* 17:30-34.

Jones, J.H. (1981) *Bad Blood: The Tuskegee Syphilis Experiment.* New York: Free Press.

Jonsen, A. (1984) Public policy and human research. Pp. 3-19 in J. Humber and R. Almeder, eds., *Biomedical Ethics Reviews.* Clifton, N.J.: Humana Press.

Jonsen, A.R. (1991) *Old Ethics, New Medicine.* Cambridge, Mass.: Harvard University Press.

Katz, J. (1984) *The Silent World of Doctor and Patient.* New York: Free Press.

Katz, J., and A.M. Capron (1975) *Catastrophic Diseases: Who Decides What?: A Psychological and Legal Analysis of the Problems Posed by Hemodialysis and Organ Transplantation.* New York: Russell Sage Foundation.

Kinsella, J. (1989) *Covering the Plague: AIDS and the American Media.* New Brunswick, N.J.: Rutgers University Press.

Kolata, G. (1991) U.S. weighs release of an AIDS drug before tests are completed. *New York Times* June 19:A-11.

Levine, C. (1988) Has AIDS changed the ethics of human subjects research? *Law, Medicine & Health Care* 16:167-173.

Levine, C. (1990) Women and HIV/AIDS research: the barriers to equity. *Evaluation Review* 14:447-463.

Marks, H.M. (1990) Historical Perspectives in Clinical Trials. Working paper prepared for the National Research Council Committee on AIDS Research and the Behavioral, Social and Statistical Sciences, Washington, D.C.

Martin, J.M., and H.S. Sacks (1990) Do HIV-infected children in foster care have access to clinical trials of new treatments? *AIDS & Public Policy Journal* 5:3-8.

Merton, V. (1990) Community-based AIDS research. *Evaluation Review* 14:502-537.

Mintz, M. (1967) *By Prescription Only*, rev. ed. Boston: Beacon Press.

Mitchell, J.L. (1988) Women, AIDS, and public policy. *AIDS and Public Policy Journal* 3(2):50-52.

National Commission for the Protection of Human Subjects of Biomedical and Behavioral Research (1978) *The Belmont Report: Ethical Principles and Guidelines for the Protection of Human Subjects of Research.* Washington, D.C.: U.S. Department of Health and Human Services.

National Commission on AIDS (1991) *America Living with AIDS: Transforming Anger, Fear and Indifference into Action.* Washington, D.C.: National Commission on AIDS.

National Institutes of Health (NIH) (1990) Instruction and information memorandum OER 90-5, December 11, NIH, Bethesda, Md.

Nolan, K. (1990) AIDS and pediatric research. *Evaluation Review* 14:464-481.

Nussbaum, B. (1990) *Good Intentions: How Big Business and the Medical Establishment are Corrupting the Fight Against AIDS.* New York: Atlantic Monthly Press.

Office of Technology Assessment (1983) *The Impact of Randomized Clinical Trials on Health Policy and Medical Practice: Background Paper.* Washington, D.C.: U.S. Government Printing Office.

Okun, M. (1986) *Fair Play in the Marketplace: The First Battle for Pure Food and Drugs.* DeKalb, Ill.: Northern Illinois University Press.

Palca, J. (1990) Conflict over release of clinical research data. *Science* 247:374-375.

Quirk, P. (1980) Food and Drug Administration. In J.Q. Wilson, ed., *The Politics of Regulation.* New York: Basic Books.

Rothman, D.J. (1987a) Ethical and social issues in the development of new drugs and vaccines. *Bulletin of the New York Academy of Medicine* 63:557-568.

Rothman, D.J. (1987b) Ethics and human experimentation: Henry Beecher revisited. *New England Journal of Medicine* 317:1195-1199.

Rothman, D.J. (1991) *Strangers at the Bedside: A History of How Law and Bioethics Transformed Medical Decision Making.* New York: Basic Books.

Ruskin, J.N. (1989) The cardiac arrhythmia suppression trial (CAST). *New England Journal of Medicine* 321:386-388.

Rutstein, D.D. (1970) The ethical design of human experiments. In P.A. Freund, ed., *Experimentation with Human Subjects.* New York: George Braziller.

Schaefer, A. (1982) The ethics of the randomized clinical trial. *New England Journal of Medicine* 307:719-724.

Silverman, W.A. (1985) *Human Experimentation: A Guided Step into the Unknown.* New York: Oxford University Press.

Silverman, M., and P. Lee (1974) *Pills, Profits, and Politics.* Berkeley, Calif.: University of California Press.

Sinclair, U. (1906) *The Jungle.* New York: Doubleday Page & Company.

Steinbrook, R., and B. Lo (1990) Informing physicians about promising new treatments for severe illnesses. *Journal of the American Medical Association* 263:2078-2082.

Thomas, S.B., and S.C. Quinn (1991) The Tuskegee syphilis study, 1932-1972: implications for HIV education and AIDS risk education programs in the black community. *American Journal of Public Health* 81:1498-1505.

U.S. Congress, House of Representatives (1991) *Drugs for Opportunistic Infections in Persons with HIV Disease.* Hearing before the Human Resources and Intergovernmental Relations Subcommittee of the Committee on Government Operations, House of Representatives, 2nd session, August 1, 1990. Washington, D.C.: U.S. Government Printing Office.

U.S. Department of Health and Human Services, Advisory Committee on the Food and Drug Administration (1991) *Final Report.* Washington, D.C.: U.S. Government Printing Office.

U.S. General Accounting Office (1990) *National Institutes of Health: Problems in Implementing Policy on Women in Study Populations.* Testimony, June 18, Mark V. Nadel, Human Resources Division. Subcommittee on Health and the Environment, House Committee on Energy and Commerce. GAO/T-HRD-90-38. Washington, D.C.: General Accounting Office.

Valdiserri, R.O., G.M. Tama, and M. Ho (1988) The role of community advisory committees in clinical trials of anti-HIV agents. *IRB: A Review of Human Subjects Research* 10(4):5-7.

Wastila, L.J., and L. Lasagna (1990) The history of zidovudine (AZT). *Journal of Clinical Research and Pharmacoepidemiology* 4:25-37.

Weiss, R., and L. Mazade (1990) *Surrogate Endpoints in Evaluating the Effectiveness of Drugs Against HIV Infection and AIDS.* Roundtable for the Development of Drugs and Vaccines Against AIDS, Institute of Medicine. Washington, D.C.: National Academy Press.

Wolfe, S., and C. Coley (1980) *Pills That Don't Work.* Washington, D.C.: Public Citizen's Health Research Group.

Young, J.H. (1990) *Pure Food.* Princeton, N.J.: Princeton University Press.

Zelen, M. (1990) Randomized consent designs for clinical trials: an update. *Statistics in Medicine* 9:645-656.

5

Religion and Religious Groups

Religion, manifested in personal belief and in organized denominations, is a large part of American life. The responses of major religious denominations and of religiously identified individuals to AIDS have been an important feature of the epidemic. Many religious groups have interpreted the AIDS epidemic in the light of their beliefs and teachings. Those interpretations have often led to public pronouncements on AIDS education, prevention, and care, as well as to the shaping of public attitudes toward those afflicted by or at risk of HIV infection. In addition, individuals who identify themselves with particular religious denominations or express particular religious viewpoints have taken positions about AIDS in light of their beliefs. Their positions have often been within the realm of private attitudes, but sometimes they have been manifested in public comments and actions. Given the broad influence of religion in the United States, the response of religious organizations and individuals is a factor in the effort to control the epidemic and to care for those affected by it.

In this chapter, *religion* is used as a general term to describe the positions and policies of major religious denominations in the United States and the views of individuals or groups that associate themselves with a professed religious belief. The chapter begins with a brief overview of religion and the ways in which the religious traditions that are influential in the United States have historically viewed epidemic disease and sexuality, which are key to understanding the reactions of religious groups to the AIDS epidemic. The chapter then turns to those reactions, first in the early years of the epidemic and then in more recent years. The chapter relates the responses of some of the larger denominations to the epidemic and reports what can be reliably ascertained about the responses of individuals and groups that express their views in religious terms.

The chapter is about responses to the epidemic by religious institutions and individuals. Those responses have not taken the form of changes in doctrines, beliefs, or adherents. However, the responses of religious institutions affect their activities, which in turn influence health policy, public education, care of the sick, and attitudes toward HIV-infected people. In this way, religious institutions are an important factor in the social response to the HIV/AIDS epidemic in the United States.

The influence of religions and religious belief on the HIV/AIDS epidemic in the United States is difficult to fully discern. Official statements, media reports, and other published accounts provide one source of information. Another source, perhaps a more important one, is beyond the easy reach of researchers: the history of personal attitudes and actions of individuals who are informed and motivated by religious beliefs. Certainly, such individuals have expressed both compassion and discrimination, reception and rejection, involvement and indifference. Many stories have been told of such reactions, but the stories are ephemeral. Similarly, collective reactions of communities of religious people at the level of parishes, synagogues, and other local organizations have also spanned the range of responses. This form of religious response, embodied in the private attitudes and actions of individuals and in isolated activities of small communities, is often hidden from or lost to scientific inquiry. This loss is distressing. The institutions of organized religion can take positions, issue statements, and influence the consciences of their adherents. But it is through individuals, with and without public disclosure, that religion finds expression and evolves in response to changing conditions.

It is also difficult to sort out a "religious" response from the myriad of other attitudes and motivations that surround any human reaction. Even official pronouncements of religious bodies, written in the idiom of religion and invoking its traditions and beliefs, may be influenced by secular and political concerns. The words and actions of individuals who present themselves as religiously affiliated or as representatives of religion may also reflect other interests. None but the most naive observer will accept every word and action by religious organizations and individuals as a pure reflection only of creeds and canons; none but the most skeptical will scorn all religious affirmations as disguised self-serving.

The chapter does not attempt to capture the entire response of American religious denominations to the HIV/AIDS epidemic. It is limited to selected Jewish and Christian groups because of their size or perceived influence within American culture. Buddhism and Islam in the United States

and the religions of Native Americans are not discussed. Although powerful forces in the personal lives of their adherents, these religions are not
ordinarily given to public statements from official representatives about
their beliefs.

The primary objective of this chapter is to describe how organized
religion has responded to the epidemic and to note the ways in which that
response has affected the broader public response and the formation of
public and health policy. Many Americans have strong feelings about religion and its place in public life. It is difficult to write about religion
without making, or suggesting, value judgments, and even strenuous efforts
to avoid such judgments will sometimes be interpreted by some readers as
condemnatory or complimentary. In this chapter, the panel has made such
efforts to avoid judgments on various religious responses to the epidemic
and also to avoid any prescriptions of how religion should respond or what
religions should teach. Rather, the intention is to elucidate the role that
religious organizations have played in the epidemic and, in so doing, stress
the importance of taking that response into account in efforts to understand
the impact of AIDS in American society.

The response of religion to the epidemic has been multifaceted. Not
only are there many religious communities with their distinct traditions, but
within the traditions themselves various themes intertwine with varying
emphases. This complexity makes generalization difficult and simplifica-
tion perilous. As discussed in this chapter, certain themes from certain
traditions were more noticeable in the early years of the epidemic, which
led to the impression that religion in general was unsympathetic toward
those touched by the epidemic and hostile toward preventive efforts. Un-
questionably, many people in the gay community strongly believe this is so,
as evidenced by two events sponsored by the AIDS Coalition to Unleash
Power (ACT-UP): a disruption of Sunday Mass at St. Patrick's Cathedral in
New York, where demonstrators desecrated the communion wafers and chained
themselves to pews while 4,500 protested outside, and a demonstration outside Boston's Holy Cross Cathedral during an ordination ceremony, where
ACT-UP members, some of them "in drag," tossed condoms at newly ordained priests as they left the building. A broader view of the religious
response shows these negative reactions, to be sure, but also a more complex picture of religion and AIDS in the United States.

The important role that religious organizations can play in the HIV/
AIDS epidemic has been recognized by the lead federal agency in the effort
to contain the epidemic, the Centers for Disease Control (CDC). Realizing
that its resources are limited and that the widest possible cooperation with
other social institutions is needed, the CDC, through the National Partnership Program of its National AIDS Information and Education Program,
began in 1989 the development of programmatic relationships with the business

and religious sectors of society. Relationships with 30 religious organizations that represent a spectrum of denominations and interests were established. The CDC provides the organizations with technical assistance, referrals, conference support, and information on use of the national AIDS information clearinghouse database. The participant organizations are expected to enhance the CDC's educational outreach by using this information in their own educational and media endeavors. According to the Centers for Disease Control (1990:10) the organizations are considered particularly appropriate:

> [they] have broad access to significant populations; have influence and control significant resources; are widely respected and have great credibility with very large segments of the population; and have communications and other networks in place to focus on HIV issues and needs.

One consequence of the partnership with religious organizations has been an expanded and positive coverage of HIV issues in the religious press (Centers for Disease Control, 1990). Also, some religious groups are collaborating with public health agencies to provide HIV prevention education to their members. Thus, CDC has recognized the importance of religious organizations as sources of communication and cooperation in the difficult task of devising and implementing educational programs. If the collaboration of religion is to be fostered in the fight against the epidemic, the nature and dynamics of the religious response to the epidemic must be understood.

RELIGIOUS DOCTRINES AND TRADITIONS

The Nature of Religion

The words *religion* and *religious* are extremely difficult to define. One distinguished scholar of religion wrote of "the striking lack of unanimity among modern students of religion regarding the nature of the concept under analysis" (Bertholet, 1934:xiii,237; see also Spiro, 1968). Every attempt to define these terms will miss some important feature or will misrepresent one or another of the many forms religion takes. For the purposes of this chapter, *religion* and *religious* refer to those organized communities of people who express adherence to an explicit canon and creed about the ultimate nature of human life and its transcendent source.

In a general way, religion in Western societies has taken the form of communities of people identified by some title, such as Roman Catholic, Reform Jew, Southern Baptist, Mormon, and so on. Those communities are structured in quite different ways, some with an authoritative hierarchy, others as consensual gatherings. The communities usually espouse a canon, that is, a set of ideas, often committed to writing, that express the origins and the most salient images, concepts, and histories with which the communities identify. For Christians of all denominations, the Old and New Testaments make up this canon; for Jews, the Torah and the Talmud. Finally, almost all religious communities have statements of principal beliefs, sometimes called creeds, that express the ideas and commitments that define the community from others.

The diverse religious communities with which American society is familiar give varying authority to their canonical scriptures and their creeds: some permit and even encourage broad interpretation; others insist on strict and even literal readings and application to belief and practice. Consequently, within the broad groupings of Christianity and Judaism are many communities that fall along a spectrum from literal and strict interpretation to liberal and figurative interpretation of their basic canons and creeds. These differences are frequently referred to with rough and often inaccurate terms. Despite the difficulty of describing these different positions in a completely accurate way, the differences are real, and they have significant influence on the way in which American denominations have responded to the AIDS epidemic.

Religion, as presented here, differs from most other social and cultural institutions in two significant ways. First, the canons and creeds almost always refer to a transcendent, supernatural power, God or Yahweh, whose relationship to the world and to humans is described in the canons and creeds with some specificity. Second, the canons and creeds explicitly contain certain directions about moral behavior on which religious communities have built moral codes and interpretations of conduct for the faithful. The forms of conduct that are prescribed are, for all faiths, vitally related to the meaning, ends, and purposes of human existence in relation to God. Serious adherence to a faith implies dedicated acceptance of its canons, creeds, and codes, even though believers will admit that they may sometimes, perhaps often, fail to live up to their professed beliefs. Although distinct faiths require adherence to their creeds, canons, and codes with greater or less literalness, religion, almost by definition (the word comes from the Latin for "bound" or "tied to"), requires adherence and fidelity to those features. At the same time, religion displays remarkable adaptability. The survival of many religious communities through very diverse, and often adverse, cultural situations is proof of that adaptability. Thus, when organized religions encounter new situations and experiences, their adherents will often interpret them in light of their beliefs. Conversely, when beliefs are challenged as outmoded or inadequate to new circumstances, religions will seek to preserve them or will modify them to the extent that modification does not violate the basic beliefs. It is rare to find a religious denomination deliberately abandoning or radically changing its beliefs: if change comes, it usually comes slowly and in less than obvious forms.

Religious institutions, then, perhaps more than any other institution, respond to unprecedented situations through defining features of their traditions. This sometimes means that a religious response will take the form of hard-line resistance to a new situation judged incompatible with its faith. Sometimes the religious response will consist of a reinterpretation of the tradition that enables it to coexist with a new situation. The doctrines and practices of religious institutions are not static, but even as they undergo change in response to new situations there is usually a strong urge to identify and preserve essential elements of the past. Thus, religion is almost always traditional and adaptive at the same time; its responses to new situations will be a mix of the dogmatic and doctrinal with the practical and pragmatic. These features of religion are important in understanding how religious groups in the United States have responded to the HIV/AIDS epidemic.

Religion in the United States

Religion was a powerful force in the origins and growth of the American republic. From colonial beginnings, Protestant and Catholic Christianity, and later Judaism, provided vital ideas, communal energy, and spiritual enthusiasm for the formulation of American institutions and public life (Clebsch, 1968; Reichley, 1985; Wuthnow, 1988; Butler, 1990). During much of the twentieth century, however, the place of religion in American culture was anomalous. The dominant cultural view was that religion has lost its influence among Americans and had moved to the margins of American life. The constitutional prohibition of establishment of religion erected a wall of separation between church and state higher than it had ever been, leading policy makers to steer clear of anything that might appear to breach that wall. Many aspects of public life, from education to entertainment, are carried on without reference to religion and, indeed, often seem antithetical to traditional religious teachings. In many respects, American life seems thoroughly secular (Clebsch, 1968).

By the late 1980s it became clear that that view was no longer tenable (Marty, 1987). Religion simply cannot be ignored as a social force in U.S. society. The sheer number of people who associate themselves with religion and who participate in its activities are testimony to the presence of religion. The constitutional wall may effectively separate governmental and ecclesiastical structures, but it does not keep ideas and influences of the world of religion from filtering into the world of public affairs. In the realm of health alone, current debates over the legality of abortion, the permissibility of fetal research, toleration of assisted suicide, and the rights of parents of religious persuasion to withhold from their children certain therapeutic and preventive health measures are recent examples of the constant interplay between religion and public affairs.

The vitality of religious life in the United States is remarkable. In 1989 there were more than 200 religious denominations in the United States. The 15 largest religious bodies encompassed 80 percent of the estimated 144 million total membership of congregations. The Roman Catholic church reports the largest membership (approximately 53.5 million), and the Southern Baptist Convention claims the largest Protestant Christian membership (approximately 14.75 million); the largest African American denomination is the National Baptist Convention, U.S.A. (an estimated 5.5 million); Reform Judaism is the fifteenth largest religious group (slightly fewer than 2 million) (Jacquet, 1989). Although reports of membership from denominations cannot be easily compared due to different definitions of membership, by self-report approximately 90 percent of Americans identify with a denomination (Goldman, 1991). Frequency of attendance at services provides another measure of religious commitment. The 1988 General Social Survey found that 27 percent of respondents attended services once or more per week, 17 percent attended more than once a month, and 20 percent attend from once a month to several times per year. By most measurable indices, the United States is a more religious country than all European nations except Ireland and Poland (Gallup Organization, 1985; Reichley, 1985).

Claims of religious affiliations and reports of church attendance are not, of course, measures of religious dedication or fervor, and there are several indications of an increase in deeply personal affirmations of religious belief. Among Christians, the number of persons expressing "commitment to Jesus Christ" indicates the importance of religious faith to many individuals. The Gallup Organization recently reported that 74 percent of adult U.S. citizens claimed such a commitment, compared with 66 percent in a 1988 survey and 60 percent in a 1978 survey (*Christian Century*, 1990). Even though many of America's 6 million Jews are not religiously observant or are only occasionally so, scholars note the emergence of a "committed minority . . . whose conscious choice of religious involvement has infused all branches of American Judaism with new energy and passion . . . that has virtually transformed American Judaism within the last two decades" (Wertheimer, 1989).

Religious affiliation and personal commitment to religious belief also find expression in patterns of charitable giving. Individual donors, who accounted for 84 percent of all giving in 1988, favored religious charities over all others. Of all households making contributions, 53 percent gave to religious organizations; human services and health were distant runners-up at 24 percent each. Religious organizations also ranked first in terms of average contribution per household: $375 to religious, $50 to human services, $44 to education, and $31 to health organizations (Independent Sector, 1990).

The place of religion in social life is indicated further by the ubiquitous presence of places of worship and religion-related educational, health, and social service organizations. Indeed, many social and cultural institutions, and even many commonly accepted "secular" beliefs, have migrated from the world of religion into the secular world and remain there, invisible but indelible (Douglass and Brunner, 1935; Clebsch, 1968; Wuthnow, 1988).

Like other huge organizations, national religious organizations can be slow to act or change. Local congregations, less burdened with bureaucracy, and individual members can be sentinels to identify emerging issues and be more immediately responsive. Yet when the national bodies speak and act, the whole nation becomes the audience and, at least theoretically, every neighborhood with a local congregation exists is affected. And political boundaries generally are not barriers to religious bodies and their institutions of education, health care, and social service.

Religion and Epidemic Disease

Christianity and Judaism retain within their traditions memories of epidemic disease. Those memories have become powerful images in the religious imagination and have influenced theological interpretations of the way God deals with humanity. The Hebrew scriptures (Old Testament), also revered by Christian faiths, contain many references to plague and pestilential disease, often in the context of divine wrath and punishment (Gen. 12:17; Lev. 26:6, 26:21, 26:25; Num. 8:19, 11:33, 15:37, 25:8, 31:16; Deut. 7:15, 28:22; II Sam. 4:8, 5:6; II Sam. 25; Jer. 21:6, 33:36). In the Book of Exodus, for example, God speaks the terrible words, "For now I will stretch out my hand, that I may smite thee and thy people with pestilence" (9:14). At the same time, God protects from the ravages of pestilential disease (Ps. 106:29). The Lord of the Hebrews and Christians is described as intimately involved in the lives of humans and brings both disease and deliverance as signs of anger and love. Undoubtedly, this idea of a God who has power over good and of evil is a difficult one: How can God be omnipotent and good and yet evil exist? The attempt to understand and answer this question, the so-called problem of theodicy, is a perennial endeavor for believers and nonbelievers alike. Still, the belief of a God who is involved in human life remains deeply embedded in the major religious traditions of American culture (Berger, 1967).

The belief that pestilence came from God was given "scientific confirmation" by contemporaneous medical explanations of the causation of disease. Greek medicine explained epidemics as the result of the conjunction of astral, meteorological, and terrestrial influences that, under certain circumstances, created a "climate" for disease. They named this the "epidemic constitution," a theory that prevailed in various forms until the nineteenth century. Since theological and philosophical views alike held that physical forces were, in some sense, under the guidance of Divine Providence, it was logical to see pestilential diseases as caused by God. The sixteenth-century surgeon, Ambroise Pare, for example, described the plague as "the coming of the wrath of God, furious, sudden, swift, monstrous, dreadful," and he devoted an entire chapter of his book to supporting this view with many scriptural quotations. He went on, however, to explain at length "the human and natural causes . . . the infection and corruption of the air and the visitation of the humours of the body that dispose them to take the plague from the air" (quoted in Winslow, 1943:177). Thus, both religious and scientific beliefs coincided to support the common contention that pestilential disease was an act of God. How that act of God was to be interpreted has always been a matter of debate.

In the Christian Middle Ages, the most common interpretation asserted that plague was punishment for the sins of humans. Religious authorities prescribed prayer and penance; at the same time, they insisted that measures be taken to prevent and stop the ravages of disease and that the sick be cared for. The sins being punished by God were usually viewed less as the particular sins of individuals than as the collective and pervasive sinfulness of all human beings. Even the most fervent preachers could not help but notice that the virtuous and the vicious, the religious and the irreligious, and the innocent child and the old villain were all stricken together. Indeed, it seemed to some observers who noted the deterioration of morals and social life consequent on great epidemics that the good were taken while the bad were spared. One early Christian historian (Gasquet, 1893:260) wrote of the plague in the reign of Emperor Justinian (A.D. 527-565): "whether by chance or providential design, it spared the most wicked." Thus, it is rare to find a link between sin and sickness, so common a theme, focused on one or another kind of sin—although an imaginative preacher could certainly seize on plague as punishment for his favorite vice (Numbers and Amundsen, 1986; Slack, 1988).

Epidemic disease regularly evoked this moral response of condemnation of sin and the call for repentance. The "great mortality" (bubonic plague) that devastated London in 1665 was commonly seen as a "visitation of God's hand," wrathful against sin in bringing the plague and merciful in removing it (Shrewsbury, 1970). Preachers and physicians alike warned the populace that plague was a judgment of God against such transgressions as "Lust, Pride and whoredom, wantonness and prophaneness" and advised them to avoid such worldliness as "profit, pleasure, usury, feasts and plays, censure, blasphemy and hypocrisy" (Leasor, 1961:68). Yellow fever, which attacked the U.S. eastern seaboard from the late eighteenth century through the first quarter of the nineteenth, inspired not only the first efforts at organized public health in the United States, but also repeated calls from clergy and public officials for prayer and repentance. In the particularly bad year of 1799, for example, the New York Common Council decreed a Day of Thanksgiving, Humiliation and Prayer. "The Hand of the Lord had lain heavily on New York, and whether its citizens had been guilty of sins of commission or omission, it was hoped that through prayer they could search their hearts and come to see the error of their ways" (Duffy, 1968:109).

The social response to the cholera epidemics in the United States in 1832, 1849, and 1866 reveals the first break in this long tradition of theological interpretation of epidemic disease. In the first two epidemics, the tradition prevailed intact. As Rosenberg (1962:40-42) notes, medical and theological opinions were in agreement that "the intemperate, the imprudent, and the filthy were particularly vulnerable." Sin, if not the primary cause of disease, was at least the "predisposing cause." Even when a respectable person died of cholera, suspicion was aroused that "this ordinarily praiseworthy man either had some secret vice or had indulged in some unwonted excess." Most Americans had no doubt that cholera was a divine punishment on sinful mankind and a divine exhortation to repentance. The governor of New York, in an official proclamation, declared that "an infinitely wise and just God has seen fit to employ pestilence as one means of scourging the human race for their sins, and it seems to be an appropriate one for the sins of uncleanliness and intemperance." Sins, it might be noted, were thought to fester among "the huddled urban masses."

By the time of the last serious cholera invasion in 1866, however, the religious interpretation and its attendant rhetoric had considerably softened. In the intervening years, the previously disdained theory of contagion had been given dramatic support by Dr. John Snow's identification of particular urban water sources as the sources of contagion. By 1866, "there were few intelligent physicians who doubted that cholera was portable and transmissible" (Rosenberg, 1962:195). In addition, the epidemiology of the disease was better understood. The ravages among the poor were better explained by the unsanitary conditions in which they were condemned to live than by their addiction to "the seven deadly sins." Rational measures of control could be put in place; theological explanations, though still relevant to the presence of any evil in the world, were relegated to the background. It appears that as scientific advance provided better explanation of the nature of communicable disease and better means of prevention, the tendency to resort to theological explanations dissipated. Only in one sort of disease, that communicated by sexual contact, did the theological reference continue to prevail—not as a substitute for the scientific causality, but as a reminder that the scientific cause, a microbe, was transmitted by human behavior that could be blamed as sinful (Brandt, 1987). In later epidemics, such as the influenza epidemic of 1919 and the polio epidemic of the 1940s, the traditional theological commentary was hardly heard in public discourse.

Christianity and Judaism, then, have long and deep traditions that interpret disease within the scope of Divine Providence. At the same time, these religious traditions contain powerful imperatives to care for the sick. The Talmud "gave permission to the physician to heal; moreover, this is a religious precept and it is included in the category of saving life," one of the most stringent of religious obligations (Shulhan Arukh, cited by Jakobovits, 1978:793). Similarly, Jewish ethics ranks "as the noblest form of charity—'loving kindness of truth' in the language of the rabbis—services rendered to those who can no longer fend for themselves, including the utmost consideration for the dignity of the dying" (Jakobovits, 1978:797). In the New Testament, Jesus tells the story of the Samaritan who "had compassion" on a wounded Jew and cared for him at his own expense (Luke 10:29-37). This image became paradigmatic for Christians; early Christian literature is filled with admonitions to care for the sick. Records of epidemic disease in the third century tell of Christians who devoted themselves to caring for Christians and non-Christians alike, even at risk of their lives: they were named "the reckless ones" (Numbers and Amundsen, 1986:48). Even when they were theologically convinced that plague was punishment for human depravity, ecclesiastical leaders organized medical care and enforced preventive efforts: quarantine and penitential processions were endorsed as protection from plague. Desertion of the sick by physicians and clergy alike was branded as shameful. Thus, historically, Christianity and Judaism strongly urged their adherents to care for the victims of epidemic disease. This profound tradition has also influenced the response of religious organizations to the HIV/AIDS epidemic.

Sexuality

The AIDS epidemic is marked by one feature that has made it particularly problematic for religion, namely, the group initially hardest hit and still numerically the group with the largest number of cases is men who have sex with men. This fact has posed a problem to those religions that explicitly condemn homosexual activity as sinful. Christianity and Judaism have historically been critical of homosexuality. Several texts of the Hebrew scriptures (Gen. 19; Lev. 18:22, 20:13) and several in the New Testament writings of St. Paul (I Cor. 6:9; I Tim. 1:10; Rom. 1:26-7) are interpreted by many to condemn homosexual activities. Early Christian writers, however, rarely alluded to them, and modern scholars debate their interpretation (Boswell, 1980; Lemay, 1980; Weeks, 1980; Adams, 1981). Still, from its beginnings, Christianity has generally considered sinful all forms of sexual expression other than procreative intercourse, although it appears that sexual acts between persons of the same gender were not singled out as more sinful than adultery or fornication. In the thirteenth century, however, church leaders began to see homosexual behavior as particularly heinous and, for the first time in Christian history, ecclesiastical, legal, and public intolerance of those who practiced such behavior became common. Since that time, Christian denominations have generally judged same-gender sex harshly and have often been supportive of legal penalties against it (Brundage, 1987). However, some Protestant and Jewish groups have adopted the more tolerant interpretation that some scholars give to the scriptural texts referring to homosexuality.

Some adherents of Christianity and Judaism were inclined to link the earlier tradition that saw plague as a divine punishment for sinfulness in general with the single sin of male homosexuality. The first civil legislation (in A.D. 533) that flatly outlawed homosexual behavior and made it subject to the death penalty, along with adultery, was associated by its enactor, the Christian Emperor Justinian, with the occurrence of plagues and earthquakes. During subsequent centuries, this association was cited from time to time when civil and ecclesiastical laws imposed penalties on homosexuality (Boswell, 1980:170-173; Brundage, 1987:398-399). Even though forgotten by most modern Christians, this ancient association seems to echo in the collective memory of some who were ready to view AIDS as divine punishment visited on homosexuals. When it became evident that the infection touched others as well, that position became more difficult to maintain, and many denominations, including major ones in the United States, have not endorsed that position (see below). Nevertheless, the association between homosexuality and infection has complicated the response of many religious people. For one major denomination, Roman Catholicism, the reaction to AIDS has also been complicated by its condemnation as sinful the use of almost all methods of birth control, and this doctrine was stated in such a way as to prohibit the use of condoms in any sexual activity (Noonan, 1970). Thus, as discussed below, the position of the Roman Catholic church regarding one of the most commonly recommended methods for preventing the spread of HIV has been the subject of intense debate.

The HIV/AIDS epidemic, then, comes to religion as an old nemesis in new guise. Religious tradition and teaching have had, from time immemorial, a place for pestilential disease. This new pestilence, however, arrives at a time when popular religious belief and theological views are different in many ways than in the past. They are more diverse, for religious traditions have separated into many branches. In addition, the relation between theological and scientific understanding is more complex; even those who believe that divine causality stands behind the events of the world do not always see that relationship in a direct, unambiguous way. Thus, today, religions have reacted to this modern epidemic in a complex way. They have almost inevitably done so with some reference to the powerful beliefs of the past, but with the more subtle and nuanced interpretations of the present. Some denominations have closely followed what they believe is the proper, literal interpretation of the relationship between disease and Divine Providence. Other denominations, open to broader interpretation of texts and to limited historical modification of doctrine, have found room in their theological traditions for a more expanded view. Roman Catholicism, for example, which in the past preached vigorously the lesson of pestilence as God's punishment, has explicitly repudiated an interpretation of divine retribution in its pronouncements about the HIV/AIDS epidemic. One bishop (Clark, 1988) wrote: "There are some misguided individuals who have declared AIDS to be a punishment from God. Deep in the Judeo-Christian tradition, however, is the knowledge that our loving God does not punish through disease."

EARLY RESPONSE TO THE EPIDEMIC

Official and Unofficial Response of Clergy and Lay People

Between 1981 and 1983 the record shows no official response from religious denominations to the nascent AIDS epidemic. In those years, AIDS was perceived as a gay disease. Since homosexuality was generally disapproved by religious groups and gay life was lived largely outside the sphere of religious congregations, the advent of tragedy among gay people drew little attention—and none at the level of official recognition. It appears that for religious groups, as for journalists, AIDS, as it was to be known, was a gay story and, as such, need not, perhaps ought not, to be told (Bazell, 1983; Kinsella, 1989).

The official silence was broken in 1983. The National Council of Churches of Christ in the U.S.A. issued a resolution that took note of the incidence of AIDS among gay men and affirmed its commitment to advocate for lesbians and gay men as a preface to calling for increased funding for research and education (Melton, 1989:115-116). The Universal Fellowship of Metropolitan Community Churches, which has a predominantly gay membership, also spoke early. Its 1983 "Resolution on AIDS" committed the denomination to pastoral care and leadership, education, political activism, and social responsibility (Melton, 1989:154-155). The Roman Catholic Diocese of San Jose, California, appears to have issued the first statement by a Catholic church official recognizing the epidemic and its implications for ministry to gay men. "Guidelines for Pastoral Ministry to Homosexuals," issued in 1984, included the following message (quoted in Melton, 1989:2):

> Ministry to the sick, dying and bereaved requires special attention and sensitivity in this context because the misunderstanding and hostility surrounding homosexuality has been grievously aggravated by the uncertainty and fear surrounding Acquired Immune Deficiency Syndrome. Afflicted

individuals, their families and friends have a special claim on the ministry of the church.

The Union of American Hebrew Congregations (Reform Judaism) issued a statement on AIDS in 1985 calling for increased funding for research, education, and the prohibition of discrimination against people with AIDS (Melton, 1989:169-170). Except for the Roman Catholic church, these groups were generally tolerant and supportive of sexually active homosexual people.

These early statements were the exception. Most major religious bodies preserved official silence during the early 1980s. At the same time, those clergy and lay people who, in accord with the tradition of caring for the sick, were drawn into ministry to people touched by AIDS, developed their own approaches, applying teaching and talent to a new challenge and need. People in denominations with stringent doctrines against homosexuality often carried out their ministries under suspicion and constraints. Still, their creative responses would become a resource for the many resolutions, declarations, and position papers that emerged across the American religious landscape later in the decade.

In contrast to this official silence and quiet ministry, some clergy and television preachers revived in strong tones the ancient association between disease and God's judgment on sin. According to Melton (1989:xvii):

> [the notion that AIDS is divine retribution on sinful people] struck a responsive cord in many religious people, especially those with a conservative traditional theology who, having wrestled with the issues of homosexuality through the 1970s, had concluded that homosexuality was a sin and that all sin stood under the judgment of God.

The epidemic appeared at the height of the popularity of televangelism, and the public prominence of some of the preachers gave their sermons high visibility (Horsfield, 1984).

Moral judgments about high-risk behavior, particularly male same-gender sex, and fears of contagion seemed to dominate the public religious response during the first 5 or 6 years of the epidemic. Stories about people with AIDS who lost jobs, apartment homes, insurance coverage, friends, family, pastoral care, and medical services did not move religious institutions to compassion or advocacy in any measurable manner. Although these implicit judgments and attitudes were not universal within religious denominations, few counter voices were heard in a nation being swept by a conservative political and religious movement in which "moral behaviors" were promoted and portrayed as the sole solution to the spread of HIV disease.

The scientific uncertainty about HIV transmission became a reason to avoid contact with people known to be infected or thought to be at risk for infection. A Roman Catholic retreat center denied use of its facilities by a

Church of the Universal Fellowship of Metropolitan Community Churches unless other groups were informed that people with AIDS would be present. "What about the bathrooms?" the center coordinator asked (quoted in Cherry and Mitulski, 1988:86). Children with AIDS did not escape rejection and isolation. Schools and neighborhoods were closed to them and their families (Kirp et al., 1989). Members of a Florida church advocated the exclusion of several hemophiliac children with AIDS from public school and banned persons with HIV infection from their Sunday school and church services (*Florida Baptist Witness*, September 17, 1987; Sider, 1988). A respected minister was asked to resign his ministry because his wife and child were infected by transfusion; several churches even refused to admit his family for worship (Hilts, 1992). There was little enthusiasm within religious communities to befriend and defend this new class of social outcast, despite the moral instruction of their traditions.

Fear was a significant factor in the religious response to the epidemic in its early years, and the fear was not restricted to contagion, disease, and death. It extended to association and was exacerbated by attitudes and feelings about sexuality and behaviors unfamiliar in the milieu of most religious communities, such as intravenous drug use. Some highly visible Christian pastors used fear of contagion as a means to isolate people with AIDS and to justify a particular standard of sexual morality. For example, the Reverend Jerry Falwell, an independent Baptist minister, in a sermon titled "How Many Roads to Heaven?" delivered on his nationally televised "Old Time Gospel Hour" (May 10, 1987), stated that God was bringing an end to the sexual revolution through the AIDS epidemic. He also said: "They [gay men] are scared to walk near one of their own kind right now. And what we [preachers] have been unable to do with our preaching, a God who hates sin has stopped dead in its tracks by saying 'do it and die.' 'Do it and die.'" Falwell's political organization, Moral Majority, opposed governmentally funded research to find a cure for AIDS because the disease was a gay problem (*Christianity Today*, 1985; *U.S. News & World Report*, 1985). He promoted the idea that AIDS was not only God's judgment on gay men, but also that divine judgment extended to all of society: "AIDS is a lethal judgment of God on America for endorsing this vulgar, perverted and reprobate lifestyle" (Falwell, 1987:5). Strong condemnations of gay sexuality, as the cause of AIDS and God's vengeance, also appeared in some religious journals. One of them affirmed (Boys, 1987:44, 45):

God warned mankind about AIDS in Numbers 32:23 when He said, "Be sure your sin will find you out." . . . Maybe the AIDS plague will educate the world that the Bible is still the bedrock of civilization, and it should be learned, loved and lived in our daily lives.

It is impossible to measure the effect of these claims on the faithful, on others who grant more or less deference to religious authority, or on the people living with an HIV diagnosis and their loved ones. It can be surmised that at least some people who listened to the condemnatory message of the preachers were persuaded to see the epidemic as the direct result of the evil practices of those affected by HIV/AIDS (Palmer, 1989). The message may have fallen on predisposed minds and reinforced preexisting attitudes, but it had an undeniable appeal. It has been reported that an appeal on the Christian Broadcasting Network to write the Justice Department in opposition to any relaxation of the rule against immigration of HIV-infected persons elicited 40,000 letters (McCarthy, 1991).

A 1985 study of intolerance of AIDS victims interviewed 371 residents of "Middletown," asking among other questions their denominational preference, extent of church attendance, attitude toward literal interpretation of the Bible, and whether America has appreciated the contributions of Christian Fundamentalists (Johnson, 1987). In response to specific AIDS-related questions, 38 percent of the interviewees said schools should exclude children with AIDS, and 49 percent thought there should be a law prohibiting people with AIDS from jobs involving close contact with others. Analysis of the answers indicated that only "failure to recognize the contributions of Christian Fundamentalists" related significantly and independently to intolerance of persons with AIDS. The author noted other sociological studies that reveal the prevalence of negative attitudes toward homosexuals and surmised (Johnson, 1987:109):

> The Christian Right sees such people as secular humanists, abortionists and homosexuals, not only as deviants but their activities as being major causes of the breakdown in America's moral standards. Thus, homosexuals, and by association AIDS victims, may serve as scapegoats for conservative Fundamentalists, so that they might blame someone for the moral decay they see all around them.

This suggestion is given further empirical support by a series of studies showing that hostile attitudes toward gay men and lesbians are consistently and positively correlated with certain religious behaviors and attitudes, such as literal belief in the Bible and frequency of church attendance (Herek, 1984, 1987a,b, 1988).

A similar conclusion was reached by the Reverend Andrew Greeley, a sociologist at the University of Chicago's National Opinion Research Center (NORC), in an analysis of the 1988 General Social Survey data, which contained a battery of questions about AIDS and an extensive series of questions about religion (Davis and Smith, 1988). The AIDS items asked whether respondents would prohibit children with AIDS from attending public school, support government programs on safe sex, permit insurance companies to test for HIV, have government pay for AIDS health care, conduct mandatory premarital AIDS tests, require identification tags for persons with HIV, and make persons with AIDS eligible for disability benefits. The survey showed high favorable response on the questions that supported restrictive or repressive practices. Greeley (1991) correlated the responses with data about denominational affiliation, frequency of church attendance, and religious imagery. On one item, for example, Greeley found that 70 percent of Protestants in the sample favored identification tags for persons with HIV/AIDS, in contrast to 54 percent of Catholics. Much of this difference was concentrated among members of fundamentalist and conservative denominations—73 and 72 percent of their members, respectively, supported tags. Factoring out these groups, 61 percent of Protestants supported tags, a proportion not significantly different from that of Catholics. Further analyses suggested that the difference between fundamentalist and conservative Protestants and Catholics could be accounted for in terms of explicit beliefs about the Bible, early formal relationship to the church, and region of origin. Church attendance did not correlate with attitudes toward tags, but it did correlate negatively with attitudes toward sex education. Greeley then attempted an analysis to determine whether more supportive, compassionate responses were correlated with the images of God cultivated in the more liberal denominations, which led him to this conclusion (Greeley, 1991:12):

> The religious correlation with negative attitudes toward AIDS victims or AIDS education is the result of moral and religious narrowness among certain members of the more devout population . . . this finding establishes that it is not religion as such but a certain highly specific type of religious orientation which tends to induce hostility on the subject of AIDS. While this religious orientation represents a strong component of American culture and society (38 percent of Americans believe in the strict literal interpretation of the Bible), it is not a majority orientation; and even among fundamentalists the majority support AIDS education programs . . . . One would predict that the greatest resistance to attitudinal change . . . would come from those with rigid religious orientations and the highest likelihood of attitudinal change from those with the most gracious images of God.

The wide spectrum of theological positions on the epidemic among individual Americans is also shown in the work of Herek and Glunt (1991). Based on a telephone survey with a national probability sample of 1,078 English-speaking adults, they conceptualized AIDS-related attitudes on two principal psychological dimensions, pragmatism/moralism and coercion/compassion. The first dimension was tested with questions about responses to certain public health measures, such as distribution of condoms and clean needles. Those falling on the pragmatic side endorsed such policies, and those on the moralistic side rejected them as condoning conduct they considered immoral. The second dimension, coercion/compassion, contrasted

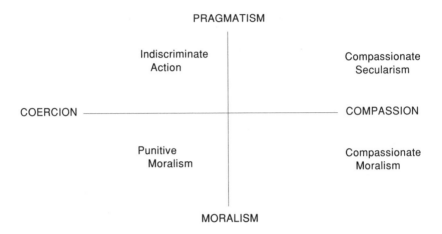

FIGURE 5-1   A Tentative Typology of AIDS-Related Attiudes. SOURCE: Herek and Glunt (1991:118).

approaches to HIV-infected persons. People with a coercive orientation viewed AIDS as punishment from God or nature, blamed individuals for being infected, and endorsed coercive measures, such as quarantine, to control the epidemic; people with a compassionate orientation tended to reject such views. On the basis of the results of this survey, the authors proposed a four-part typology for understanding AIDS-related attitudes (Figure 5-1).

Although Herek and Glunt's typology was developed to categorize the attitudes of individuals, it can be applied by analogy to the responses of religious organizations. On the first dimension, the official responses of religious institutions have generally stressed moralism over pragmatism. That is, they have tended to reject such policies as widespread distribution of condoms and sterile needles, and they have been unwilling to impart nonjudgmental information about techniques for safer sex. They have emphasized moral prohibitions against certain types of sexual expression (e.g., homosexuality) rather than practical strategies for avoiding infection while engaging in such sexual behavior. Thus, their responses do not fit in either the compassionate-secularism or indiscriminate-action quadrants of the typology.

Religious institutions have shown greater divergence on the coercion/ compassion dimension. As already described, Fundamentalist groups such as the Moral Majority have advocated punitive policies toward persons with AIDS and toward groups affected by the epidemic, such as gay men and lesbians. Herek and Glunt (1991) labeled this a pattern of punitive moralism. Other institutions, in contrast, have adopted a stance of compassionate moralism. The Catholic church, for example, has officially urged compassion for people with AIDS although it rejects education about condoms as promoting immoral behavior. The response of the nation's largest Protestant denomination, the Southern Baptist Convention, exemplifies the dimension of compassionate moralism. The denomination affirms the autonomy of local congregations and the integrity of an individual member's conscience, so any resolution passed during its annual meeting represents only the majority opinion of the delegates and is not binding on local churches. Still, it can be surmised that the majority opinion probably accurately portrays the attitudes of the majority of members in local congregations. In 1987 the Southern Baptist Convention passed a resolution (quoted in Melton, 1989:130) that did not call for any specific action by the denomination or by the government; rather, it sought to infuse the public discussion of the epidemic with "biblical standards of decency and morality." The resolution urged Christians to be compassionate in their contact with people affected by AIDS, and it expressed opposition to "safe sex" programs "which appear to accept infidelity, adultery, and perversion." Finally, the resolution stated that, "obedience to God's laws of chastity before marriage and faithfulness in marriage would be a major step toward curtailing the threat of AIDS."

Individual commentators from more conservative religious perspectives have stated positions that, while clearly falling within the moralism category, waver between punitive and compassionate moralism. Ronald Sider, for example, the executive director of Evangelicals for Social Action, repudiates the link between God's punishment for the sin of homosexuality and HIV/AIDS. He insists, however, that Christians must continue to view homosexuality as sinful. He writes (Sider, 1988:11-14): "There is no Biblical basis for linking specific sicknesses with kinds of sin. . . . Evangelicals should be able, however, to condemn homosexual practice as a sinful lifestyle without being charged with homophobia." He goes on to urge Evangelical Christians to provide ministry to people with AIDS, to educate and counsel, and to avoid intolerant acts toward those with HIV/AIDS. "If Christians offer compassionate, costly care to people with AIDS, they will . . . bring glory to God." At the same time, they must affirm their belief in God's law regarding sexuality. While deploring the "vicious" attacks by some conservative Christians on "fellow evangelical [then] Surgeon General C. Everett Koop," Sider stated that the promotion of condoms would encourage promiscuity.

Boys (1987), also an evangelical Christian, takes a much more punitive position than Sider, maintaining strongly that AIDS is clearly God's punishment for "sodomites." He inclines toward the compassionate dimension only once in a long article (Boys, 1987:52): "People of good will and Christians should not endorse 'gay bashing' . . . however, there is no doubt that such atrocities (and much worse) will continue to accelerate as greater numbers of innocent people die of AIDS."

As this brief sampling of opinion suggests, many persons with a religious commitment find themselves perplexed: they are caught between the traditional condemnation of same-gender sex and the traditional admonition to be compassionate toward those with a disease, in this instance one commonly contracted through same-gender sexual activity. Some religious people and institutions, grounded in a tradition and a psychology that fears sin above all, incline toward coercive, punitive moralism; others, without repudiating sin, respond more strongly to the call for compassion. Many others struggle to affirm both sides of the dilemma: they honestly condemn intolerance as well as sexual sin but exhort the faithful to concern and compassion. The fear of being perceived as "soft on sin" was and remains a barrier to more supportive care by some religious groups for people with HIV disease and to vigorous education on HIV risk prevention and reduction. It requires a difficult psychological and homiletic balancing act to follow the ancient maxim, "hate the sin and love the sinner."

Isolation of Homosexuals from Religious Communities

The early religious response to the epidemic occurred in the context of a virtual absence of gay people from the life of religious communities. Because of the common religious opposition to homosexual activity, most gay men and lesbians either did not participate in organized religious activities or, if they did, were careful not to be identified. As such, they were, and are generally, an unacknowledged presence in religious institutions. Other gay people who wanted to be open about their sexuality either aligned with the Universal Fellowship of Metropolitan Community Churches, joined the few mainline congregations that would accept them, or organized caucuses to seek standing and acceptance by their religious groups of preference: Dignity (Roman Catholic), Integrity (Episcopalian), Affirmation (Methodist), and similar groups. Some groups of this sort have been welcomed within the larger congregations; others have been repudiated. After the Congregation for the Doctrine of the Faith (1986) of the Vatican issued a strong reaffirmation of the traditional Catholic doctrine condemning homosexuality and ordered the hierarchy to sever relationships with groups that did not accept this position, Dignity responded by asserting the morality of same-gender physical sex (Dignity USA, 1989); in turn, many dioceses denied Dignity the use of church facilities (Ostling, Harris, and Witteman, 1988).

This situation allowed clergy and laity to assume that gay men at risk for HIV infection were not part of congregational life. With low visibility, congregations not only overlooked gay men and their spiritual needs, but also failed to consider that gay men had families who were active members of the congregations and who could be drawn into the HIV/AIDS epidemic through the diagnosis of a family member. The perception existed almost across the spectrum of religious groups that the HIV epidemic was somebody else's problem, beyond the walls of the sanctuary and of little immediate relevance to what goes on within the sanctuary.

This perception of insulation, together with notions of AIDS and divine retribution, contributed to the feeling within congregations that they would not be affected by the epidemic. The disease, according to this view, would run its course through the high-risk populations of gay men and intravenous drug users. Little attention was given to the prospect that people active in the daily life of the congregation, including the clergy, might be engaging in activities that would put them at risk for HIV infection. Furthermore, congregations are constantly invited by their pastors to be concerned about a variety of human needs and causes for social justice. Peace, hunger, homelessness, poverty, health care, education, joblessness, and other concerns vie for attention and compensatory action. AIDS was a new need joining an already overcrowded list. Other issues directly affected more people than did AIDS in the early 1980s. The immediacy of many of the other problems gave them an urgency and priority over the unknown scope of AIDS, despite the intensity of the suffering AIDS imposed on people and the unknown length of time that AIDS would remain a problem, given the hope for a cure. These considerations are particularly important in understanding the response of African American religious communities to the epidemic (discussed below). Many competing priorities—joined with a settled moral viewpoint and a reluctance to enter the world of people whose life-styles were perceived as different, distasteful, and dangerous—provided a convenient rationalization either for official neglect or for strident pulpit oratory.

In sum, the two viewpoints described above, one that held closely to the tradition that saw all epidemic disease as divine retribution for sin and one that represented the tension between that viewpoint and the religious imperative of compassion, seemed to dominate public discourse during the first phase of the epidemic. These positions, often broadcast by journalists, offered a platform and appearance of credibility to a conservative political administration in Washington. As a result, the impression was given to the public, and especially to gay people, that all religions were hostile toward those most at risk of infection and opposed to programs for research, education, prevention, and care. That impression was certainly justified by the words and actions of a portion of the religious community, but not by the majority of organizations and individuals with religious affiliations. The majority were rather silent during the first years of the epidemic: very few compassionate articles appeared in the religious press or in theological journals before 1985. With the few exceptions mentioned above, no official statements were issued until 1986.

A Changing Climate of Views and Actions

A few theologians began to prepare the way for official policy statements. They emphasized such religious themes as service, compassion for the poor and the sick, justice, mercy, and redemption in ways that deemphasized the condemnatory aspects of the traditions. One such early article, for example, made the following observation (Shelp and Sunderland, 1985:800):

> For the church to ignore the needs that cluster around AIDS, to fail to express itself redemptively, and to abandon a group of people who have almost no one to cry out in their behalf for justice and mercy, would constitute a failure in Christian discipleship.

In the next several years, many theologians stressed this point of view (Bohne, 1986; Stulz, 1986; Schaper, 1987; Evans, 1988; Green, 1988; Hale, 1988; McCormick, 1988; Spohn, 1988a,b; Street, 1988; Vaux, 1988; Wiest, 1988; Washofsky, 1989). Their themes, one can presume, influenced the words of the preachers, the policy statements of many denominations, and probably, the attitudes of congregations   The voices of the hierarchy were added to those of the theologians. Episcopal Bishop William E. Swing (Diocese of California) entered the public discourse about AIDS on January 18, 1986, with an open letter to the Reverend Charles Stanley, a well-known Fundamentalist Southern Baptist pastor and president of the Southern Baptist Convention. It was reported that Stanley had claimed in a speech that AIDS was created by God in order to express displeasure toward the nation's acceptance of homosexuality. Bishop Swing responded:

> When I read about Jesus Christ in Scriptures and try to understand something of the mind of God, I cannot identify even one occasion where he pictures his Father as occasionally becoming displeased and then hurling epidemics on nations. Especially in relation to sexual matters! Rather than hurling wrath when dealing with an adulteress, Jesus said, "Whoever is without sin, cast the first stone." . . . Thus I do not believe in the God who becomes displeased and decides to show his anger by murdering large numbers of people, or in this case homosexual people.

John R. Quinn, Roman Catholic archbishop of San Francisco, also offered a more compassionate view of the obligation of the Christian church (Quinn, 1986:505-506):

> The Christian—the church—must not contribute to breaking the spirit of the sick and weakening their faith by harshness. . . . The presence of the church must be a presence of hope and grace, of healing and reconciliation, of love and perseverance to the end . . . [AIDS] is a human disease. It affects everyone and it tests the quality of our faith and of our family and community relationships. Persons with AIDS and ARC are our brothers and sisters, members of our parishes . . . . As disciples of Jesus who

healed the sick and is Himself the compassion of God among us, we, too, must show our compassion to our brothers and sisters who are suffering.

These statements from two respected religious leaders, both of whom presided over churches in a city where the epidemic was most devastating, were telling. Cardinal Joseph Bernardin of Chicago spoke in the same vein in October 1986 (Congregation for the Doctrine of the Faith, 1986). In the spring of 1987, all of the Catholic bishops of California issued a pastoral letter reminding their faithful that all who suffer from AIDS should be treated with the same love shown by Jesus for the lame, lepers, the blind, and others he healed. They offered their support and fellowship to "members of the homosexual community, some of whom have been separated from the church and its spiritual life" (Bishops of California, 1987).

To words were joined actions. Individual hospital chaplains and congregation-based clergy who had somewhat quietly provided pastoral care to people with AIDS and their loved ones began to form interfaith groups to provide professional ministry to affected people. The testimony of these compassionate ministries contrasts with stories of rejection and condemnation. Some health care and social service agencies sponsored by religious groups participated in the care of people with AIDS as they could. During the middle 1980s, individual congregations began to offer organized and generally interfaith ministries of care. The first program that placed lay people as helpers in the homes of people with AIDS appears to have originated in Houston, Texas, during a divisive municipal political campaign in 1985 in which AIDS and homosexuality were issues. Teams of congregation-based, trained lay people provided home-based social, emotional, physical, and spiritual care to people with AIDS (Shelp, DuBose, and Sunderland, 1990; Sunderland and Shelp, 1990).

The middle years of the decade were a time in which supportive lay people and ordained clergy emerged from private, one-to-one contact to a public and organized response in several cities. In 1985 the Roman Catholic Archdiocese of New York opened a shelter for AIDS patients and a telephone line for information and referral (*New York Times*, 1985). In January 1986 Mother Theresa's order, the Missionaries of Charity, opened a hospice in New York City's Greenwich Village, and in the following year it opened others in Washington, D.C. and San Francisco (*Christian Century*, 1986). In the last half of 1986 in San Francisco, Holy Redeemer Catholic parish raised $500,000 to convert an unused convent into an AIDS hospice; Temple Emmanu-El raised $30,000 for hospital beds for AIDS patients; and the United Methodist Church developed counseling and support programs (Godges, 1986). Many other local activities also began (*Health Progress*, 1986). In early 1987 Cardinal Bernardin appointed a diocesan coordinator for AIDS ministry in Chicago, a post that was also created in San Francisco,

Washington, D.C., Los Angeles, Seattle, and many other Catholic dioceses. Gradually, denominations began to set up national offices to assist local efforts in sharing information, resources, and programs. The AIDS National Interfaith Network was organized in 1988 to perform this service and to foster a more extensive religious response to the epidemic. And a group of religious leaders meeting under the auspices of the Carter Center in Atlanta in December 1989 issued "The Atlanta Declaration," in which they affirmed the dedication of their respective churches and synagogues to "compassionate, non-judgmental care, respect, support and assistance" (AIDS National Interfaith Network, 1989:8). They also endorsed broad educational, preventive, research, and care programs.

OFFICIAL STATEMENTS AND LOCAL ACTIVITIES

The accumulating knowledge, experience, and concern described thus far provided a background for numerous official statements from religious bodies that appeared in increasing numbers in 1987 and 1988. It has become common in many denominations to issue occasional statements about matters of interest to both the denomination and the public. The status of the statements varies with the denominational structure, but in general they are intended to guide and inform adherents rather than to impose doctrines or duties. As public declarations, they influence religious agencies and administrators responsible for the implementation of programs. They also speak to people outside the denomination's membership in an effort to influence public policy, opinion, or legislation. Finally, they can be focal points for debate within and outside the denomination. It must be noted, however, that many denominations and religious organizations do not speak in this way; rather, they leave such matters to individuals and local congregations (Melton, 1989:ix).

Statements about HIV/AIDS can generally be best understood if they are viewed in the context of the discussions about homosexuality that have taken place within many of the denominations. Conservative denominations remained outside that debate, standing squarely on the biblical texts, which they take to be clear condemnations of same-gender sex. The Southern Baptist Convention, for example, judges homosexuality an abomination. Gay men and lesbians are expected to change their sexual orientation or remain celibate as a condition for membership. Certain liberal denominations, such as Reform Judaism, the United Church of Christ, and the Unitarian Church, passed beyond the debate and opened pastoral ministry to all people, including homosexuals. Many major denominations in the middle of the liberal-conservative spectrum, however, struggled to reconcile the traditional condemnation of homosexuality with the universal call to fellowship. Vigorous debates have attended proposals that gay persons be admitted to the sacraments or ordained to the clergy. Many of the major denominations had gay caucuses, which articulated their concerns and advocated their interpretation of the relationship between sexuality and historic religious beliefs. A report of a committee of the Presbyterian Church, USA, for example, recommended that gay and lesbian people be eligible for ordination whether or not they are celibate, but the report was rejected in April 1991 by the national synod of the church. A report of a similar study group of the Episcopal church recommended that the decision to ordain be left to each diocese, on consideration of the merits of the candidates (Steinfels, 1991); this proposal suggests a departure from the rule that denies ordination to noncelibate gay and lesbian people. The Roman Catholic church, the Eastern Orthodox church, and the United Methodists and most other Protestant denominations remain opposed to ordination of noncelibate gay and lesbian people.

While doctrinal positions on same-gender sex strongly influence denominational positions on AIDS, the other major risk behavior, intravenous drug use, is not a matter of debate. It is not often mentioned in religious statements and, when it is, it is simply assumed to be a moral evil, harmful to individuals and to society. There has been no debate about this conclusion. Intravenous drug use is seen as a contemporary instance of the ancient vice of intemperance, and religious organizations generally deal with drug users as individuals, not as an organized community that promotes a social or political agenda. Intemperate individuals, from a religious standpoint, can repent and abstain from the offending behavior. The "cure" for intemperance is personal, not corporate. Moreover, people who use intravenous or other drugs generally do not agitate for social change or recognition, in contrast to gay men and lesbians who speak and act as a community and challenge the social order and the religious sanctions attached to it. These differences may explain, in part, the greater attention given to sexual behaviors than to drug-use behaviors in denominational statements.

Almost without exception, the denominational resolutions and statements, in contrast to highly publicized statements by popular preachers, do not affirm the claim that AIDS is God's punishment on gay men. Rather, they treat the epidemic as a human problem and provide factual information. Moreover, their theological content tends to focus on the opportunity the crisis presents for compassion, care, and education about morality and risk avoidance and reduction, as well as the protection of the civil rights of infected individuals.

The official statements mark a culmination of the initial learning process of major religious groups as the facts, fears, and issues associated with a new epidemic were sorted out. Moral and theological perspectives were formulated with respect to high-risk behaviors (particularly sexual) and obligations to minister to people who are sick, dying, or bereaved. With national organizations officially recognizing and speaking about AIDS, local congregations, denominational agencies, and individuals were validated in their existing compassionate ministries and approved to create ministries of education, care, and advocacy where none existed.

Clearly, local congregations are closest to people facing AIDS on a personal level. The response to the epidemic of religious groups at this level would appear to have the greatest impact, in terms of care and prevention. Activity at this level in certain locations "filtered up" during the early years of the epidemic to inform and help shape national statements and AIDS-related program commitments. It is equally reasonable to expect that time will be required for these proclamations and programs to "filter down." The relative slowness with which the process occurs in either direction dismays people who want a more vigorous and extensive compassionate response. In addition, congregations and agencies at local levels are free, according to the governing rules of many if not most groups, to set their own priorities and implement their own programs. Authorization at a national level does not necessarily result in activity at a local level. Still, the authoritative voice of major denominations, speaking clearly and at a national level, has presumably had a real effect on their local congregations. The remainder of this section summarizes, in alphabetical order, the official statements of some major U.S. religious groups and then offers some examples of local congregational activities.

African American Churches

African American churches and religious leaders are powerful influences in their communities. Hence, involvement of the clergy and their congregations would be important for HIV prevention and support services. Like other national religious bodies, these churches with exclusively or predominantly African American membership tended to be officially silent during the early years of the epidemic. African American religious congregations, however, appeared to give the epidemic lower priority than other urgent problems besetting their predominately urban communities, such as unemployment, crime, family disintegration, discrimination, and drugs (Lambert, 1989). Part of their reluctance to address the epidemic was explained by Angela Mitchell (1990:32):

> AIDS is still considered by many to be a gay white man's disease, and most blacks with AIDS in this country are intravenous drug users (or their sex partners) and homosexuals—people whose existence many of us would rather deny. Moreover, if the black community were to embrace AIDS as our problem, we would all become associated with a disease many think is divine retribution for sexual immorality; a disease sufferers "bring on themselves" by "doing things they shouldn't have been doing anyway"; a disease of the

morally bankrupt, sexually deviant, promiscuous, hedonistic and drug affected—all stereotypes deserving our rejection.

Moreover, it has been assumed that the doctrinal fundamentalism and the social conservatism often characteristic of African American Christianity is an obstacle to acknowledgment of the epidemic. Dalton, however, does not consider the Fundamentalist doctrine or social conservatism of black churches an insurmountable obstacle to their participation in the national response to the epidemic (Dalton, 1989:211):

> these characteristics . . . are constraints not so much on what can be done in the realm of social action as on how to do it. In practice, the church has proved adaptable, pragmatic, and even crafty when need be . . . if you want to understand the black church, watch what it does, not what it says. Time and again, the church has demonstrated its awareness of the variability of human existence and the fragility of the soul under siege. Time and again, the church has been responsive to the needs, spiritual and nonspiritual, of the community.

During the end of the 1980s, some black religious leaders and congregations publicly acknowledged the threat of the HIV/AIDS epidemic and began to develop educational and compassionate responses. The full extent and content of those activities are difficult to document, however, because most are locally organized and responsive to local conditions.

In February 1988 the National Black Church Consortium on Critical Health Care Needs was convened to address and develop "strategies to confront the AIDS crisis in the Black Community." The consortium consists of representatives of many black religious denominations, including the National Baptist Convention U.S.A. (5.5 million members), National Baptist Convention of America (2.7 million), and the African Methodist Episcopal Church (2.2 million). Recognizing that African Americans are disproportionately affected by AIDS—12 percent of the nation's population but 29 percent of cumulative AIDS cases reported through December 1991 (Centers for Disease Control, 1992)—the consortium's statement agreed that churches could be silent no longer. Acting in their historical role of conscience for their communities, the denominations resolved "to call upon all members of Black Churches, nationwide to mobilize an immediate response to this epidemic which threatens the very existence of our community" (National Black Consortium on Critical Health Needs, 1988).

Church of Jesus Christ of Latter-Day Saints

The Church of Jesus Christ of Latter-Day Saints, the Mormon church, is not numerically a major denomination, but it has significant influence, particularly in the western United States. In a press release, the Office of the First Presidency has urged members to be compassionate toward people with AIDS, "particularly, those who have received the virus through blood transfusions, babies afflicted from infected others, and innocent marriage partners who have been infected by a spouse." The church's message of prevention recalls "time-honored revelations from God, including the principle of chastity before marriage, total fidelity in marriage, and abstinence from all homosexual behavior" (Church of Jesus Christ of Latter-Day Saints, 1988).

Evangelical Lutheran Church

The Evangelical Lutheran Church in America has a membership of approximately 5.3 million. The denomination's Church Council issued a message of concern regarding AIDS in November 1988, urging members to support and participate in ministry to people suffering as a consequence of AIDS. The statement made no specific mention of homosexuality or intravenous drug use. However, an awareness that judgments about those behaviors might affect the church's response is implied in the theological basis for the call to service (quoted in Melton, 1989:86):

> The church's ministry of caring is a grateful response to God's caring for us. The undeserved love of God announced for all in the Gospel of Jesus Christ is our reason for standing with our neighbor in need. Jesus responded graciously to persons who were sick without assessing their merit. In the same way we are called to "be Christs" for all in our midst who suffer and are ill. Our calling summons us to compassion for, acceptance of and service with people affected by AIDS both within and outside of our congregations.

Various program units within the denomination have developed print and video resources for use by pastors and congregations for education and assistance in providing ministry to people touched by HIV/AIDS. Directories of specialized services have been created and revised. The church has incorporated concerns about HIV/AIDS into existing programs and agencies, as well as creating a national steering committee on AIDS and task forces at lower administrative levels and a planned synodical network to share information, resources, and activities.

Adele Stiles Resmer, assistant executive director of the church's Division for Social Ministry Organizations, reports that the HIV epidemic has had a minimal impact of the church's national structure (personal communication, 1990). The real impact, in her opinion, has been at the local or congregational level, especially in areas where the AIDS caseload is very high. The presence of people with disease who are seeking ministry seems to be necessary to move a congregation or pastor beyond intellectual awareness to actual engagement.

Judaism

Reform Judaism did not participate in the debate about AIDS as a punishment from God. The theological and moral issue for the denomination was the Jewish tradition's obligation to offer healing and comfort to the sick (Melton, 1989). Conservative Judaism agreed in 1987, calling for a compassionate response to people with AIDS, including visitation and care (Melton, 1989). Respected Orthodox rabbis have emphasized healing as the biblically mandated human response to AIDS (Freundel, 1986-87). Although AIDS is not regarded as punishment, it is seen in Orthodox Judaism as "a consequence of a form of life that is morally unacceptable" (Jakobovits, 1987:22). Nevertheless, in 1988 the Union of Orthodox Jewish Congregations of America called for increased funding and research to combat AIDS (Orthodox Union, 1988).

Presbyterian Church, U.S.A.

The Presbyterian Church, U.S.A. has a membership of nearly 3 million. Its General Assembly, the highest governing body of the church, adopted a "Resolution on Acquired Immune Deficiency Syndrome" in 1986, in which it declared that AIDS is an illness, "not punishment for behavior deemed immoral." It called Presbyterians to prayer for healing and congregations to nonjudgmental ministry.

The denomination promoted the provision of factual information about AIDS and required that people be protected from discrimination. AIDS-related activity at the denominational level is located in the ministry unit of the social justice and peacemaking program. Two consultants funded for 15 days a year work with a full-time person with a 10 percent time commitment to provide models of AIDS-related ministries and consciousness raising. Conferences for representatives of synods (intermediate organizational level) introduce examples of local church and institutional ministry. The expectation is that activities will be initiated within the synod following the conferences. Interest in AIDS-related ministries by pastors and other church leaders seems to be growing as more congregations and neighborhoods are affected by the epidemic. In addition, an information, referral, and resource registry, the Presbyterian AIDS Network, was created, and in 1990 the General Assembly mandated that AIDS educational material for youths be created and used in congregations.

Dave Zuverink, the church's associate for human services, reports that compassion for people with AIDS is increasing among Presbyterians (personal communication, 1990). The association of HIV infection with male homosexuality has tended, in his opinion, to polarize existing sentiment (against or tolerant) regarding homosexuality, however. Furthermore, he suggests that compassion for drug users may increase if the perception of this behavior as a disease grows.

Roman Catholic Church

The story of the efforts of the Roman Catholic hierarchy to formulate a statement on the HIV/AIDS epidemic is complex. In the summer of 1987 a number of Roman Catholic bishops suggested to their national organization, the U.S. Catholic Conference, that a position paper on AIDS be prepared. An ad hoc committee of the conference, with Cardinal Bernardin of Chicago as chair, drafted a document that recognized the devastating nature of the epidemic and its impact on those who contracted the disease, and it endorsed in clear, theologically supported terms the obligation of Catholics to care for those who suffered from AIDS and to avoid discrimination against the infected. The document also addressed the problem of prevention quite specifically. In the context of general Catholic teaching about sexuality, it recommended abstention from sexual relations as the primary preventive measure. It also acknowledged, however, that not all persons would observe this moral injunction and, thus, that in educational programs about prevention, the mention of condoms could be tolerated. This position was justified by reference to a traditional doctrine of moral theology—the toleration of a lesser evil in order to prevent a greater evil. The document, "The Many Faces of AIDS," was adopted by the Administrative Board of the conference in December 1987 (U.S. Catholic Conference Administrative Board, 1987; Place, 1988).

Certain leading figures of the Roman Catholic hierarchy not involved in drafting the document were severely critical of it. In addition, Cardinal Ratzinger, prefect of the Vatican Congregation for the Doctrine of the Faith, sent a letter to the American bishops in which he affirmed "unequivocal witness of effective and unreserved solidarity with those who are suffering" and insisted on "witness of defense of the dignity of human sexuality which can only be realized within the context of moral law" (quoted in Tonucci, 1988:117-118). He criticized "compromises which may even give the impression of trying to condone practices which are immoral, for example, technical instructions in the use of prophylactic devices."

In June 1988 the entire membership of the U.S. Catholic Conference (1989) issued a second statement on AIDS, "Called to Compassion and Responsibility: A Response to the HIV/AIDS Crisis," which reiterated the obligation to care for persons with HIV/AIDS without discrimination. It urged abstention as the sole mode of prevention and criticized safe sex as contrary to the ideals of true human sexuality, and it mentioned condoms only to assert their unreliability as a preventive measure. It did not, however, explicitly refer to, nor repudiate, the position of the earlier document.

Thus, at this writing, Catholic teaching on AIDS takes official form in two documents: one permits education about condoms and the other affirms abstinence as the sole mode of prevention but does not explicitly condemn education about condoms.

A long-standing tradition in Catholic moral theology allows individuals freedom of conscience in moral matters when solid theological and moral authority supports alternative positions. Thus, some Catholic educators accept the more liberal position of "Many Faces of AIDS"; others follow the more conservative position that is suggested, though not explicitly mentioned, in "Called to Compassion" (Reverend Michael Place, research theologian, Archdiocese of Chicago, personal communication, 1991). One priest, who is in a leadership position in AIDS education, stated (Reverend Rodney J. De Martini, director of AIDS education, Archdiocese of San Francisco, personal communication, 1990): "Both are operative documents, but in order to be honest educators and counsellors, we must mention not only the moral issues but the relevant scientific and medical facts. Among these is the relative efficacy of condoms." The *Teacher's Manual for AIDS: A Catholic Educational Approach*, issued by the National Catholic Educational Association (1988), provides a plan for wide-ranging and frank discussion of HIV/AIDS, in the course of which it states: "Basically, research is showing that, while condoms may provide some barrier to AIDS infection, they are often unreliable" (p. 130). *AIDS: Ethical Guidelines for Healthcare Providers*, issued by the Catholic Health Association of the United States in a second, revised edition of 1989, speaks of condom education in almost the exact phrases of "Many Faces of AIDS," but in the spirit of "Called to Compassion," notes their unreliability (p. 12).

Pronouncements of the U.S. Catholic Conference have moral authority but are not binding on individual bishops. Thus, dioceses headed by conservative bishops may enforce the more conservative position on AIDS education. This has happened, for instance, in the Archdiocese of New York, where Archbishop O'Connor has insisted that AIDS services within the church's jurisdiction refrain from distributing condoms and from education about safe-sex reproductive behavior in any way that violates the church's doctrines. In other dioceses, such as Cleveland, the bishop has authorized the more liberal approach taken in "Many Faces of AIDS." After emphasizing the church's doctrine on extramarital sexuality, the guidelines recommend that those who disagree with the church's position may be informed that public health advice includes condoms as prevention against AIDS (Spohn, 1988b:108).

United Methodist Church

The United Methodist Church is the second largest Protestant denomination in the United States with a membership of about 9 million. The denomination has a history of social activism. Its statement, "AIDS and the Healing Ministry of the Church," adopted in 1988, sets forth an extensive agenda for service, education, and support activity within the church and public advocacy for resources, protection of human and civil rights, education beginning at the elementary school level, and support for policies that permit people with AIDS to work to the greatest extent possible (reprinted in Melton, 1989:148-151). The church's Council of Bishops also spoke in 1988 to the church's members and beyond. The bishops stated that they "are certain that it [HIV] is not sent as a curse from God upon those whose life style is called into question." Furthermore, they cautioned against associating the epidemic with gay men (Council of Bishops, 1988):

> There is almost no category of the human family where the deadly virus does or has not appeared. Therefore, it is the better part of wisdom not to categorize the disease as only that of a certain element or group in the society. To do so will only delude us into believing that it is "their" problem not ours. Nothing could be further from the truth and nothing will more hamper responsible efforts to arrest and hopefully one day control this disease. It is our problem.

All people are called to "engage in behavior that can prevent and/or minimize the spread of Acquired Immune Deficiency Syndrome."

The church's teaching was restated by the bishops: heterosexual, monogamous sexual relations within marriage is the standard expected of United Methodists, and the practice of homosexuality is not condoned and is considered incompatible with Christian teaching. For people unable or unwilling to follow this standard, use of condoms is urged, as is avoiding intravenous drugs and needle sharing. The bishops' statement concluded by calling for the denomination at all levels and individuals to compassionate ministry, education, and public advocacy (Council of Bishops, 1988).

The denomination has created an interagency task force on AIDS to provide a coordinated and conscientious approach to the epidemic and to develop AIDS-related resources. In addition, an AIDS Ministries Network has been created to list resources, provide information and examples of ministry, and give voice to people with HIV infection. The denomination has begun to incorporate the special human needs and educational challenges raised by the epidemic within its multifaceted mission. The pace and extent to which this occurs are affected, however, by the fact that the church's agencies are controlled by local boards whose thinking often reflects the local values and cultural mores, conservative or liberal. Although it is doubtful that the epidemic will effect a change in the church's teaching regarding risk behaviors, there appears to be some moderation of attitudes "when AIDS comes home" in the person of a family member or friend (Cathie Lyons, associate general secretary, Health and Welfare Ministries, General Board of Global Ministries, United Methodist Church, personal communication, 1990).

Activities in Local Congregations

As official statements were being formulated at the national level of various denominations, more members of religious congregations became willing to discuss how the epidemic was reaching into their homes and within the walls of their sanctuaries. As members disclosed how AIDS was affecting them and called on their congregations for care and support, the magnitude of the epidemic became more difficult to deny, and harsh judgments tended to wane when the person infected or the family affected was loved or respected. Congregations and their leaders, thus, had to decide how to respond to the needs generated by an individual AIDS diagnosis (Amos, 1988). Some congregations have elected to say and do nothing, effectively denying the epidemic and the people affected by it. Others have responded to AIDS as they would to any other life-threatening disease and taken care of their own. Still others have developed specialized ministries and programs, often in cooperation with secular service agencies and on an interfaith basis, directed to members and nonmembers alike. By January 3, 1989, the *Washington Post* could run an article headlined, "AIDS Epidemic Is Slowly Gaining Attention in Local Pulpits" (Stepp, 1989).

The Second Presbyterian Church in Kansas City, Missouri, provides an example of local AIDS activities. The church organized an AIDS Ministry Group following a weekend seminar in the fall of 1989. Some members volunteer at secular AIDS agencies. Others make quilts for AIDS patients at a local hospice and collect materials for a quilt to be made by state prisoners to honor other prisoners who have died. The group educates the full congregation about the disease and how it should respond. It also helped a local nursing home establish an AIDS wing (William Tammeus, Elder, Second Presbyterian Church, Kansas City, Missouri, personal communication, 1990).

In Seattle, volunteer Catholic religious and lay persons created the Catholic AIDS Spiritual Ministry, a team of people trained to give spiritual assistance to individuals with AIDS. The group occupies office space in a parish and is funded by Dignity. Although it receives no financial support from the archdiocese, it is, says its director, "supported in spirit" (*Health Progress*, 1986:61).

Glide Memorial Church in San Francisco, led by a prominent African American pastor, has initiated AIDS projects to provide education, individual counseling, support groups, and buddy programs, in addition to spiritual ministries (Mitchell, 1990:40). Throughout the country, other congregations have started support groups, joined with other congregations to field teams of volunteers to help people in their homes, financially supported people with AIDS and AIDS-related community-based organizations, and engaged in other special activities.

In several cities, the African American religious community has formed alliances with the health department in order to educate a large number of people and to stimulate a compassionate response to people with AIDS from religious leaders (Jennings, 1989). In Philadelphia, the city gave Blacks Educating Blacks about Sexual Health Issues (BEBASHI)—an organization founded by Rashidah Hassan, a Muslim nurse—$100,000 for education on sexually transmitted diseases, including HIV. During 1985 BEBASHI distributed up to 20,000 condoms a month. African American clergy appear visibly in the fight against AIDS, according to Hassan, when they conduct the funeral of a person with AIDS and minister to the surviving family (Eisenstadt, 1988).

It would be a mistake, however, to conclude that these sorts of responses at the congregational level are typical. Only a small fraction of congregations have chosen to make special commitments to serving people with AIDS, even though sanctioned to do so by their national organizations. But these social ministries, relatively few as they are, are significant because they generally involve lay people on an organized basis. Ministries of visitation, sacrament, prayer, and worship characteristically are offered to anyone suffering illness, but in many denominations, these ministries have traditionally belonged to ordained clergy and other professional church workers. Hospital chaplains, individual clergy, and others have provided these traditional services to people with HIV/AIDS from the beginning of the epidemic (Eisenstadt, 1988), and more clergy have been drawn to these ministries as the cumulative AIDS caseload has grown. Lay people, on the other hand, are not under the strict regimen of church authorities. They generally are free to select where and how to commit themselves in ministry. As such, the mobilization of lay people on an organized basis signals an important event: their appearance in direct compassionate ministries suggests that congregations on a broader scale have experienced the epidemic and begun to have a compassionate response to those who are affected by the epidemic. As Elizabeth Eisenstadt (1988:78) observed regarding the religious response in Philadelphia:

> Lay people have often been the spur for AIDS ministries; most couldn't be done without them. So often, clergy feel that they need to educate their flocks. More often than not, it's the sheep who turn around and push the shepherd back into the road.

Given the size and the organizational strength of the Roman Catholic church, its participation in AIDS activities is important. Relatively little empirical research has been done, however, on the response of pastors and local congregations to the epidemic and the official pronouncements of the hierarchy. One study consists of a number of interviews with Catholic clergy and educators in the Los Angeles archdiocese, the largest in the United States. The author, after describing the various discussions and documents of the hierarchy, states (Horrigan, 1988:88): "While the Church is still debating what to say, its lower echelons have already plunged into action. According to Church officials, there are an estimated three million Catholics in the Archdiocese of Los Angeles—about fifty percent with Spanish surnames." The action consisted of a broad and programmed approach in three realms: spiritual support, practical care, and educational outreach. In 1986 Archbishop Mahoney established the Office of Pastoral Ministry to Persons with AIDS and commissioned 40 priests to this ministry. According to Horrigan, although spiritual support flourishes, educational efforts are limited in scope and in content, particularly with regard to condoms. However, priests and nuns engaged in educational works often express a willingness to collaborate with others not under direct church authority in providing the full scope of education about prevention. Despite these activities, the major segment of the Catholic population that is at risk, the Latino community, is largely unserved. Clergy and AIDS educators alike state that they would hope to see the significant organizational power of the church brought to bear in that community, but there is reluctance to do so, motivated by many reasons, including the desire not to stigmatize that population. Horrigan's study appears to be the only sociological inquiry into the actual response of Catholics at the level of social services and education.

Despite the controversy concerning condoms, both U.S. Catholic Conference documents and several other pastoral statements stress the social responsibility of the Catholic church in caring for those afflicted with HIV/AIDS. In response, Catholic health care facilities and service organizations have expanded existing programs and created new services aimed at helping HIV/AIDS patients and their families. In *AIDS: Ethical Guidelines for Healthcare Providers* (Catholic Health Association of the United States, 1989:8), health care institutions are urged "to develop clear, coherent policies based on the principle of justice to guide them in their responsibilities to patients and employees, and toward preventing the spread of HIV." Thus, most policy efforts in Catholic health care institutions have been directed at promoting infection control and dealing with personnel who refuse to care for patients with AIDS and with employees who test positive for HIV or who have AIDS. According to Dennis P. Andrulis, president of the National Public Health and Hospital Institute, the experience of Catholic hospitals in caring for AIDS patients has paralleled that of other private hospitals in the United States (Catholic Health Association of the United States, 1990:1,5). Catholic hospitals in the Northeast have felt the greatest impact from the AIDS crisis because of the large number of AIDS patients in the region.

A 1988 survey by the national office of Catholic Charities reported that many Catholic charities had converted existing programs to respond to the HIV/AIDS epidemic. Such programs and services include education and prevention programs, drug treatment programs, housing, legal services (advocacy for people with AIDS), financial assistance, information and referral services, hospice and home health care, psychological and emotional support for patients and family members, meals and groceries, and transportation (Lightbourne, 1989). An annual survey by Catholic Charities showed that AIDS health clinics and hospices were among the top three areas to receive attention from agencies in 1989; AIDS advocacy ranked second in social action activities. Several agencies reported the development of new programs in AIDS education and prevention during 1989.

It seems fair to say that the Roman Catholic church's vast network of health care and social services agencies have made notable efforts to provide assistance to persons with HIV disease or AIDS. This has been done despite a deeply ingrained doctrinal, and sometimes personal, antipathy to homosexual behavior and life-style. One Catholic official commented (personal communication, Don Hardiman, public affairs officer, AIDS/ARC Services, Catholic Charities of San Francisco, 1990) that the biggest impact is that AIDS has caused the church to consider people who don't sit in the front pew or don't sit in the pews at all; those who even though they might be Catholics, have been ignored and often disdained, such as gay persons and drug users.

CONCLUSIONS

The response of American religion to the AIDS epidemic has been notable and nuanced. It has been notable because, on the whole, it has followed the religious imperative to provide compassionate care and has repudiated discrimination. It has been nuanced because, in following that imperative, many religious denominations have had to accommodate the tradition of an epidemic as divine visitation on sin, as well as traditional doctrinal teachings on sexuality.

The response of U.S. religious organizations to AIDS must be seen as mixed, as is to be expected, given the diversity of religion in America. Two broad patterns can be discerned, however, and should be taken into account in the 1990s. In the first pattern, religious groups are a "restrained" ally in the fight against the epidemic; this is seen in those churches that have declared the imperative of compassion as the most suitable religious response. Taken seriously by the faithful, this response has mobilized considerable personal and institutional energies in the work of care. At the same time, many of these religious institutions have doctrinal commitments that, to a greater or lesser extent, restrain their involvement, particularly in education and prevention. These doctrinal commitments, primarily teachings about homosexuality, sexual relations outside marriage, and contraception, may mute the response of even those religious groups that are viewed as allies.

The second broad pattern can be seen among those religious groups in which doctrinal commitments, usually about sexuality, are so strong as to prevent the faithful from engaging in an active program of compassionate care. These groups continue a stance of condemnation of the causes of infection and, in so doing, contribute to what they consider the most, and only morally, effective message about prevention, namely, sexual restraint and abstinence from addictive substances.

It would be a mistake for policy makers to fail to enlist the support of religious groups of the first sort in the fight against the epidemic. Even with their constraints, many can contribute significant energies and resources. At the same time, any alliances that can be formed must be entered with a clear awareness of the limits imposed by traditional doctrinal positions and communal attitudes. It would also be a mistake for policy makers to assume that the second form of response represents the uniform and universal response of religious groups. The formulation of policies for HIV/AIDS care, research, education, and prevention should be sensitive to the diversity of the response to the epidemic by the U.S. religious community.

REFERENCES

Adams, J. du Q. (1981) John Boswell, Christianity, social tolerance, and homosexuality. *Speculum* 56:350-355.

AIDS National Interfaith Network (1989) *We Are Living with AIDS: An Interfaith Call to Hope and Action* (The Atlanta Declaration). New York: AIDS National Interfaith Network.

Amos, Jr., W.E. (1988) *When AIDS Comes to Church*. Philadelphia, Pa.: Westminster Press.

Bazell, R. (1983) The history of an epidemic. *New Republic* August 1:14-18.

Berger, P. (1967) *The Sacred Canopy: Elements of a Sociological Theory of Religion*. Garden City, N.Y.: Doubleday.

Bertholet, A. (1934) Religion. In *Encyclopedia of Social Sciences*. New York: Macmillan.

Bishops of California (1987) A pastoral letter on AIDS. *Origins* (NC Documentary Service) 16:786-789.

Bohne, J. (1986) AIDS: ministry issues for chaplains. *Pastoral Psychology* 32:173-192.

Boswell, J. (1980) *Christianity, Social Tolerance and Homosexuality*. Chicago: University of Chicago Press.

Boys, D. (1987) AIDS: reason for responsible anger. *The Evangelist* December:44-55.

Brandt, A. (1987) *No Magic Bullet: A Social History of Venereal Diseases in the United States from 1880*, expanded ed. New York: Oxford University Press.

Brundage, J. (1987) *Law, Sex and Christian Society in Medieval Europe.* Chicago: University of Chicago Press.

Butler, J. (1990) *Awash in a Sea of Faith: Christianizing the American People.* Cambridge, Mass.: Harvard University Press.

Catholic Health Association of the United States (1989) *AIDS: Ethical Guidelines for Healthcare Providers.* St. Louis, Mo.: Catholic Health Association of the United States.

Catholic Health Association of the United States (1990) Catholic experience in caring for PWA's matches that of other private hospitals. *Catholic Health World* 6(20):October 15.

Centers for Disease Control (CDC) (1990) Developing national partnerships for HIV and AIDS education. *CDC HIV/AIDS Prevention 1* December: 10-11, 14.

Centers for Disease Control (CDC) (1992) *HIV/AIDS Surveillance Report.* Atlanta, Ga.: Centers for Disease Control.

Cherry, K., and J. Mitulski (1988) We are the Church alive, the Church with AIDS. *Christian Century* 05:85-88.

Christian Century (1986) Help for AIDS victims. *Christian Century* February 26:201.

Christian Century (1990) Record commitment. *Christian Century* October 10:896.

Christianity Today (1985) The church's response to AIDS. *Christianity Today* 29(Nov. 22):50-52.

Church of Jesus Christ of Latter-Day Saints (1988) First Presidency Statement on AIDS. Press release. Salt Lake City, Utah, May 27.

Clark, M. (1988) Pastoral Instruction on the AIDS Crisis. New York, Diocese of Rochester, February 29.

Clebsch, W.A. (1968) *From Sacred to Profane: The Role of Religion in American History.* New York: Harper & Row.

Congregation for the Doctrine of the Faith (1986) The pastoral care of homosexual persons. Letter to the world's Bishops from Cardinal Joseph Ratzinger. *Origins* (NC Documentary Service) 16:377, 379-382.

Council of Bishops (1988) Unpublished document, Secretary, Council of Bishops, United Methodist Church, San Francisco, April 18.

Dalton, H.L. (1989) AIDS in blackface. *Daedalus* 118:205-227.

Davis, J., and T. Smith (1988) *General Social Surveys 1972-1988: Cumulative Codebook.* Chicago: National Opinion Research Center.

Dignity USA (1989) Statement of Position and Purpose. Dignity USA, San Francisco.

Douglass, H.P., and E. Brunner (1935) *The Protestant Church as a Social Institution.* New York: Russell and Russell.

Duffy, J. (1968) *A History of Public Health in New York, 1625-1866.* New York: Russell Sage Foundation.

Eisenstadt, E. (1988) *AIDS and Religion: The Philadelphia Response.* Philadelphia, Pa.: The Philadelphia Commission on AIDS.

Evans, A. (1988) Bearing one another's burdens. *Religious Education* 83:170-187.

Falwell, J. (1987) AIDS: the judgment of God. *Liberty Report* April 5.

Freundel, B. (1986-87) AIDS: a traditional response. *Jewish Action* Winter:48-57.

Gallup Organization (1985) *Gallup Report* May 23:39-56.

Gasquet, F.A. (1893) *The Great Pestilence.* London: Simpkin, Marshall, Hamilton, Kent and Co.

Godges, J. (1986) Religious groups meet SF AIDS challenge. *Christian Century* September 10:771-775.

Goldman, A.L. (1991) Portrait of religion in U.S. holds dozens of surprises. *New York Times* April 10:A1.

Greeley, A. (1991) *Religion and Attitudes Toward AIDS Policy.* Chicago: National Opinion Research Center.

Green, R. (1988) The perspective of Jewish teaching. *Religious Education* 83:221-229.

Hale, J.P. (1988) The Bishops blunder. *America* 6:156-171.

Health Progress (1986) AIDS: responding to the crisis. *Health Progress* (special section) 67.

Herek, G.M. (1984) Beyond "homophobia": a social psychological perspective on attitudes toward lesbians and gay men. *Journal of Homosexuality* 10:1-21.

Herek, G.M. (1987a) Can functions be measured? A new perspective of functional approach to attitudes. *Social Psychology Quarterly* 50:285-303.

Herek, G.M. (1987b) Religious orientation and prejudice: a comparison of racial and sexual attitudes. *Personality and Social Psychology Bulletin* 13:34-44.

Herek, G.M. (1988) Heterosexuals' attitudes toward lesbians and gay men: correlates and gender differences. *Journal of Sex Research* 25:451-477.

Herek, G.M., and E.K. Glunt (1991) AIDS-related attitudes in the United States: a preliminary conceptualization. *Journal of Sex Research* 28:99-123.

Hilts, P.J. (1992) Minister's ties to church are sundered by AIDS. *New York Times* Sept. 8:A1.

Horrigan, A. (1988) AIDS and the Catholic Church. In R. Berk, ed., *The Social Impact of AIDS in the United States.* Cambridge, Mass.: Abt Books.

Horsfield, P. (1984) *Religious Television: The American Experience.* New York: Longman.

Independent Sector (1990) *Giving and Volunteering in the United States. Findings From a National Survey.* Washington, D.C.: Independent Sector.

Jakobovits, I. (1978) Judaism. In *Encyclopedia of Bioethics*, Vol. 2. New York: Free Press.

Jakobovits, I. (1987) *AIDS: Jewish Perspectives.* London: Office of the Chief Rabbi.

Jennings, V.T. (1989) Black churches allying against AIDS. *Washington Post* July 3:B1, B4

Johnson, S.D. (1987) Factors related to intolerance of AIDS victims. *Journal for the Scientific Study of Religion* 26:105-110.

Kinsella, J. (1989) *Covering the Plague: AIDS and the American Media.* New Brunswick, N.J.: Rutgers University Press.

Kirp, D.L., S. Epstein, M.S. Franks, J. Simon, D. Conaway, et al. (1989) *Learning by Heart: AIDS and Schoolchildren in America' Communities.* New Brunswick, N.J.: Rutgers University Press.

Lambert, B. (1989) Black clergy to address AIDS threat to race. *New York Times* June 10:B29, B32.

Leasor, J. (1961) *The Plague and the Fire.* New York: Avon Books.

Lemay, H.R. (1980) Homosexuality in the Middle Ages. *Cross Currents* Fall:352-358.

Lightbourne, W. (1989) Meeting the needs of persons with AIDS. *Charities, USA* (March-April):1-9.

Marty, M. (1987) *Religion and the Republic. The American Circumstance.* Boston: The Beacon Press.

McCarthy, S. (1991) Unappealing appeal to fear and prejudice. *New York Newsday* August 5:8.

McCormick, R.A. (1988) AIDS: the shape of the ethical challenge. *America* 6:147-154.

Melton, J.G. (1989) *The Churches Speak On: AIDS.* Detroit, Mich.: Gale Research Inc.

Mitchell, A. (1990) AIDS: we are not immune. *Emerge* November:30-44.

National Black Consortium on Critical Health Needs (1988) *Resolution on AIDS.* Washington, D.C.: National Urban Coalition.

National Catholic Educational Association (1988) *Teacher's Manual. AIDS: A Catholic Educational Approach.* Washington, D.C.: National Catholic Educational Association.

New York Times (1985) AIDS center run by Archdiocese. *New York Times* November 28:B3.

Noonan, J. (1970) *Contraception.* Boston: Harvard University Press.

Numbers, R.L., and D.W. Amundsen, eds. (1986) *Caring and Curing: Health and Medicine in the Western Religious Traditions.* New York: Macmillan.

Orthodox Union (1988) Resolutions of the Union of Orthodox Jewish Congregations of America. New York, New York.

Ostling, R.N., M.P. Harris, and P.A. Witteman (1988) Gays vs. the Vatican. *Time* December 5:60.

Palmer, S.J. (1989) AIDS as metaphor. *Society* January/February:44-50.

Place, M. (1988) The many faces of AIDS: some clarifications of the recent debate. *America* 6:135-141.

Quinn, J.R. (1986) The AIDS crisis: a pastoral response. *America* June 28:505-511.

Reichley, A.J. (1985) *Religion in American Public Life.* Washington, D.C.: The Brookings Institution.

Rosenberg, C.E. (1962) *The Cholera Years: The United States in 1832, 1849, and 1866.* Chicago: University of Chicago Press.

Schaper, R.L. (1987) Pastoral care for persons with AIDS and their families. *The Christian Century* 104:691-694.

Shelp, E.E., and R.H. Sunderland (1985) AIDS and the Church. *The Christian Century* September 11-18:797-800.

Shelp, E.E., E.R. DuBose, and R.H. Sunderland (1990) The infrastructure of religious communities: a neglected resource for care of people with AIDS. *American Journal of Public Health* 80:970-972.

Shrewsbury, J.F.D. (1970) *A History of the Bubonic Plague in the British Isles.* Cambridge, England: Cambridge University Press.

Sider, R.J. (1988) AIDS: an evangelical perspective. *Christian Century* 105(1):11-14.

Slack, P. (1988) Responses to plague in early modern Europe: the implications of public health. *Social Research* 55:433-453.

Spiro, M.E. (1968) Religion: problems of definition in explanation. In M.P. Banton, ed., *Anthropological Approaches to the Study of Religion.* London: Tavistock Publications.

Spohn, W. (1988a) AIDS and the Catholic Church. *America* 158:142-146.

Spohn, W. (1988b) The moral dimensions of AIDS. *Theological Studies* 44:107-109.

Steinfels, P. (1991) Two churches weigh clergy proposals: Presbyterian and Episcopal panels push for the lifting of ordination obstacles. *New York Times* March 1:A20.

Stepp, L.S. (1989) AIDS epidemic is slowly gaining attention in local pulpits. *Washington Post* January 3:D1.

Street, J.L. (1988) A shared praxis approach. *Religious Education* 83:234-242.

Stulz, J. (1986) Toward a spirituality for victims of AIDS. *America* 28:509-511.

Sunderland, R.H., and E.E. Shelp (1990) *Handle with Care: A Handbook for Care Teams Serving People with AIDS.* Nashville, Tenn.: Abingdon Press.

Tonucci, G. (1988) Cardinal Ratzinger's letter on AIDS document. *Origins* (NC Documentary Service) 18:117-118.

U.S. Catholic Conference (1989) Called to compassion and responsibility: a response to the HIV/AIDS crisis. *Origins* (NC Documentary Service) 19:421, 423-434.

U.S. Catholic Conference Administrative Board (1987) The many faces of AIDS: a gospel response. *Origins* (NC Documentary Service) 17:482-489.

U.S. News & World Report (1985) Jerry Falwell: circuit rider to controversy. *U.S. News & World Report* 99:11.

Vaux, K. (1988) Learning fidelity: the pedagogy of watchful care. *Religious Education* 32:212-220.

Washofsky, M. (1989) AIDS and ethical responsibility: some Halachic considerations. *Journal of Reform Judaism* 36:53-65.

Weeks, J. (1980) In the days of yore when knights were gay? *History Today* 30:49.

Wertheimer, J. (1989) Recent trends in American Judaism. Pg. 162 in D. Singer and R. Seldin, eds., *American Jewish Yearbook.* Philadelphia: The Jewish Publication Society and New York: The American Jewish Committee.

Wiest, W.E. (1988) God's punishment for sin? *Religious Education* 83:243-250.

Winslow, C.E.A. (1943) *The Conquest of Epidemic Disease.* Princeton, N.J.: Princeton University Press.

Wuthnow, R. (1988) *The Restructuring of American Religion. Society and Faith Since World War II.* Princeton, N.J.: Princeton University Press.

6

Voluntary and
Community-Based Organizations

From the early Christians who cared for the victims of third century plagues and earned the name *parabolani* or "reckless ones" to the gravediggers of the Black Death and even to the volunteer "sanitary monitors" of the influenza epidemic of 1919, epidemics have always called forth volunteer helpers. With the rise of governmental public health agencies and organized health care, however, the role of volunteers in epidemics became less prominent: it was expected that existing social and government institutions would respond to the needs of the sick and the protection of the well.

The AIDS epidemic once more pushed to the fore the importance of volunteers. Already stigmatized by homophobia, distrustful of governmental intrusions and angry over the slowness of those same government agencies to take action, the gay community quickly began to organize volunteer efforts to help their own. At the same time public health officials and providers of care, frustrated by governmental inaction at high levels and aware of their limited ability to gain the trust of the communities most affected, encouraged the active participation of volunteers. Thus, one of the prominent features of the HIV/AIDS epidemic has been the growth and influence of volunteer groups in providing education, support, and care, as well as advocacy. Even before AIDS had a name, there were volunteers: community-based organizations (CBOs) rapidly appeared, devoted to serving persons with AIDS, raising money for care and for research, fighting discrimination, and providing education to those at high risk.

Observers of the American scene dating back to de Tocqueville and as recently as Bellah and colleagues (1985) have described Americans' penchant for forming voluntary associations as a way of coping with social problems. As de Tocqueville said (1835-1839 [1945:115-116]): "Americans of all ages, all conditions, and all dispositions constantly form associations . . . associations of a thousand other kinds, religious, moral, serious, futile, general or restricted, enormous or diminutive . . . . I have often admired the extreme skill with which the inhabitants of the United States succeed in proposing a common object for the exertions of a great many men and inducing them voluntarily to pursue it". AIDS has been no exception. Community-based organizations are a key component in the care of persons with AIDS. In many communities they play an important role in reducing the length of hospital stays for persons with AIDS by enabling them to be cared for at home by friends and family to the greatest extent medically appropriate.

Little of the research on the costs of providing care for persons with HIV disease or AIDS has looked explicitly at the contribution of volunteers. Arno's studies (1986, 1988) are among the few exceptions. In the 1985 fiscal year, Arno (1986) estimated the value of AIDS-related volunteer labor to be $1.2 million. Some researchers have attributed a drop of more than two-thirds in the annual cost of caring for persons with AIDS in San Francisco (from $150,000 to $40,000) to the contribution of volunteers. According to Arno (1988:57):

> [An] important reason to determine the value of volunteer labor is that it is not equally available in all regions of the country or to all groups at risk. Further, as the nature of the epidemic shifts, the supply of volunteers may prove inadequate. Thus, full market value may have to be paid if services now provided by volunteers are to be available, and it is therefore vital to know what those services actually cost.

The volunteer and community-based organizations that formed in response to the epidemic appear to have reached a crucial crossroads as the epidemic moves into its second decade. Doubts have arisen about whether CBOs will be able to meet the needs of increasing numbers of persons with AIDS and about whether the needs of intravenous drug users, their sexual partners, and their offspring can be addressed in ways that replicate the response of the more affluent and organized gay community from which the volunteer movement arose.

THE ORIGINS OF COMMUNITY-BASED
SERVICE ORGANIZATIONS

It is often said about AIDS that it shines a harsh light to expose the cracks and flaws in the U.S. system of delivering and financing health care.

The community-based volunteer organizations that sprang up in high-incidence urban centers such as New York City and San Francisco were in part
a response to a lack of sensitivity to the health care needs of gay men and
lesbians by mainstream medical establishments. Their lineage can be traced
to the human rights and consumer movements of the 1960s.

One of the earliest groups formed to respond to AIDS was New York
City's Gay Men's Health Crisis. It grew out of meetings in gay playwright
Larry Kramer's living room in the summer of 1981, during which a group
of gay men discussed the rumors about a new disease that was striking
down previously healthy young gay men. In San Francisco, the Kaposi's
Sarcoma Foundation was formed in 1981 to respond to the crisis, and by
early 1982 volunteers began to staff hotlines, distribute literature, and provide advice to help individuals confront a disease about which very little
was known except its fearsome potential consequences.

Two years into the AIDS epidemic, 45 self-help groups had been formed
in the United States, mostly organized by gay men (Chambre, 1989). By
the end of the first decade of the AIDS epidemic, more than 600 community-based AIDS service-providing organizations had sprung up around the
country. A handful of the oldest and largest of those organizations now
have annual budgets in the millions of dollars, scores of paid staff, and
hundreds of volunteers. Other groups are considerably more modest, yet
they make a large difference in the lives of persons with AIDS. Among the
hundreds of groups organized in the past few years is a proliferation of
AIDS-specific volunteer organizations, many seeking to address targeted
needs of persons with AIDS, such as food, health education, housing, income support, or hospice care.

By the time AIDS appeared, the consumer movement had matured, and
there was a new-found willingness to confront and question professional
authority of all types, including the traditional "paternalism" of medical
care. These attitudes were embraced by those with AIDS. Many resented
being labeled as "victims" or even "patients," preferring instead "persons
with AIDS," so as not to convey the same flavor of dependency as "patient"
(Grover, 1988; Navarre, 1988; Gayle, 1989).

The decades prior to 1980 had also witnessed a remarkable shift in
attitudes toward death and dying on the part of patients and health care
practitioners. Earlier, an age-old taboo had precluded the discussion of
impending death between patients and their doctors was reflected in the
practice of many doctors. A 1961 survey of physicians, for example, showed
that 90 percent of them preferred not to inform patients of a cancer diagnosis; they were more likely to disclose a terminal diagnosis to the spouse or
other family member and even to enlist them in the deception of the patient.
By 1977, however, 97 percent of physicians surveyed said they routinely
disclosed cancer diagnoses to patients (President's Commission for the Study

of Ethical Problems in Medicine and Biomedical and Behavioral Research, 1982:76, n. 14). The significant shift in attitudes toward death and dying was partly a result of the writings of Elisabeth Kubler-Ross (1969, 1987), who encouraged an open discussion of death and popularized the ideas that there are stages in the dying process and that it is healthy and therapeutic for dying persons and their loved ones to struggle together toward acceptance of death. This development prepared the way for caring for those dying of AIDS. According to Chambre (1988:15-16):

> The sustained response of citizens to care for the dying evident in this epidemic is an historically unique event; in the past caring for the sick and the dying was restricted to plague doctors, to priests and nuns, and to a few heroic and later sainted individuals who were sometimes forced to live in isolation until the epidemic ended. . . . Actual care of the dying evident in the AIDS epidemic has one precedent, the influenza epidemic of 1918-19, when there was a better understanding of disease transmission and infection control. Unlike AIDS, the response was a short-term collective response to a disaster, quite different from the sustained, long-term efforts that have been required for AIDS [footnotes omitted].

WHO VOLUNTEERS AND WHY

A number of studies of altruism, volunteer motivation, social movements, and volunteer organizations have been conducted in recent years independently of the HIV/AIDS epidemic (Jenkins, 1983; Bellah et al., 1985; Ayers, 1989). Also of interest are studies of gift giving in various cultures. It was the work of anthropologists, dating back to the classic studies of gift exchanges among the people of Melanesia and Polynesia by Mauss (1925), that began to unravel the complexities of the gift relationship. Those studies show that gifts are rarely given without engendering an obligation of reciprocity. Gift givers and receivers are intertwined in a cycle of giving and receiving. Gifts are often given out of a feeling of perceived obligation, and they frequently impose substantial obligation, in turn, on the recipient. Similarly, volunteering is not a unilateral act, a charity that flows only in one direction. Although volunteers may feel uncomfortable admitting that their motivations are not purely altruistic, it should not be surprising, or embarrassing, to find that this is true. Studies of volunteering and giving to charities have revealed a complicated welter of emotions and motivations.

When Titmuss (1970) studied blood donors in the United States and Great Britain, he found that volunteer donors were not spontaneous or purely altruistic. In interviews, donors expressed a wide array of reasons for making a donation of blood that would eventually be transfused into a stranger.

Respondents mentioned reciprocity, gratitude, awareness of need, and response to a personal or public appeal as reasons for giving. More recently, Murray (1991:238) concluded, "AIDS does not appear to have altered in any fundamental way the meaning of gifts of blood for giver or recipient."

Chambre (1988) and Kobasa (1991) have suggested some particular factors that motivate AIDS volunteers. Chambre describes volunteering as "bearing witness," a complex blend of secular and religious responses to a frightening epidemic before which one feels powerless: volunteering is a way of coping with the uncertainty posed by an incurable illness. To understand volunteers' motivations, according to Chambre (1988:7), it is necessary to understand such diverse topics as "cultural definitions of disease and terminal illness, social responses to natural and man-made disasters, social movements, the search for meaning of community, and changes in the meaning of death and dying." Chambre's research calls attention to the parallels between the creation of new organizations and the mobilization of volunteers. She notes (Chambre, 1991:278) that: "although actual concerns or grievances are important in understanding how a social movement evolves, it is also important to point to the historical and cultural context and to an organization's ability to mobilize two key resources: money and people." The rapid growth of the Gay Men's Health Crisis (GMHC) in New York is consistent with mobilization theory. GMHC served as the entry point for large numbers of men into volunteer associations dealing with AIDS, and it also provided access to the funds needed to support such organizations.

Chambre (1991) has examined volunteerism specifically in the context of the AIDS epidemic and drawn some interesting observations regarding the mobilization of volunteers. She notes that volunteering reveals collective behavior during a period of turmoil or social change and the apparent differences between recruitment of volunteers for a new social cause as opposed to recruitment for long-standing and more persistent problems (Chambre, 1991:276):

> . . . it's easier to find volunteers to do difficult work than it is to find volunteers to do easy work. . . . Most people who volunteer want to do something meaningful, where they know they're making a difference. And in some ways they want to be challenged by what they're doing . . . they don't hesitate to do something that's going to be hard. In fact, they seek something that's going to be hard.

The trauma of the AIDS epidemic in gay communities fits the model of volunteering for a major natural or man-made disaster—the sense of shock and total devastation motivated the level of response normally found only in extreme emergencies.

In addition to being a way to cope with fears about getting AIDS, and to create or reconstruct a sense of community, Chambre (1991:277) found that volunteering "entails a complex and broad range of motivations that merit consideration." Almost universally, she found an important reward "was the privilege of working with truly exceptional people. In some settings, this was defined as a transformative experience." She suggests new directions for understanding the meaning of volunteer work and the process of burnout, including a "conscious effort by the organization to clarify the powerful impact that volunteering could have on the volunteers' lives."

Other students of AIDS volunteers have identified similarly complicated motivations. There is, of course, the unalloyed desire to help someone in need. Many volunteers describe the privilege of volunteering and talk about what they learn from those they help. For those who are infected or at risk of HIV, volunteering may be perceived as a way to keep from getting ill. Individuals who are fearful of AIDS may find volunteering a way of coping with and confronting their own fears and mortality. Sometimes the bargaining is explicit: volunteers may seek preferential treatment when they themselves become ill and look to the organization for which they volunteered for support.

The demographics of AIDS volunteers is also interesting. Kobasa (1991) studied 600 new volunteers at New York City's Gay Men's Health Crisis from 1988 to 1990 and found that although most of the earlier volunteers had lost friends or lovers to AIDS, many new recruits simply wanted to help. Gay male volunteers are being supplemented by increasing numbers of lesbians and heterosexual women, whose motivations may be somewhat different.

VOLUNTEERS AND WHAT THEY CONTRIBUTE

It is not immediately obvious what is meant by "volunteer work." In fact, much unpaid work on behalf of persons with AIDS may not even be thought of as volunteering because it takes place in the context of kinship or other personal relationships. A spouse taking care of a dying partner or a gay man taking care of his lover is seldom regarded as volunteering. In fact, in certain contexts there may be more social support for strangers than for family members in caring for individuals. In the foster care setting, strangers are paid for the care of children placed with them, whereas aunts, uncles, or grandparents who take care of young family members might not be eligible for the same type of payments as nonrelated foster care parents (see Chapter 8). What if an individual regularly goes shopping or does housework for a neighbor or friend who is ill? This kind of activity, outside the family circle, may be closer to what is generally thought of as volunteering, although such informal helping is not likely to be captured in surveys.

What is most often meant by "volunteering" in the AIDS epidemic is work performed under the aegis of churches, health care institutions, or local community-based AIDS service organizations. Hospitals have long made use of the services of unpaid volunteers, although before the advent of AIDS, volunteers mostly performed functions unrelated to direct patient care, such as staffing gift shops and information desks or handing out passes to visitors. Paid administrators of volunteer services tend to be quite low in the hospital hierarchy, and their departments are peripheral in planning for and providing services. In many hospitals the impetus for bolstering volunteer resources for patients with AIDS came from the outside, and funds were provided by foundations or hospital auxiliary agencies. Chambre (1991: 283) noted a "gap between the rhetoric of voluntarism and hospitals' commitment to ensuring success of volunteer programs, even in organizations that view themselves as depending on volunteers."

Outside of hospitals, the voluntary, community-based response to AIDS has included an array of health education, social support, and counseling activities. At the beginning of the epidemic in the early 1980s there was a great deal of uncertainty as to the nature of the disease and its etiology, how it might be treated, and how and the extent to which it could transmitted. These uncertainties, combined with the stigma of the association of AIDS with homosexuality and drug use, made it difficult for those afflicted to obtain adequate and dignified social services and medical care (National Commission on AIDS, 1991). The lack of services and the discrimination experienced by persons with AIDS led to the establishment of a host of local, community-based organizations, often comprising mostly gay men.

AIDS telephone hotlines were among the earliest services provided by volunteers. Another noteworthy service development is the "buddy system," in which a volunteer is paired with a person with AIDS to provide emotional and social support services, such as providing transportation to health care appointments and helping with house chores. Buddies are given training and the latest information on AIDS by their organization, and they usually meet in support groups to help each other cope with the experience of working with a dying person, with whom they are likely to establish a strong bond.

The array of services offered by CBOs is designed to ensure that a person with AIDS can remain outside the hospital to the greatest extent possible. Some local AIDS groups are purely service oriented; other, newer groups have political goals and agendas (see below). Many of the local CBOs, as noted, were formed to meet specific needs of persons with AIDS, such as housing, hospice care, or direct financial assistance. In a number of cities, organizations are devoted primarily to providing "meals on wheels"— food for homebound persons with AIDS: God's Love We Deliver in New York City, Cure AIDS Now in Miami, the Chicken Soup Brigade in Seattle, and Project Open Hand in San Francisco exemplify this type of group.

Some CBOs that were in existence prior to the AIDS epidemic have adjusted their goals and expanded their services to include persons with

AIDS. The Shanti Project in the San Francisco Bay Area was formed in the mid-1970s to provide counseling to the dying and the bereaved; its member quickly turned to the needs of those dying from AIDS, and it played a prominent role in San Francisco's strongly volunteer approach to AIDS care. Other hospice projects also initiated in the decade before the epidemic took similar steps to assist with the death and dying of persons with AIDS (Arno, 1986). The Whitman-Walker Clinic in Washington, D.C., which was established in the late 1970s to offer gay-sensitive health care focused on sexually transmitted diseases, has expanded its activities to provide a number of AIDS-specific services. Other, more broadly focused organizations that rely on charitable contributions and volunteer support, such as the Red Cross and the United Way, have incorporated AIDS services into their agendas—although not always painlessly (Perrow and Guillen, 1990).

A survey of the contributions of AIDS volunteers at Cook County Hospital in Chicago provides a representative sampling of volunteer job categories: educator/speaker, legal aid, telephone aid, donation coordinator, crisis intervention, event coordinator, art therapy, pastoral care, hair stylist, and clowns (Boyd, Kuehnert, and Sherer, 1990). In many cases the services are provided by lay volunteers with a modicum of training. In other cases the services are closer to what ancillary medical personnel usually provide. It is not uncommon for family members or lovers of persons with AIDS to perform fairly invasive and complicated medical procedures, including starting and maintaining intravenous lines. As noted in Chapter 3, interventions that used to entail hospitalization are now often provided for persons with AIDS on an outpatient basis or at home.

Although AIDS-related CBOs may have been created by volunteers, the volunteers are not necessarily amateurs. Nor are volunteer services limited to the medical arena. Many AIDS volunteers come from backgrounds in management, accounting, public relations, or community organizing. In many large cities, cadres of volunteer lawyers have been organized under the auspices of CBOs or bar association groups to provide low- or no-cost legal services to persons with AIDS, such as drafting wills, trying to obtain insurance coverage, or filing discrimination claims (Barnes, Greenberg, and Pinksy, 1989; Rivera, 1989; Hansell and Calabrese, 1990).

The provision of psychological support services raises particular concerns about lay versus professional authority and responsibilities. One case in point is "rational suicide" or "assisted suicide." The incidence of suicide among persons with AIDS or HIV disease has been higher than among individuals facing other chronic or terminal illnesses (Marzuk et al., 1988). In fact, many persons with AIDS have asserted their belief in their right to die in a manner of their own choosing, even if it involves enlisting friends, lovers, or caregivers in finding and using the appropriate means. A few people who have assisted persons with AIDS in taking their lives have gone public in an effort to gain legalization of the practice of assisted suicide (Johnson, 1988). If anything, the role of volunteer service providers in advising clients about taking their own lives is more complicated than for professional health care providers because reciprocal duties and obligations between clients and volunteers may be less clearly defined than the relationship between patients and health care providers. AIDS volunteer organizations, in their volunteer training and program manuals, embrace a wide spectrum of views about the appropriate behavior when a client requests advice or assistance with suicide.

THE RISE OF ADVOCACY

For some people affected by the HIV/AIDS epidemic, traditional volunteering through social service organizations has not provided enough of an outlet. Caring for others has not allowed them to express their anger or vent their frustration at what they believe to be a federal government without a plan to confront the epidemic or a leader to take charge. According to Maddocks (1989:1):

> If volunteers operate only within existing government frames, they will tend to support the *status quo*. If they are encouraged to work outside official bodies, they will begin to develop an independent approach. Within the urban programmes, many young persons become "radicalized," and begin to express negative comments about government, and a greater commitment to change. This may be uncomfortable for governments but it is probably good for society.

In 1987 a loosely organized group of persons with AIDS and their friends and supporters was formed to mount a political challenge, largely at the behest of playwright Larry Kramer. By 1990 the group, known as the AIDS Coalition to Unleash Power (ACT-UP), had about 65 chapters throughout the country (Krieger, 1990). Larry Kramer, in characteristically unvarnished prose, described his reason for helping to found the new group: "I helped found Gay Men's Health Crisis and watched them turn into an organization of sissies. I founded ACT-UP and have watched them change the world" (quoted in Kolata, 1990:A-11). Others who have eschewed social volunteering in favor of political activism have concluded that the continued growth of voluntary organizations allows government to abdicate its responsibilities, crossing the "line separating civic duty and community solidarity from overdependence and governmental irresponsibility" (Arno, 1988:69).

ACT-UP had its roots in the white gay male community, but it soon attracted black and Hispanic gay men, lesbians, and heterosexual women. The largest and most visible ACT-UP chapter is in New York City, where members' talents in politics, media relations, advertising, and law have been harnessed in an effort to bring public attention to the needs of persons with AIDS and to change the direction of AIDS policy. The tactics of ACT-UP, which frequently involve civil disobedience leading to arrest and the individuals ACT-UP has chosen to target and vilify as enemies of persons with AIDS have sparked an ongoing debate within and without the activist community (see Cohen, 1989; Spiers, 1989). ACT-UP protests— "zaps"—have been mounted against government and public health officials, church leaders, drug company executives, clinical researchers, and science reporters. ACT-UP attacks can be scathing; prominent government clinical researchers, for example, have been labeled Nazis by some ACT-UP protestors.

ACT-UP has waged its fight on a variety of fronts, frequently garnering national attention in the electronic and print press. Protests have included picketing the offices of *Cosmopolitan* magazine to protest the publication of what was claimed to be misleading information on heterosexual transmission of HIV; campaigning for needle and syringe distribution to intravenous drug users; protesting "mainstreaming" persons with HIV infection into New York City homeless shelters; and demonstrating against sodomy laws in Atlanta, Georgia. Some protests have been directed at particular policies, others at general consciousness raising. Two examples of the latter in San Francisco were protesters' snarling traffic on the Golden Gate Bridge, keeping commuters stranded for hours and disrupting the opening night of the 1989 opera season. In perhaps the most notorious ACT-UP zap, protestors disrupted a mass being celebrated by Cardinal John J. O'Connor at New York City's St. Patrick's Cathedral. During the protest, one activist crushed a communion wafer, which provoked a cry of protest and condemnation from a range of commentators, including New York Governor Mario Cuomo and President George Bush. The President decried ACT-UP tactics in an interview with religious broadcasters.

Much of ACT-UP's energy has been focused on the Food and Drug Administration, where protestors have charged that outmoded regulations and bureaucratic intransigence have impeded the development, licensing, and marketing of drugs to treat HIV infection and associated opportunistic infections. ACT-UP members have also locked themselves in the offices of Burroughs-Wellcome, accusing the drug company of gouging in the pricing of zidovudine (AZT), and they have occupied the offices of clinical researchers at the National Institutes of Health in Bethesda, Maryland.

Such very public protests have been supplemented by more quiet, "inside" work in policy-making councils. A few ACT-UP members have become exceedingly well schooled in the complex and often arcane details of drug development and regulation and the design of clinical trials. ACT-UP representatives have participated in the Institute of Medicine's Drug and

Vaccine Development Roundtable and testified at meetings of the National Commission on AIDS. ACT-UP's Treatment and Data Committee has produced lengthy and detailed critiques of drug development strategies. Members have been influential in provoking biostatisticians to rethink issues of clinical design and in encouraging federal regulators to reconsider how drugs are approved for patients with terminal illnesses. In an unprecedented way, volunteers have become effective participants in this most professional of enclaves, the world of scientific research (see Chapter 4).

An examination of ACT-UP's organizational structure, goals, and tactics raises profound questions about how individuals whose lives are touched or threatened by AIDS ought best respond to the epidemic (Elbaz, 1990). AIDS activists share many dilemmas with other social and political movements in which passions run deep and moral outrage soars, such as the civil rights movement and the pro-life and pro-choice movements in the abortion debate. When is civil disobedience warranted? When is it effective? When do protests cause a counterproductive backlash from policy makers or the public? Ad hominem attacks on clinicians and researchers, for example, have reportedly discouraged some people from participating in AIDS research and treatment efforts. In 1991, the protests took place in the context of tight budgets that dampened increases in funding for AIDS research and treatment, and the public debate on the allocation of money for AIDS versus other diseases has grown louder (see Cimons, 1990; Murphy, 1991). For example, a syndicated journalist and television commentator observed (Krauthammer, 1990:80):

> AIDS is now riding a crest of public support, won in the rough and tumble of politics. All perfectly legitimate, and a tribute to the passion and commitment of AIDS activists. But that passion turns to mere stridency when they take to the streets to protest that a homophobic society has been ungenerous and stinting in its response to the tragedy of AIDS.

> It is hard to see from where [those who have contacted AIDS from sex or drug abuse] derive the claim to be first in line—ahead of those dying of leukemia and breast cancer and stroke—for the resources and compassion of a nation.

VOLUNTEERS AND COMMUNITY-BASED ORGANIZATIONS IN THE SECOND DECADE

A number of CBOs with roots in the gay culture have faced an identity crisis. AIDS has focused attention on the gay community as never before (Altman, 1988). In some communities, AIDS service organizations and volunteer opportunities for gay men and lesbians have provided a catalyst for a social and cultural network that did not exist previously. Yet AIDS has also tended to overwhelm other issues, such as gay civil rights, political recognition, and lesbian health. AIDS service groups have on many occasions downplayed their gay roots and links in order to secure funding and support from the wider community. An intense debate continues in the gay and lesbian communities about the appropriate balance between AIDS and other issues of concern (Rist, 1989). The Gay Men's Health Crisis in New York encourages name recognition by the public of its acronym alone, GMHC, and it certainly serves a broader clientele: slightly more than one-half of GMHC's clients are white gay men; approximately 25 percent are black or Hispanics and 15 percent are white women; 10 percent of the clients are intravenous drug users (Perrow and Guillen, 1990). Many leaders of gay-identified AIDS service organizations fear that a stronger stance on gay rights issues will jeopardize funding for AIDS programs. For some programs, this has meant problems in deciding how to address issues of gay sexuality and how far to go in eroticizing safer sex educational materials or in making them relevant to the needs of gay clients.

These conflicts were also reflected in the debates among health and government officials. One outcome was the decision to portray AIDS as an ecumenical, equal opportunity disease, and not a "gay disease." In some quarters, this has provoked criticism from those who have suggested that scientific attention to the risk of heterosexual transmission of AIDS was disproportionate to the real risk and merely a stratagem to garner greater attention and funding (Fumento, 1990). Yet HIV is a risk to many heterosexuals, especially those who have sex with intravenous drug users.

The rapid expansion of CBOs as they try to keep pace with caseloads has resulted in some serious growing pains. It is difficult to plan and develop an infrastructure to support an organization that has doubled its staff and caseload every year for several years. The development skills and energies necessary to get new organizations off the ground may be quite different from the managerial skills necessary to maintain them. Managing an organization with a multimillion dollar budget requires a certain degree of bureaucratization and the development of a corporate culture, which may be at odds with the ethos of volunteering.

Burgeoning caseloads and client needs are posing many planning challenges for AIDS service organizations. Some have responded to the growing need with risky decisions to maintain low reserve balances and make hiring and program decisions based on projected, but unconfirmed, increases in funding (Howell, 1991). In designing programs, there is also the danger that the availability and prospects for obtaining certain types of funding will drive program choices, independent of the actual needs of those to be served. Pediatric AIDS, for example, has a unique cachet, and funds are often available in amounts that are considerably disproportionate to the number of cases of pediatric AIDS (Kirp, 1990; see also Chapter 8). Limited resources also means making allocation decisions involving hard choices between services to those already infected with HIV and education and prevention efforts to prevent further spread of the virus. This conflict has been complicated by the misperception of some that there is no further need for prevention efforts to foster and maintain behavioral change among gay men. The prospect of achieving beneficial effects through earlier intervention with asymptomatic HIV-infected individuals also forces similarly difficult tradeoffs—how to allocate services among those who are already sick and others who may be able to live healthier longer with the proper support.

The fundraising activities of local AIDS organizations have grown increasingly sophisticated. Perhaps the earliest example of the ability to raise funds on behalf of AIDS charities was a circus sponsored by GMHC at New York's Madison Square Garden in April 1983, which was attended by about 18,000 people. Many cities have a number of annual events to raise funds. A 1990 New York AIDS walk, for example, raised more than $3 million for GMHC, a quarter of its budget for the year (Seltzer and Galvin, 1991).

The private sector has played a significant role in supporting the work of CBOs and other AIDS organizations. Private foundations and corporations have contributed an estimated $120 million to efforts to combat AIDS since 1983 (Seltzer and Galvin, 1991). Initially, many funders were reluctant to get involved in AIDS work because of the stigma associated with the disease. In addition, many foundations have strictures on providing money to "single disease entities," aware that such a policy would open them up to entreaties from scores of national health charities. The Robert Wood Johnson Foundation made an exception to that policy; to date it has contributed more than $20 million to HIV-related efforts, a large share of which has gone to community organizations. The foundation sought to stimulate groups and agencies with no prior contact with the foundation to submit proposals for innovative programs in HIV prevention. Many other major foundations followed Robert Wood Johnson's lead. Led by the Ford Foundation, the National Community AIDS Partnership was formed in 1988 and it has involved more than 50 foundations and contributed more than $5 million to technical assistance and project funds to encourage the establishment and growth of AIDS-related CBOs.

Groups that have managed to diversify funding streams so as not to become dependent on a single source of money are most likely to continue to thrive. This is especially important because federal and private foundation support for AIDS services has often been "seed money" or a "demonstration grant," not intended to sustain the organization. Many local groups have benefited from seed grants from private foundations, as well as the federal Health Services Research Administration (Howell, 1991; Seltzer and Galvin, 1991). The most successful groups have been able to put together funding packages with contributions from various levels of government, private donations, and money raised from fund-raising events and direct mail. Newer groups that are starting up in minority communities must compete for a slice of what is often too small a pie. In addition, experience in fund-raising and technical skills are critical, and such experience may not always be readily shared with others. A description in a report on the adequacy of the response to AIDS in Philadelphia contains a passage that would apply in many localities (Philadelphia Commission on AIDS, 1988:26):

> A . . . problem hampering the growth of community-based organizations in Philadelphia has been the existence of conflicts among the groups. The lack of adequate and stable funding has served to intensify their history of philosophical and personal conflicts. . . . Fragmentation within CBOs has led to some reluctance among some foundations, health care organizations, and others to become involved in what they see as squabbles.

With the number of persons with AIDS on the rise, and with greater opportunities for therapies to delay the onset of symptoms in otherwise healthy HIV-infected individuals, CBOs and local AIDS-specific volunteer organizations need more volunteers and broader sources of funding. AIDS advocates have pressed governments at all levels to increase funding for health care and social support services provided at home. Reimbursing individuals for services provided in the home, however, will depend on the development of uniform standards and quality control mechanisms.

Community-based organizations active in the HIV/AIDS epidemic face some special problems not shared by other organizations that depend on volunteer labor. These problems range from burnout and sickness and death to difficulties in finding rental space for offices or clinics due to unfounded fears of HIV transmission and neighborhood resistance to having gay men or intravenous drug users congregating nearby. Flexible work schedules may be needed for staff and volunteers who are themselves suffering from HIV-related illnesses (Carbine and Lee, 1988). A number of AIDS organizations have experienced problems in obtaining or maintaining health insurance benefits for their employees as a result of the insurance underwriting practices for small groups.

Community-based organizations formed to respond to AIDS among middle-class, white, gay men have recently been forced to reexamine their roles. As the proportion of AIDS cases grows among minorities in poor urban areas and among intravenous drug users and their sexual partners, the need has grown for organizations that reflect and can respond sensitively to these people's needs. This is of critical importance because minorities make up a disproportionate number of persons with AIDS: African Americans account for 12 percent of the U.S. population, yet 29 percent of AIDS cases; Hispanics account for 9 percent of the population, but 16 percent of AIDS cases (Centers for Disease Control, 1992). There have been significant limitations in the ability of AIDS service organizations to respond to their needs, however. Particular problems have been the lack of minority input in program design and implementation, insufficient minority representation on boards of directors, and inadequate sensitivity to the needs of minorities in training programs for staff and volunteers. To help address these issues, a National Minority AIDS Council was formed by minority-based CBOs in 1987.

The difficulty of tapping volunteer resources to meet the needs of minorities with HIV and AIDS is manifest. Poverty and unemployment make volunteering difficult or impossible for many people in poor communities. AIDS is only a single instance of the "synergism of plagues" that confront poor, minority individuals (Wallace, 1988; see Chapter 1). There are political fears that efforts to direct further attention to AIDS in minority communities will only subject those communities to additional racism and neglect. The stigma associated with homosexuality and intravenous drug use in the Hispanic and African American communities has also stifled the participation of what otherwise might be the most natural place to turn for help in times of need—the church (see Chapter 5). Community organizations also face special barriers in meeting the needs of intravenous drug users and their sexual partners and children (Winkle, 1991). In addition to the exigencies of drug addiction, poverty, unemployment, and poor education, Friedman and colleagues (1987) identified a number of barriers to mobilizing drug users. These include a lack of historical precedent for collective self-organization, criminal penalties for possession and use of drugs, and competition and conflict within the drug subculture. The chaotic lives and social settings of the drug subculture can frustrate the most sincere efforts of outsiders to help.

Despite the particular difficulties faced by intravenous drug users, a few groups, such as New York City's Association for Drug Abuse Prevention and Treatment, have been organized to provide outreach to drug users and to influence drug prevention and treatment policy. Former drug users who are enlisted as street and outreach workers play a special role because they may be able to reach drug users who are inaccessible to health care or public health workers. The stress of such work is substantial, however. Outreach workers must maintain relations with the drug subculture and current users, and they must deal with people who may be sick or dying from AIDS or other health complications of drug use.

As the epidemic settles into communities in which volunteer efforts from the outside may be distrusted as well as difficult to implement and in which volunteer efforts from within are either inhibited by cultural values or impossible to organize, one of the important features of the HIV/AIDS epidemic—the rallying of volunteers to care for their own may be imperiled. The volunteer efforts that have been so significant in providing care, support, and education may not emerge in these communities, leaving these activities to already overburdened and sometimes collapsing social and health care agencies. In addition, the crucial advocacy that has come from CBOs may be absent, leaving the threatened communities without voice in the places of power.

CONCLUSIONS

The involvement of volunteers and voluntary organizations has been one of the defining characteristics of the AIDS epidemic. Although a substantial fraction of Americans has always participated in formal or informal volunteer activities in health, social service, and religious organizations, the contributions of volunteers in the AIDS epidemic have been unique. Individual volunteers and the formation of hundreds of community-based volunteer organizations were a principal way in which society responded to the outbreak of an epidemic disease in a stigmatized population.

The AIDS epidemic created a great demand for volunteer labor and in the process gave rise to questions about the proper role of government and private citizens in responding to a public health crisis. It also gave rise to questions about the proper roles and functions of volunteers in relation to paid or "professional" workers. As a collective behavior, volunteering has been a way of coping with the epidemic; on an individual level, it has proven meaningful not only to those receiving services, but also to the volunteers, people whose complex motivations are only beginning to be recognized and understood.

In the second decade of the HIV/AIDS epidemic, volunteers are likely to continue to play an important role, but the capacity of the voluntary sector to respond to continuing and new needs will be sorely tested. The increasing bureaucracy of the volunteer groups may hinder their flexibility; the decreasing flow of philanthropic funds will limit their efficacy; the growing number of HIV-infected persons who will develop AIDS in this decade will strain their resources; and the heavy emotional demands of the epidemic will exhaust their strength. Above all, the difficulties—social, cultural, and psychological—of moving into, or emerging from, those marginalized and deprived communities where the epidemic is now rapidly spreading, may render the valuable contribution of volunteers futile, precisely where they are most needed.

REFERENCES

Altman, D. (1988) Legitimation through disaster: AIDS and the gay movement. In E. Fee and D.M. Fox, eds., *AIDS: The Burdens of History*. Berkeley, Calif.: University of California Press.

Arno, P.S. (1986) The non-profit sector's response to the AIDS epidemic: community-based services in San Francisco. *American Journal of Public Health* 76:1325-1330.

Arno, P.S. (1988) The future of voluntarism and the AIDS epidemic. In D. Rogers and E. Ginzberg, eds., *The AIDS Patient: An Action Agenda*. Boulder, Colo.: Westview.

Ayers, T.D. (1989) Dimensions and characteristics of lay healing. *American Journal of Orthopsychiatry* 59:215-225.

Barnes, M., D.M. Greenberg, and L. Pinsky (1989) Providing high quality, low cost legal services to people with AIDS: an antidiscrimination law project. *AIDS Care* 1:297-306.

Bellah, R.N., R. Madsen, S.M. Sullivan, A. Swindler, and S.M. Tipton (1985) *Habits of the Heart: Individualism and Commitment in American Life*. New York: Harper & Row.

Boyd, L., P. Kuehnert, and R. Sherer (1990) Serving, hope, humor and compassion: implementation of a widely diverse volunteer support program for persons with AIDS/HIV infection at Cook County Hospital, Chicago. Paper presented at the Sixth International Conference on AIDS, San Francisco, June 20-24.

Carbine, M.E., and P. Lee (1988) *AIDS into the 90's: Strategies for an Integrated Response to the AIDS Epidemic*. Washington, D.C.: National AIDS Network.

Centers for Disease Control (1992) *HIV/AIDS Surveillance Report*. Atlanta, Ga.: Centers for Disease Control.

Chambre, S. (1988) *Responding to Uncertainty by Bearing Witness: Volunteering as Collective Behavior in the AIDS Epidemic, 1981-1988*. Center for the Study of Philanthropy, Bernard M. Baruch College. New York: City University of New York.

Chambre, S. (1989) Kindling points of light: volunteering as public policy. *Nonprofit and Voluntary Sector Quarterly* 18:249-268.

Chambre, S.M. (1991) The volunteer response to the AIDS epidemic in New York City: implications for research on voluntarism. *Nonprofit and Voluntary Sector Quarterly* 20:267-288.

Cimons, M. (1990) AIDS: a funding backlash surfaces. *Los Angeles Times* June 18:A-1.

Cohen, C. (1989) Militant morality: civil disobedience and bioethics. *Hastings Center Report* 19:23-25.

de Tocqueville, A.D. (1835-1839) *Democracy in America*, Vol. II. New York: Alfred A. Knopf, 1945.

Elbaz, G. (1990) ACT-UP survey. Paper presented at the Sixth International Conference on AIDS, San Francisco, June 20-24.

Friedman, S.R., D.C. Des Jarlais, J.L. Sotheran, J. Garber, H. Cohen, et al. (1987) AIDS and self-organization among intravenous drug users. *The International Journal of the Addictions* 22:201-219.

Fumento, M. (1990) *The Myth of Heterosexual AIDS*. New York: Basic Books.

Gayle, J.A. (1989) The effect of terminology on public consciousness related to the HIV epidemic. *AIDS Education and Prevention* 1:247-250.

Grover, J.Z. (1988) AIDS: key words. In D. Crimp, ed., *AIDS: Cultural Analysis/Cultural Activism*. Cambridge, Mass.: MIT Press.

Hansell, D., and T. Calabrese (1990) Community-based legal service delivery to HIV-affected communities of color. Paper presented at the Sixth International Conference on AIDS, San Francisco, June 20-24.

Howell, E.M. (1991) The role of community-based organizations in responding to the AIDS epidemic: examples from the HRSA service demonstrations. *Journal of Public Health Policy* 12(2):165-174.

Jenkins, J.C. (1983) Resource mobilization theory and the study of social movements. *Annual Review of Sociology* 9:527-553.

Johnson, T. (1988) A "humane and dignified death." ABC News "Nightline" transcript, March 31. Journal Graphics, New York.

Kirp, D. (1990) The politics of pediatric AIDS. *The Nation* May 14:666-668.

Kobasa, S.C. (1991) AIDS volunteering: links to the past and future prospects. In D. Nelkin,

D.P. Willis, and S.V. Parris, eds., *A Disease of Society: Cultural and Traditional Responses to AIDS*. New York: Cambridge University Press.

Kolata, G. (1990) AIDS advocates find a decline in private funds. *New York Times* August 7:A-11.

Krauthammer, C. (1990) AIDS: getting more than its share? *Time* June 25:80.

Krieger, L.M. (1990) Ideology clash underlies split within ACT-UP. *San Francisco Chronicle* October 14:B-1.

Kubler-Ross, E. (1969) *On Death and Dying*. New York: Macmillan.

Kubler-Ross, E. (1987) *AIDS: The Ultimate Challenge*. New York: Macmillan.

Maddocks, I. (1989) Volunteering for the care of patients with the acquired immunodeficiency syndrome (editorial). *Medical Journal of Australia* 151:1-2.

Marzuk, P.M., H. Tierney, K. Tardiff, E.M. Gross, E.B. Morgan, et al. (1988) Increased risk of suicide in persons with AIDS. *Journal of the American Medical Association* 259:1333-1337.

Mauss, M. (1925) *The Gift: Forms and Functions of Exchange in Archaic Societies*. New York: Norton, 1967.

Murphy, T.F. (1991) No time for an AIDS backlash. *Hastings Center Report* 21(2):7-11.

Murray, T.H. (1991) The poisoned gift: AIDS and blood. In D. Nelkin, D.P. Willis, and S. Parris, eds., *A Disease of Society: Cultural and Institutional Responses to AIDS*. New York: Cambridge University Press.

National Commission on AIDS (1991) *America Living with AIDS: Transforming Anger, Fear and Indifference into Action*. Washington, D.C.: National Commission on AIDS.

Navarre, M. (1988) Fighting the victim label. In D. Crimp, ed., *AIDS: Cultural Analysis/ Cultural Activism*. Cambridge, Mass.: MIT Press.

Perrow, C., and M.F. Guillen (1990) *The AIDS Disaster: The Failure of Organizations in New York and the Nation*. New Haven, Conn.: Yale University Press.

Philadelphia Commission on AIDS (1988) *Report to the Community*. Philadelphia, Pa.: Philadelphia Commission on AIDS.

President's Commission for the Study of Ethical Problems in Medicine and Biomedical and Behavioral Research (1982) *Making Health Care Decisions: The Ethical and Legal Implications of Informed Consent in the Patient-Practitioner Relationship*. Washington, D.C.: U.S. Government Printing Office.

Rist, D.Y. (1989) Exchange. *The Nation* 248(June 19):834.

Rivera, R.R. (1989) Lawyers, clients, and AIDS: some notes from the trenches. *Ohio State Law Journal* 49:883-928.

Seltzer, M., and K.M. Galvin (1991) Organized philanthropy's response to AIDS. *Nonprofit and Voluntary Sector Quarterly* 20:249-266.

Spiers, H.R. (1989) AIDS and civil disobedience. *Hastings Center Report* 19:34-35.

Titmuss, R.M. (1970) *The Gift Relationship: From Human Blood to Social Policy*. London: Allen & Unwin.

Wallace, R. (1988) A synergism of plagues: "planned shrinkage," contagious housing destruction and AIDS in the Bronx. *Environmental Research* 47:1-33.

Winkle, C.R. (1991) Inequity and power in the nonprofit sector: a comparative analysis of AIDS-related services for gay men and intravenous drug users in Chicago. *Nonprofit and Voluntary Sector Quarterly* 20:313-328.

7

Correctional Systems

As the nation's prison population burgeons, so too does the population of inmates with HIV disease. The presence of HIV-infected prisoners within correctional facilities raises a host of issues. Some concerns relate to public health: drug use or sexual activity within prisons may contribute to the spread of HIV infection; at the same time, the prison setting provides opportunities to encourage prisoners to avoid behaviors that transmit the virus. Other concerns relate to the adequacy of medical treatment and access to experimental therapies that characterize much of AIDS care. And the stigma and fear associated with HIV pose special challenges for correctional officials charged with the day-to-day management of prisons and jails.

In seeking to gauge the impact of AIDS in a society, correctional facilities are convenient units of social analysis. Prisons and jails typify *total institutions*: they are "place[s] of residence and work where large numbers of like-situated individuals, cut off from the wider society for an appreciable period of time, together lead an enclosed, formally administered round of life" (Goffman, 1961:xiii). The ready availability of prisoners makes them easy to study, at least in some respects. Indeed, a growing literature on the impact of AIDS on prisons and corrections has emerged. Various mandatory and voluntary HIV-antibody screening programs also provide some information of the extent of HIV disease in prisons, although some prisoners' rights groups have questioned the focus on prisoners in HIV-seroprevalence studies (Hammett and Dubler, 1990:496):

Staff of the New York Prisoner's Rights Project (PRP) oppose singling out inmates for epidemiologic studies of HIV infection. Prisoners, they argue, offer no particular characteristics unavailable in the free population, except that they can be conveniently studied. According to PRP staff, convenience should not be a governing factor in the approval of such research [citation omitted].

Among the recent studies are the surveys on AIDS in correctional institutions conducted by Abt Associates under contract to the National Institute of Justice (Hammett et al., 1989; Moini and Hammett, 1990). These surveys of various prison systems provide information on policy trends related to such issues as housing and segregation of prisoners with HIV/AIDS, AIDS education, conjugal visitation, and health care access. In most cases the data compiled represent the official responses of correctional administrators, however, and actual practices within institutions may diverge from stated policy. Other sources of information are also available. The subject of HIV in prisons has been given much attention in state legislatures (Gostin, 1989). Litigation concerning HIV in prisons has continued unabated throughout the epidemic, and judicial opinions and court records tell much of the story of AIDS in prisons (see Greenspan, 1989; Gostin, 1990; Gostin, Porter, and Sandomire, 1990). Prisoners have challenged specific practices related to attempts to control the spread of HIV.[1] Prisoners with HIV disease have sued to protest their segregation from the general prison population (Branham, 1990), and HIV-negative prisoners have sued to try to force the segregation of those with HIV disease. In some lawsuits, HIV treatment has become part of larger claims related to the adverse consequences of overcrowding on environmental health and safety, medical care, and violence within institutions. In addition to court battles, journalistic accounts also offer powerful, if impressionistic, evidence of the impact of HIV on prisons (Applebome, 1989; Boodman, 1989; Lambert, 1989), as do writings of prisoners themselves (Starchild, 1989).

When evidence from all of these sources is adduced, it is not a simple matter to sort out the impact of HIV on prisons versus that of overcrowding, other threats to health and safety, and the lack of funds, equipment, and trained health care personnel. Some aspects of prison life related to transmission of HIV, such as drug use and sexual activity behind bars, are not readily subject to scrutiny. Institutional administrators, who control the access of researchers to prison facilities, are reluctant to even admit that such activities occur. Prisoners themselves are unwilling to share information about activities that might subject them to further sanctions. Information about the impact of AIDS on jails and juvenile detention centers is especially difficult to obtain, partly because of the rapid turnover of people detained in those institutions.

Finally, to focus only on what transpires *within* the prison walls as it relates to HIV is a mistake: such a perspective fails to capture the range of social impacts on prison staff, prisoners, and their families and friends. What transpires in prisons has a great deal to do with the social life of many inner-city neighborhoods, even if the prisons are located on rolling hillsides, hundreds of miles away. The correctional enterprise, through the parole system, remains involved in many prisoners' lives long after they leave the institution. For many offenders, moreover, prisons have revolving doors. HIV disease may also play a role in decisions about charging criminal defendants, determining the term of incarceration when sentencing prisoners, and deciding when to release prisoners to the community.

This chapter first presents a brief overview of the U.S. prison population and then examines the scope of HIV disease in prisons and its impact on prisoners and prison administration. Among the issues addressed are prison policies regarding HIV testing and screening, segregation of HIV-infected prisoners, prisoner access to routine health care and to experimental treatment, and policies regarding the transfer and release of prisoners with HIV disease.

WHO ARE THE PRISONERS

Approximately 1 million individuals are currently confined in prisons and local jails in the United States (Associated Press, 1991; Mauer, 1991).[2] The prison population has grown every day since 1974; recent growth is the largest since the federal government began keeping annual records in 1926 (Johnson, 1990). Of every 100,000 U.S. residents, 426 are incarcerated; among black men, the number is 3,109 per 100,000.[3] Spending on federal and state prisoners in the United States approaches $25 billion annually (Malcolm, 1991). Since the beginning of the HIV epidemic (approximately 1980), the population in federal prisons and in prisons in the District of Columbia and 18 states has doubled; in California and New Jersey, two states particularly hard hit by the HIV/AIDS epidemic, the number of inmates tripled during the same period (National Commission on AIDS, 1991).

Most commentators have attributed the dramatic increase in the U.S. prison population to mandatory minimum sentences (commonly associated with drug and weapons offenses and sexual assaults and other violent crimes) and restrictive parole eligibility criteria. Langan (1991) holds that the most important factor has been higher imprisonment rates (prosecutors obtaining more felony convictions and judges meting out more prison sentences), which Langan says account for 51 percent of the increase in state prison populations from 1974 to 1986. By contrast, imprisonment for drug offenses accounts for only 8 percent of the increase (although the increase may be greater in recent years, and many property crimes are drug related).

The growing prison population has resulted in significant overcrowding, which may be the most intractable problem in all jurisdictions. Difficulties in maintaining tolerable living conditions, delivering health care, and establishing security follow in the wake of overcrowding—problems that can undermine the efforts of even the most well-intentioned administrators. Nearly 40 states are operating prisons under court orders concerning overcrowding (Malcolm, 1991).

The incarcerated population in the United States comprises in large part impoverished individuals from urban areas. Almost one-half of all prisoners are African American (48 percent, compared with 11 percent in the population at large). In a report based on data from the Justice Department's Bureau of Justice Statistics, the Sentencing Project, a sentence reform organization based in Washington, D.C., noted that 23 percent of African American men between the ages of 20 and 29 are under the control of some component of the criminal justice system (Mauer, 1990). This compares with 6 percent for white males and 10.4 percent for Hispanic men, and 3 percent, 1 percent, and 2 percent, respectively for black, white, and Hispanic women in the same age group. The majority of prisoners are not only members of racial and ethnic minority groups, they are also overwhelmingly poor. It is difficult to find a simple indicator of inmates' socioeconomic level, but some estimates have put the proportion of inmates who are poor at as high as 90 percent (Montefiore Medical Center, 1990). They are also less educated than the general population. In New York City jails, where as many as 25 percent of the inmates are estimated to be HIV positive, about 50 percent of the inmates have completed high school, 30 percent are high school dropouts, and 16 percent have finished only elementary school or have no formal schooling (Montefiore Medical Center, 1990).

Women are also a growing proportion of the nation's prison population. Often overlooked because, historically, small number of women have been incarcerated, the situation is changing. In 1980 13,000 women were in federal and state prisons; by 1989 the number had grown to approximately 41,000. In 1989 alone the female prison population grew by 25 percent, nearly twice the rate of the male prison population. The traditional role of women in caring for children raises special concerns when they are incarcerated: 80 percent of female prisoners have children, and of those, 70 percent are single parents. Prior to their incarceration, 85 percent of female prisoners had custody of their children (compared with 47 percent of male prisoners). A significant proportion of women, moreover, give birth just prior to or during incarceration. In New York City jails, approximately 8 percent of female inmates are pregnant at the time of incarceration (National Commission on AIDS, 1991).

THE BURDEN OF HIV DISEASE IN PRISONS

A first step in examining the impact of AIDS on prisons and jails is to determine the extent of HIV/AIDS among inmates. As with studies of HIV seroprevalence in general, a mosaic of seroprevalence studies can be pieced together that depict HIV prevalence in prisons (Glass et al., 1988; Vlahov et al., 1989, 1990, 1991; Hoxie et al., 1990; Singleton et al., 1990). Systematic overviews and comparisons of HIV prevalence in prisons, however, are very limited by methodological and temporal differences among the studies.[4]

States that have conducted mass screening programs with mandatory, identity-linked testing of all incoming or current inmates or releasees have largely been the ones with relatively low rates of HIV seropositives. For example, positive seroprevalence rates among inmates entering correctional facilities conducting mass screening in 1986 and 1987 was 0 percent in Idaho, 0.1 percent in South Dakota, 0.2 percent in Nebraska and Indiana, 0.3 percent in Wisconsin, 0.4 percent in Colorado, and 0.9 percent in Michigan (Moini and Hammett, 1990). In contrast, seropositivity rates were 7.0 percent in Maryland and 17.4 percent in New York, where surveys involved anonymous, blinded testing.

Vlahov and colleagues (1991) surveyed inmates at 10 correctional facilities, chosen for geographical diversity and to allow comparisons between prisons and jails. The individual institutions were not identified. Their sample of 10,994 entrants between June 1988 and March 1989 revealed positive seroprevalence rates ranging from 2.1 to 7.6 percent for men and from 2.5 to 14.7 percent for women. In 9 of the 10 facilities surveyed, the rate was higher among women than men, especially among those aged 25 or younger (5.2 percent for women and 2.3 percent for men). The overall HIV seropositivity rate for nonwhites was nearly twice that for whites, 4.8 and 2.5 percent, respectively.

The geographical distribution of AIDS cases in prisons and jails is also severely skewed; some prison systems have few or no cases, and others are overwhelmed.[5] As of 1989, 45 of 50 state correctional systems reported at least one inmate with AIDS, but 79 percent of the inmates with AIDS were concentrated within 7 of 51 prison and jail systems (14 percent) surveyed by Hammett and colleagues (Moini and Hammett, 1990). By late 1989, 5,411 confirmed cases of AIDS had been reported by federal prisons, state prisons, and a sampling of county and city jail systems.

Correctional institutions in California, Florida, New Jersey, New York, and Texas have been particularly hard hit by AIDS. It is in these states that the impact of AIDS has been most palpable and where the numbers tell a good part of the story. For example, New York State prisons currently house more than 54,000 inmates, approximately 17 to 20 percent of whom are HIV positive. Of the 9,000 or so HIV-positive prisoners, at least 800 show symptoms of AIDS. Since the beginning of the epidemic, 850 people have died of AIDS while in the custody of New York's prison system (Potler, 1988; National Commission on AIDS, 1991).

Testing and Screening Controversies

The question of whether to screen inmates for HIV antibodies has arisen with particular urgency in the prison setting, and considerable resources have been expended in legislative debate and in court challenges of testing and screening practices. Prison administrators have been under pressure from legislators, city and county officials, correctional officers, and inmates themselves to conduct mandatory screening of all inmates and to identify seropositive inmates. Many actors in the prison drama have asserted a "need to know" information about HIV serostatus.

As in the outside world, proposals for mandatory, identity-linked screening of prisoners have raised questions related to the accuracy of test results and the appropriate balance between resources expended for screening and other educational activities. Critics of mandatory HIV-antibody screening of prisoners have been skeptical of the public health, clinical, or behavioral justification for such programs, although the advent of efficacious early therapeutic intervention is muting some of the criticisms. Critics of mandatory screening have also pointed to the special difficulties in keeping health information confidential in a prison setting. In some instances, HIV-positive inmates have been forced to disclose their status to parole boards, family members, sexual partners, and in at least one state (Alabama), potential employers (Freeman, 1991).

A number of prison systems, as noted, have conducted blinded, anonymous seroprevalence studies from which data are available only in the aggregate and individual inmates are not told the results (Hammett and Dubler, 1990). Informed consent is generally not sought, and inmates are often not told a study is being conducted. Most HIV seroprevalence and transmission studies in prisons have used portions of blood drawn from all inmates for independent purposes, such as entry or annual physicals. Some commentators have raised ethical concerns about blinded seroprevalence studies (Bayer, Lumey, and Wan, 1990). Under the design of blinded studies, seropositive individuals cannot be apprised of their status, a practical concern now that there is evidence of efficacious treatments that can be administered before symptoms develop. Others have suggested that blinded epidemiologic studies "risk stigmatizing the entire [prison] population" (Hammett and Dubler, 1990:496).

In some states, prison officials have had to rethink their approach to identity-linked HIV antibody screening when the results began to come in. A few states (e.g., New Mexico and South Dakota) abandoned their programs when they found low seropositivity rates. Other states (e.g., Arkansas and Texas) screen on the basis of apparent risk factors, testing intravenous drug users, prostitutes, self-identified gay men, and those with clinical symptoms of sexually transmitted diseases, tuberculosis, or HIV infection. According to Jan Diamond, a physician at the California Medical Facility at Vacaville State Prison (quoted in Smith, 1991:29):

> The prison administration knows they do not have the capacity to handle everyone who is infected, so they are not eager to find out. For a long time the California legislature wanted to institute mandatory testing of prisoners, followed by quarantine of the infected, ostensibly to stop transmission. But when AZT became accepted therapy for treating asymptomatics, they quickly figured out how much it would cost to really know who had the virus and they dropped their push.

Most prison systems offer HIV antibody testing on a voluntary basis. In Oregon's program, which is characterized by aggressive educational efforts and individualized risk assessments, two-thirds of the inmates volunteered to be tested in a study conducted from September 1987 to January 1988 (Andrus et al., 1989). In a sample of 977 newly incarcerated inmates, only 1.2 percent (12) were HIV positive, despite the fact that 63 percent (611) of the sample reported having engaged in risk behaviors. For each inmate who had engaged in a risk behavior and seroconverted, 53 had not, which underscores the potential of education and counseling in preventing HIV transmission.

Transmission Within Prisons

Very little data are available on how many prisoners become infected *while* in prison. Even when retesting is conducted among prisoners who were seronegative at intake, the "window" period of seroconversion (during which HIV-infected individuals test negative with available screening methods) makes it impossible to tell whether those who later test positive actually became infected while in prison. Impressions from fragmentary data gathered in Maryland and Nevada suggest that transmission rates among inmates while in prison may be quite low (Horsburgh et al., 1990). In an analysis of AIDS cases in New York State and Florida, only a small percentage of the inmates had been incarcerated for more than 2 years prior to their diagnosis in prison, which makes it unlikely that the majority became infected while in prison. Another transmission study is being conducted among male Illinois prison inmates, using blinded blood samples collected at two sequential annual physicals (Hammett and Dubler, 1990), but no data are yet available.

Data from the Federal Bureau of Prisons based on time-interval tests indicate extremely small rates of seroconversion while in prison. Of approximately 98,000 HIV-antibody tests, 14 previously seronegative inmates were positive on retesting. All of the 14 inmates seroconverted within the first 6 months of incarceration, which suggests they had become infected prior to imprisonment. Moreover, seroprevalence rates for releasees from federal prisons continue to be lower than for incoming inmates, which also suggests little, if any, seroconversion within federal prisons. This is not to say that transmission of the virus never occurs in correctional settings. The fact that inmates acquire sexually transmitted diseases with incubation periods of days or weeks is evidence that sex occurs in jails, and the sexual transmission of HIV is possible.[6]

Prison sex is a particularly sensitive issue, and it has received more attention since the AIDS epidemic began (A Federal Prisoner, 1991). Both in the popular imagination and in actuality, sex in prisons includes violent, forcible rape.[7] Prison sex may also be "consensual," although consent is always suspect in the prison context (Lockwood, 1980; Propper, 1981). Submission to sexual overtures may involve outright intimidation or bargaining in exchange for protection, commissary items, or other favors. New inmates and openly gay or effeminate inmates may be particularly vulnerable to forced sex. The prevalence of all types of sexual activity most likely varies from institution to institution. There have been few studies of sexual activity in prisons. The most frequently cited involve anecdotal evidence collected prior to the AIDS epidemic (see studies reviewed in Hammett and Moini, 1988:55-56).

Perhaps surprisingly, however, it is concern about the spread of HIV by seropositive prisoners through other than sexual means that has preoccupied judges and correctional staff. Much of the focus has been on modes of transmission highly unlikely to transmit the virus, such as by casual contact or through food. There have been 40 or more criminal cases involving assaultive behavior by HIV-positive inmates, (e.g., biting, spitting, or throwing the contents of slop buckets at prison officials), but there has not yet been a case documented in the medical literature of HIV transmission to a correctional worker or inmate in such a manner. In one case a prisoner sued correctional officials for failure to isolate an HIV-positive inmate who bit him, claiming that failure to do so violated his Eighth Amendment rights to be free from cruel and unusual punishment (*Cameron* v. *Metcuz*, 705 F. Supp 454 (N.D. Ind. 1989)). In another instance, an HIV-positive inmate saved up his saliva in a bucket to pour over a particularly despised guard. Although relatively few in number, the cases involving assaultive behavior by an HIV-positive inmate have tested the ability of the courts to sort out scientific data about transmission risks from fears and prejudices (Burris, 1990).

Other potential mechanisms of disease spread are unique to prison culture. Because razor blades are difficult to acquire in prisons, inmates commonly share them and thus risk exposure to contaminated blood. Tattooing and ear piercing are also common among inmates, who are resourceful in finding sources of pigment and instruments for such purposes. Instruments used in tattooing can be a mode of disease transmission when not sterilized between use. There is also "spitback methadone," whereby a prisoner swallows and regurgitates methadone for later use.

Some commentators have urged that greater attention be given to the prison as a setting for counseling for intravenous drug users, especially those who are young and might otherwise be unlikely to seek drug abuse treatment for several years (Lampinen, Brewer, and Raba, 1991). Drug use continues within prisons, and ingenious methods and the cooperation of guards and visitors are used to smuggle drugs into the prison (Dash, 1990).

HIV Education and Prevention

Most prison and jail systems have instituted some kind of educational program for inmates and staff concerning HIV prevention. The nature and quality of these efforts vary considerably from jurisdiction to jurisdiction. Many local jails rely almost exclusively on written or audiovisual materials. Most state and federal prisons, on the other hand, conduct AIDS education sessions led by trained staff members.

Prisoners have special needs with regard to AIDS education. Materials must be geared toward the sensitivities of racial and ethnic minorities. Moreover, many prisoners are illiterate or do not speak English, and less than one-fourth of correctional systems have made special provisions for AIDS education in this regard. As one solution, the National Commission on AIDS (1991) recommended strengthening the role of community-based organizations in providing educational and support services for inmates and their families. One of the most promising solutions is the use of prisoners as peer educators, although only a few systems report having adopted such programs. One of the earliest and most successful such programs, initiated by the prisoners themselves, is at Bedford Hills prison for women in New York State. Women in prison have special needs for targeted AIDS education that have often been overlooked (Viadro and Earp, 1991), and peer educators can be expected to be sensitive to those needs and know how to communicate with women about them.

With regard to prevention, one specific aspect that continues to vex prison administrators is the propriety of distributing condoms to inmates. As noted, an undeniable, if difficult to quantify, amount of sexual activity takes place within prisons (van Hoeven, Rooney, and Joseph, 1990). Many inmates are aware of the risk of HIV and other sexually transmitted diseases, as evidenced by an illicit market for plastic wrap and similar items that can provide barrier protection when used in sexual activity. Nevertheless, the distribution of condoms continues to be resisted by prison officials, who are unwilling to admit the extent of same-gender sexual contact among prisoners or to appear to condone such behavior among prisoners. Fears have also been voiced that condoms might be used as weapons or as containers to smuggle drugs. According to the National Commission on AIDS (1991), however, condom distribution has not disrupted prison operations in the few systems that distribute them.

Vermont was the first state in which the prison system distributed condoms. Mississippi, Philadelphia, San Francisco County, and New York City are among the few other jurisdictions that allow condom distribution (Hammett et al., 1989). As one proponent graphically explained (Rooney, 1990:63-64):

> What we did [to convince officials to allow the distribution of condoms] was to prove to Corrections that sexual intercourse did take place in a correctional setting by proving to them a substantial number of cases of acquired gonorrhea, oral, urethral, and rectal.

When condoms were first introduced in New York City jails, uniquely colored condoms were used so they could be distinguished from commercially available condoms in the event they were used to smuggle drugs from visitors. Such fears about condom distribution have not been realized, however. The way in which condoms are made available has much to do with whether they are actually used. Distributing condoms under the "medical model" has proven palatable to some correctional officials who otherwise resisted allowing their use. Making them available only by prescription or only through the prison pharmacy, however, may significantly limit access and use. In Philadelphia, condoms are available to inmates on intake into the facility, at AIDS education sessions, and at "medication call." A report by the U.S. Conference of Mayors (1989:5, 8) described how the process works:

> Depending on the jail, condoms are placed in shoe boxes or buckets and left for residents to voluntarily pick up at the sick call dispensary, thus allowing for non-personal disbursal to avoid embarrassment or identification with unallowed sexual activity. . . . During education sessions, condoms are enclosed in a packet of information so as to reduce residents' anxiety about being seen taking condoms.

Housing and Segregation

Prior to the AIDS epidemic, prison officials often faced questions about where to house specific types of prisoners. Many prisons, for example, have special units for sex offenders or inmates with a propensity for violence; those convicted of capital offenses are commonly housed together on a "death row." Some prisons designate units for openly gay or effeminate inmates, and transvestites to protect them from predatory behavior. For 15 years a central Florida jail segregated homosexuals and forced them to wear pink arm bands (Associated Press, 1989).

Since the AIDS epidemic began, many jurisdictions have been faced with decisions about the advisability of segregating asymptomatic HIV-positive prisoners or those with AIDS. Segregation decisions have been justified on the grounds of inmate security, the possible risk of transmission of HIV, or availability of specialized health services. In some aspects the prison debate mirrors concerns of health care providers about the creation of AIDS-dedicated hospital wards or medical facilities (see Chapter 3). Is the creation of an AIDS-dedicated prison unit a way of delivering health care more efficiently by those with specialized training, a way of protecting the health of inmates whose immune systems are compromised, or merely an administrative convenience, which will exacerbate the stigma that attaches to AIDS?

A number of potential harms are inherent in blanket segregation of HIV-infected inmates. Isolating HIV-positive prisoners labels them in the eyes of all other inmates and staff and may put them at greater risk of assault and discrimination.[8] Segregation often limits prisoners' access to a wide range of prison activities, such as religious services, visitation, and drug treatment programs (e.g., Alcoholics Anonymous or Narcotics Anonymous). It also limits access to libraries, educational and recreational facilities, and work: many jurisdictions exclude known HIV-positive prisoners from food service positions, despite the lack of evidence of any danger in this regard.[9] In some prisons, segregation of inmates with HIV disease has resulted in harrowing conditions, some of which have been the subject of journalistic exposés and court challenges.[10] Furthermore, the segregation of HIV-positive prisoners may give a false sense of security about the risk of HIV transmission, however. Because of the window period for seroconversion, even widespread screening programs are unlikely to identify all HIV-positive entrants, and this HIV transmission may still be a possibility within the general prison population. As one official reported (Maisonet, 1990:96-97):

> [with segregation of HIV-positive inmates] the inmates themselves believe that they are now safe. My greatest problem now is having putatively heterosexual men continually solicit sexual favors from our effeminate male homosexuals. . . . Segregated housing has created a myth that we don't have to worry about HIV in the general [prison] population . . . . Most inmates who are HIV positive have not been identified and are still involving themselves in high risk behavior.

HIV status can overwhelm a wide range of relevant considerations in decisions about where to house prisoners. According to Catherine A. Hanssens, of the New Jersey Public Advocate's Office (National Commission on AIDS, 1991:23):

> In the New Jersey prison system, AIDS is the great equalizer; a prisoner's AIDS diagnosis substitutes for the system of classification based on the offense, prior record and incarcerations, institutional behavior, staff evaluations and similar factors by which all other offenders, including those with other types of chronic illnesses, are judged. Only one other group of prisoners in the New Jersey state system is subject to automatic segregation without periodic review for consideration of return to the general population—those under a sentence of death.

At least 20 state prisons segregate all prisoners with AIDS; 8 segregate those with AIDS-related complex; and 6 segregate inmates who are HIV positive but not symptomatic (Moini and Hammett, 1990). The courts have thus far rejected efforts to either compel or stop the segregation of prisoners with HIV disease. Judges have viewed isolation and segregation as matters of prison administration rather than public health and have shown a "marked propensity" to "uphold the administrative discretion of corrections officials unless their conduct is arbitrary or capricious" (Gostin, Porter, and Sandomire, 1990:18).

The trend in state and federal prisons has been away from blanket policies that segregate prisoners solely on the basis of HIV status. In a majority of state systems, individualized clinical or behavioral assessments are the basis for segregation decisions. In city and county jails, segregation of all AIDS cases is only slightly more prevalent than individualized determinations, 46 and 43 percent, respectively (Moini and Hammett, 1990).

Visitation Policies

In states with many prisoners with HIV disease, prison administrators have also had to reexamine their policies related to visitation, including conjugal visitations. Prior to the HIV/AIDS epidemic, correctional administrators advanced a number of justifications for conjugal visits: conjugal visits provide for sexual and emotional release; some believe that they reduce the level of homosexual activity in prison, although there is no definitive evidence in that regard; and conjugal visits may help provide for a smoother release back into society by helping to maintain or reestablish family ties. Their attractiveness to prisoners means that they are a significant privilege and their granting or denial can be a reward or punishment (Bates, 1989). In many states, inmates with HIV disease have been refused not only conjugal visits with spouses but also visits with parents, siblings, or children. Gay male and lesbian prisoners are never allowed conjugal visits with their lovers.

MEDICAL TREATMENT

Prisoners' Health and Access to Care

It is difficult to gauge the impact of HIV disease on the health of the prison population, in part because of the lack of epidemiologic data related to prisoners' health status. Most studies tend to focus instead on the adequacy of health services (Hammett and Dubler, 1990). The prison population, as noted, is drawn disproportionately from minority groups and the urban poor, whose overall health status has been declining in recent years. Studies of the health of prisoners prior to the AIDS epidemic cited a number of problems related to poverty, drug use, and lack of access to care that had imperiled inmates' health before they were incarcerated (Barton, 1974; Marini, Bridges, and Sheard, 1978). One study summed up the current situation by stating that "prisoners now arrive at lock up sicker than at any time in the last 50 years" (Shenson, Dubler, and Michaels, 1990:655).

A report from the Montefiore Medical Center (1990), which provides medical and mental health care services under contract to Rikers Island, a New York City jail, recently called for more systematic attention to gathering data on prisoners' health status. The report did, however, record its impressions of the health status of prisoners under the care of the Montefiore Medical Center (1990:3):

> Because many prisoners come from the most disadvantaged sectors of our population, they reflect the epidemiology of these communities. Recent trauma is often encountered in the clinical setting. . . . HIV infection, venereal diseases, hypertension, substance abuse, asthma, abnormal liver function tests, dental cavities and missing teeth are frequently seen (p. 2).

The report goes on to speculate about the impact of HIV (p. 3):

> A high prevalence of HIV infection has dramatically altered the nature of routine medical care. . . . Generalized lymphadenopathy, oral candidiasis, herpes zoster, and seborrheic dermatitis have increased in frequency and must now be evaluated in the context of HIV-related superinfections such as tuberculosis, pneumocystis pneumonia, cryptococcal meningitis, and cryptosporidial infection. Provision of medical therapies directly related to HIV infection, such as zidovudine, immunizations, and pneumocystis prophylaxis, require significant allocations of medical, nursing, and pharmacy services.

One barometer of the imperiled health status of inmates has been the resurgence of tuberculosis in correctional facilities (Braun et al., 1989; Snider and Hutton, 1989). Unlike HIV, tuberculosis can be spread through the air, and poor sanitary conditions and prison overcrowding contribute to its spread. HIV is a major risk factor for the development of tuberculosis among individuals infected with the tubercle bacillus. Intravenous drug users appear to be at higher risk for tuberculosis than other HIV risk groups. One study of a cohort of 260 HIV-positive intravenous drug users in Baltimore sought to assess the relative risk of purified protein derivative (PPD) tuberculin positivity: age, receiving public assistance, history of arrest, and duration of drug use were associated with increased relative odds of being PPD positive. The study illustrates the difficulties in sorting out the discrete impact of incarceration. Although the association between arrest and PPD positivity suggests that transmission of tuberculosis infection may be occurring in prisons, the authors' multivariate analysis actually suggests that "previous arrest is just another marker for an impoverished lifestyle, extended time using drugs, and other risk behavior" (Graham et al., 1992:373). A Centers for Disease Control (1989) survey of 29 states in 1984-1985 found inmates to be three times as likely to develop tuberculosis as age-matched controls who were not incarcerated. In 1989, all of the 70 cases of active tuberculosis identified in New York State prisons were among prisoners who were also HIV positive (National Commission on AIDS, 1991).

Prison health care embodies some distinct paradoxes. The goals of medicine and corrections are frequently at cross-purposes. Medicine seeks to heal, extend life, and relieve suffering. In furtherance of these goals, a high value is placed on the quality of the doctor-patient relationship and the confidentiality that helps to foster it. Prisons exist to confine, punish, and perhaps, rehabilitate. Many aspects of the correctional enterprise impinge on health care delivery. Moreover, according to Prout and Ross (1988:130): "Access to medical care is a loaded emotional issue for inmates who have a lot of time to think about their own physical and emotional states, who crave opportunities to test the system, and who feel isolated and alienated from normal, safe human contact."

Health workers may also find the prison system difficult to negotiate. Physicians must cede to prison administrators some of the authority and control they have in most health care settings. The milieu in which prison health care is delivered is also generally dreary. The preeminence of security concerns means that health care workers, together with the inmates, are isolated from the community while they work. These factors combine to make it difficult to recruit and retain quality medical care staff, yet dedicated and professional medical staff make a major difference in the care of HIV disease within prisons. In a few prison settings, prisoners with AIDS have been offered state-of-the-art drug therapies because individual physicians have been diligent in seeking out information from knowledgeable colleagues and pressing institutional administrators for support.

Prisons have historically been backwaters of health care, yet inmates are virtually the only group with a constitutional right to health care.[11] In 1976 the Supreme Court held that "deliberate indifference" to the serious medical needs of inmates violates the Eighth Amendment to the Constitution that bars cruel and unusual punishment (*Estelle* v. *Gamble*, 429 U.S. 97 (1976)). The Court reasoned that because prisoners are unable to seek care anywhere else while in custody, to fail to provide them care would be "unnecessary and wanton" infliction of pain. The "deliberate indifference" standard articulated by the Supreme Court and fleshed out in subsequent case law is not a very demanding one. The establishment of a constitutional right to at least some level of health care has been a useful tool in litigation, but advocates for better prison health care still have an uphill battle. Burris (1990:3, 14) provided the following interpretation of the law in the context of AIDS-related health care:

> For the most part, the law provides prisoners, as such and as people with HIV, with negative rights—rights not to be abused. The legal system is more open to a claim that a particular medical procedure was improperly denied than that inmates are entitled to the most effective medical care possible, more open to a claim that an inmate has suffered discrimination than a claim that a prison ought to be educating staff and prisoners about HIV. . . .
>
> Prison medical care is not required to be very good, and many prisons live down to that low standard. AIDS patients do not get very good treatment, but neither do heart patients or back patients. When conditions are bad enough, a general attack on medical care, or care of people with AIDS, may have a better chance of success than a single inmate's complaint, but such a case requires an enormous investment in collecting and presenting the factual evidence. On the other hand, a suit for a specific treatment known to be effective, like AZT, may be easier to conduct than a global challenge, but a judge who does not see the systemic failures in care is more likely to indulge what a prison will likely claim is an isolated failure.

Many state prisons and local jails do not have the facilities to treat sick prisoners. Often the highest level of care available is infirmary care. New York State has a total of 36 beds available for treating prisoners with AIDS; an estimated 1,200 inmates have symptoms of HIV. In New York City, the jails have access to six skilled-care nursing beds, which are always filled. According to prisoners' rights advocates, the lack of prison health facilities leads to "chaining, like dogs, sick and debilitated prisoners to their hospital beds in regular civilian wards—a practice called 'outposting'—or in being shuttled between hospital and prison infirmary—a practice referred to by City officials as 'ping-ponging'" (Wiseman, 1990:8).

The lack of appropriate, state-of-the-art health care has taken its toll on inmates' lives, at least according to some observers. A study conducted by the Correctional Association of New York found that the median time between diagnosis and death was 159 days for intravenous-drug-using prisoners with AIDS, compared with 318 days for nonprisoner intravenous drug users. Of the cases reviewed, 25 percent were not diagnosed as AIDS until autopsy (Dubler, Bergmann, and Frankel, 1990:368, n. 24). One New York study found a mortality rate of 22 percent for prisoners with a first bout of *Pneumocystis carinii* pneumonia (PCP), the most common cause of AIDS deaths, compared with 8 percent for patients in the community. The key recommendation of the Presidential Commission on the Human Immunodeficiency Virus Epidemic (1988:135) in the area of corrections was that "care and treatment available to HIV-infected inmates in correctional facilities should be equal to that available to HIV-infected individuals in the general community." The gulf between what is generally available to HIV-infected prisoners and what is available on the outside, however, appears to be widening with the advent of early intervention to treat HIV disease.

According to National Institute of Justice surveys (whose data, as noted, are admittedly incomplete and reflect official policy, not necessarily actual practice), by November 1989 (Hammett and Dubler, 1990:489) "less than one-third of correctional systems were providing AZT to all HIV seropositive inmates with CD4 . . . counts below 500," although all systems with 50 or more cumulative AIDS cases reportedly met the Public Health Service's standard for providing for AZT. PCP prophylaxis was not as readily available (Hammett and Dubler, 1990:489):

> Just over half (58 percent) of state/federal prison systems and less than half (39 percent) of city/county jail systems . . . had policies in compliance with these PHS standards . . . . Less than half of the correctional systems with more than 50 cumulative AIDS cases (four of 11 prison systems and two of five jail systems) meet new standards for aerosolized pentamidine.

In evaluating prisoners' access to care and treatment for HIV, it is important to keep in mind a critical feature of prison health care. Health care for prisoners is supported by state and federal corrections budgets. Prisoners are not eligible for conventional public entitlement health care programs, such as Medicaid or Medicare. In most instances, funds for HIV care in prisons have had to come from corrections health care budgets, and they have remained static as prison populations have skyrocketed. In New York State, for example, two-thirds of the correctional system's health care budget of approximately $100 million is earmarked for HIV care. In New Jersey, the state supreme court stopped the practice of giving hospitalized prisoners emergency releases in order to avoid putting the burden of paying for health care on public hospital programs (*Saint Barnabas Medical Center v. Essex County*, 111 N.J. 67 (1988)).

One trend of interest—although not directly related to the HIV/AIDS epidemic—is the "privatization" of prisons. Increasingly, states are contracting with private enterprise to build, staff, and operate prisons, including providing security, food, transportation, and medical care. A number of models of prison health care delivery have been developed with various combinations of public and private services. In some cases, local public health departments or nearby university hospitals are involved in delivering prison health care. In others, private companies, operating in a manner similar to health maintenance organizations, provide health care services under a fixed, annual contract. Incentives to keep costs down may have a particularly harsh impact on HIV-infected prisoners and make it especially difficult for asymptomatic, HIV-positive prisoners to obtain adequate care.

Access to Experimental Treatments

AIDS tests the limits of prison health care because treatments tend to be expensive and difficult to deliver. Often the only treatments possible are experimental and are available only through clinical trials or expanded access programs (see Chapter 4). Prisoners confront formidable barriers in trying to gain access to drugs on clinical trials, and prisoners have access to experimental drugs in early stages of development in only a handful of corrections systems.

Historically, prisoners have been favored research subjects because of their accessibility and the limited expense incurred by their participation. The practice dates back to ancient Rome, where poisonous substances were tested on prisoners. In this century, the Nazi medical experiments on prisoners of war spawned new codes of medical ethics when what had transpired in the name of science came to light at the Nuremberg trials. In the decades following World War II, prisoners in the United States were frequently the subject of medical research, sometimes without their knowledge. Exposés in the 1970s brought to public attention some of the practices involved in testing drugs and vaccines on prisoners, who in journalistic parlance, were "cheaper than chimpanzees" (Mitford, 1973). Many observers believed prisoners' consent to the research to be highly suspect. Simple inducements of decent food, clean sheets, and medical care could mean a great deal to inmates who were otherwise deprived of many necessities and amenities. A stipend of a few dollars a day for participating in research might be considered coercive when compared with the 10 to 25 cents an hour typically earned for prison work.

A new era in medical research began in the 1960s and 1970s with the heightened concern for the rights and welfare of patients and research subjects (National Commission on AIDS, 1991; see Chapter 4). In 1978 federal regulations were adopted to address such issues as informed consent and voluntariness in participation, subject selection, confidentiality, and independent review related to federally funded research (45 C.F.R. 46.301-306 (1978)). In 1983 those regulations were amended to include special provisions that made it difficult to conduct clinical research with prisoners as subjects (45 C.F.R. 46.306 (a)(2)(d)(1983)). Not all prisoners welcomed the benevolent paternalism of the regulators, however. Many prisoners had willingly accepted the risk of participation in research, welcoming both the stipends and the diversion from the daily routine. Moreover, much of the nontherapeutic drug testing in prisoners, involving initial toxicity studies of new drugs, was of minimal risk (Schroeder, 1983). Some prisoners' rights groups asked that inmates be allowed to continue to participate, but their arguments failed to win the day with prison officials, physicians, and regulators.

One lasting impact of the AIDS epidemic on prisons may be a new attitude concerning the participation of prisoners in clinical and epidemiologic research, both on HIV and other diseases of concern in correctional settings. Prior to the AIDS epidemic, most prison medical experimentation involved nontherapeutic research—toxicity assessments and studies of treatments for diseases the prisoners did not have. Today, regulations promulgated to protect prisoners from overreaching and abuse in nontherapeutic research are now perceived as obstructing their access to needed medical care. With HIV disease, the line between research and treatment has never been more blurred.

A number of policy groups have been convened in recent years to address the role of prisoners in clinical and epidemiologic research on AIDS. A group convened by the Division of Law and Ethics in the Department of Epidemiology and Social Medicine at Montefiore Medical Center in New York City concluded that a reasonable interpretation of federal research regulations currently in effect would allow participation of prisoners in clinical trials so long as use of a placebo is not part of the study design (Hammett and Dubler, 1990; Dubler and Sidel, 1991). With this understanding, most AIDS research protocols would be open to prisoners. Other groups, such as the one that met under the auspices of the Washington, D.C.-based AIDS Action Foundation in 1990, have concluded in principle that "with the proper safeguards in place—voluntary decision making, confidentiality, and protections against abuse—prisoners should be permitted access to Phase II and III trials" (Hammett and Dubler, 1990:492).

TRANSFER AND RELEASE CONCERNS

As noted above, the HIV epidemic poses serious concerns about the availability of an appropriate level of services in a system in which access to hospital beds for treatment of acute and chronic conditions is severely limited. Placing prisoners in a setting concomitant with their health care needs is a challenge. Release and transition to community health care are critical, yet often poorly handled. Often "release" is a euphemism for "transfer" (what is known in the argot of teaching hospitals as "turfing") (Pottenger, 1990:2-3):

Transfer . . . is also quite common—from one institution to another, but within the same system. Daily monitoring and treatment is vital for these inmates, and the days, or weeks, that can be lost in the transfer or release process can be fatal. . . . The medical records system in our prison system is in a shambles. Because of the overcrowding and population caps at several facilities, the "midnight special" is a commonplace. . . . These midnight specials spell an exhausting bus ride from one jail to another, and a few hours sleep on a hallway cot or mattress. For HIV-infected inmates, such midnight transfers also mean a change in medical providers—and delays of days or even weeks in shipping medical records. . . . Staying a jump ahead of the medical records [is] a deadly game of tag.

This is the description of the situation in Connecticut prisons by a prisoners' rights advocate, who provides some context for his statement (Pottenger, 1990:3): "Connecticut is unusual in that both its jails and prisons are unified in a single Department of Corrections, so its problem of frequent movements may be more serious than those facing other States."

AIDS has prompted a number of states to reexamine their policies that allow for the release of inmates suffering from a variety of terminal illnesses. Few prison health care systems have the medical, nursing, or social services necessary to take care of dying persons (Kamerman, 1991). Such services are better provided in hospitals, hospices, nursing homes, or in home settings with nursing care support. Prisoners are not a popular political constituency, however. Being perceived as "soft on crime" makes a politician vulnerable to attack, as was evidenced by the influence of the Willie Horton case during the 1988 presidential campaign. Hence, early release for prisoners on compassionate grounds has been viewed warily by politicians. In a few states hard hit by AIDS, legislative proposals to provide for "medical parole" have run afoul of such sentiments.

For prisoners believed to be terminally ill (whether as a result of AIDS, cancer, heart disease, or other illness), a variety of options for shortening their sentences are available. In most states the governor can commute a sick prisoner's sentence by a grant of executive clemency. In some jurisdictions, for some crimes, judges have the option of resentencing prisoners in the event of terminal illness. In some jail systems, detainees who are terminally ill may have their bail reduced to amounts they can afford or be released on their own recognizance under "compassionate release" programs.

There is evidence that some parole boards, rather than seeing HIV illness as a reason to reduce sentences, believe it to be a reason for denying parole (Starchild, 1988, 1989). About one-third of prison systems notify parole boards of prisoners' HIV-positive status. According to Freeman (1991:14-28): "the predictable effect is that HIV-positive prisoners appear to serve, on the average, more time on their sentences than seronegative prisoners."

CONCLUSIONS

Correctional facilities in the United States are straining to cope with unprecedented growth in numbers of inmates—the U.S. prison population has tripled in the last 16 years. Keeping pace with current growth "requires building the equivalent of a 1000-bed prison every 6 days" (Langan, 1991:1568). The influx of prisoners has come at a time when economic hardship is forcing local, state, and federal lawmakers to make difficult choices among social programs. Burgeoning prison populations and budget constraints have resulted in the most intractable problem from jurisdiction to jurisdiction—overcrowding. Overcrowding is challenging the ability of even the most well-meaning correctional officials to house and feed inmates, to maintain order, and to deliver health care.

Prisoners in the United States are disproportionately poor and members of racial or ethnic minorities, as is increasingly the case with people with HIV disease in general. A growing proportion of prisoners are women, many of whom have children. Prison life is hard. Stretches of boredom are often relieved by threats of violence, facilities are often substandard, and it is difficult to gain access to needed medical services. How much of this is changing because of the HIV/AIDS epidemic?

In particularly hard-hit jurisdictions the presence of AIDS is already palpable—prison infirmaries are full of inmates in various stages of HIV disease. Moreover, the inmates already infected are vivid reminders that the number of persons estimated to be HIV seropositive who are not yet symptomatic means there will be many more prisoners with AIDS in the future. In some jurisdictions the impact of AIDS is causing prison officials to reconsider how prison health care is delivered and paid for and to look at new ways to attract and retain quality medical staff. Lawsuits filed on behalf of prisoners to challenge standards of care often include particulars about denial of care for HIV disease although many prison inmates come from community circumstances where it may have been as difficult to obtain needed health care as it is in prison.

One of the most significant impacts of HIV disease in correctional facilities may be a sea change in the way epidemiological and clinical research involving prisoners is viewed. Regulations adopted to protect prisoners from overreaching and exploitation at the hands of drug companies or clinical investigators are now being looked at in an entirely different light when they may block prisoners from receiving experimental treatments.

The behavioral aspects of HIV disease—its spread through the sharing of contaminated injection paraphernalia and unprotected sexual intercourse—is a reminder of both the sexual and drug-using behavior that continues to take place in prisons. It is also a reminder that prisons are not totally insulated. The length of sentences served and recidivism rates mean that prisoners come and go with substantial frequency. Prisoners are also often under the jurisdiction of correctional officials even beyond the time they leave prison. Prisoners maintain links to loved ones, families, and neighborhoods. This has important implications for AIDS prevention and efforts to inculcate changes in behavior that can be maintained once prisoners are released into the community.

NOTES

1. Freeman (1991:4A-1 to 4-B-4) lists AIDS-related legal, educational, and volunteer resources available for prisoners nationwide.

2. Jails house those who are accused of crimes, individuals arraigned and awaiting trial, and those convicted of misdemeanor offenses, for which the sentence is typically less than 1 year. In some systems, individuals may be jailed for considerable lengths of time because of their inability to "make bail," although bail may be as low as a few hundred dollars. Prisons house inmates serving terms of 1 year or more for felony convictions.

3. The United States is first among nations in incarceration rates. South Africa is second, with 333 of every 100,000 incarcerated (and 729 of 100,000 black males). The former Soviet Union is third in incarceration, with 218 of every 100,000 residents (Mauer, 1991).

4. The Federal Bureau of Prisons has engaged in widespread HIV screening, but no longer tests all inmates. Currently, it tests inmates about to be discharged; inmates temporarily released through furlough or halfway-house programs; "predatory" or "promiscuous" inmates; and inmates manifesting clinical symptoms of HIV disease (Federal Bureau of Prisons, 1989).

5. Raw numbers of cases are not necessarily directly proportionate to the social impact of AIDS. As has been well documented in the context of another "total institution," a single schoolchild with AIDS can lead to massive publicity, boycotts, and lawsuits, all demanding significant attention from administrators (Nelkin and Hilgartner, 1986; Kirp et al., 1989). So too, in the prison context, a single incident of an HIV-positive prisoner attacking a guard can be traumatic for the institution as well as the guard.

6. A study of New York City jail inmates found that 10 percent of all gonococcal infections (gonorrhea cases) diagnosed between October and December 1986 were acquired while the inmate was in the correctional facility. The study used gonorrhea as a surrogate for homosexual activity. Since the normal incubation period is 2 to 6 days, any inmate diagnosed with a new case of gonorrhea more than one week after intake was considered to have become infected while in prison (van Hoeven, Rooney, and Joseph, 1990).

7. Some commentators have speculated about a possible relationship between homosexual rape and some prison suicides (Wiggs, 1989).

8. A legal advocate described the practice of one system: The Department had an official policy of labeling all HIV-positive inmates by placing "red dots, of sufficient attention size," on all their medical and prison records, their housing cards, and any transfer papers (Pottenger, 1990).

9. Courts have upheld federal policy that precludes HIV-positive inmates from serving as food service workers, based on the fear of transmission harbored by other inmates. "Inmates may perceive the presence of HIV positive inmates in food service or the hospital as a threat to their own health and well-being and might not adequately avail themselves of these services" (*Farmer* v. *Moritsugu*, DC WWisc. No. 89-C-926-S, 3/36.90); but see *Feigley* v. *Jeffes* (104 Pa. Cmmwlth. 540, 522 A.2d 179 (1987)), finding no public health justification for HIV-antibody screening of food handlers.

10. In the Capshaw, Alabama prison, 130 HIV-positive men are segregated in a building known as "Thunderdorm" (Boodman, 1989; Whitman, 1990).

11. Involuntarily committed patients in mental hospitals also have certain rights to treatment protected by the Constitution.

REFERENCES

A Federal Prisoner (1991) Prisoners of longing: sex behind bars is serious business. *San Francisco Chronicle* January 27:3.

Andrus, J.K., D.W. Fleming, C. Knox, R.O. McAlister, M.R. Skeels, et al. (1989) HIV testing in prisoners: is mandatory testing mandatory? *American Journal of Public Health* 79:840-842.

Applebome, P. (1989) For AIDS inmates, a prison in prison. *New York Times* March 5:A-22.

Associated Press (1989) Pink bracelets for homosexuals in Florida jail are challenged. *New York Times* December 3:35.

Associated Press (1991) Rate of imprisonment in U.S. is cited as highest in world. *New York Times* January 7:A15.

Barton, W.I. (1974) Drug histories and criminality: survey of inmates of state correctional facilities. *International Journal of Addictions* 15:233-259.

Bates, T.M. (1989) Rethinking conjugal visitation in light of the "AIDS" crisis. *New England Journal on Criminal and Civil Confinement* 15:121-145.

Bayer, R., L.H. Lumey, and L. Wan (1990) The American, British and Dutch responses to unlinked anonymous HIV seroprevalence studies: an international comparison. *AIDS* 4:283-290.

Boodman, S.G. (1989) HIV in prison: is isolation cruel or prudent? Alabama sued over testing, segregating those with AIDS virus. *Washington Post* April 29:A1.

Branham, L.S. (1990) Out of sight, out of danger? Procedural due process and the segregation of HIV-positive inmates. *Hastings Constitutional Law Quarterly* 17:293-351.

Braun, M.M., B.I. Truman, B. Maguire, G.T. DiFerdinando, Jr., G. Wormser, et al. (1989) Increasing incidence of tuberculosis in a prison inmate population. *Journal of the American Medical Association* 261:393-397.

Burris, S. (1990) Testimony before the National Commission on AIDS. August 17, New York City.

Centers for Disease Control (CDC) (1989) Tuberculosis and human immunodeficiency virus infection: recommendations of the advisory committee for the elimination of tuberculosis (ACET). *Morbidity and Mortality Weekly Report* 38:236-238; 243-250.

Dash, L. (1990) A system beset from within: some correctional officers worked while on crack. *Washington Post* June 10:A-1.

Dubler, N.N., and V.W. Sidel (1991) AIDS and the prison system. In D. Nelkin, D.P. Willis, and S.V. Parris, eds., *A Disease of Society: Cultural and Institutional Responses to AIDS*. New York: Cambridge University Press.

Dubler, N.N., C. Bergmann, and M. Frankel (1990) Management of HIV infection in New York State prisons. *Columbia Human Rights Law Review* 21:363-400.

Federal Bureau of Prisons (1989) Operations Memorandum No. 179-89(6100), November 30. Federal Bureau of Prisons, Washington, D.C.

Freeman, A. (1991) AIDS and prisons. In P. Albert, R. Eisenberg, D.A. Hansell, and J.K. Marcus, eds., *AIDS Practice Manual: A Legal and Educational Guide*, 3rd ed. San Francisco: National Lawyers Guild AIDS Network.

Glass, G., W. Hausler, P. Loeffelholz, and C. Yesalis (1988) Seroprevalence of HIV antibody among individuals entering the Iowa prison system. *American Journal of Public Health* 78:447-449.

Goffman, E. (1961) *Asylums: Essays on the Social Situation of Mental Patients and Other Inmates*. Garden City, N.Y.: Anchor Books.

Gostin, L.O. (1989) Public health strategies for confronting AIDS: legislative and regulatory policy in the United States. *Journal of the American Medical Association* 261:1621-1630.

Gostin, L.O. (1990) AIDS Litigation Project. A national review of court and human rights commission decisions, Part I. The social impact of AIDS. *Journal of the American Medical Association* 263:1961-1970.

Gostin, L.O., L. Porter, and H. Sandomire (1990) *AIDS Litigation Project: Objective Description of Trends in AIDS Litigation*. Washington, D.C.: U.S. Department of Health and Human Services.

Graham, N.M.H., K.E. Nelson, L. Solomon, M. Bonds, and R.T. Rizzo (1992) Prevalence of tuberculin positivity and skin test anergy in HIV-1-seropositive and seronegative drug users. *Journal of the American Medical Association* 267:369-373.

Greenspan, J. (1989) HIV infection among prisoners. *Focus: A Guide to AIDS Research and Counseling* 4:2-3.

Hammett, T.M., and N.N. Dubler (1990) Clinical and epidemiologic research on HIV infection and AIDS among correctional inmates: regulation, ethics, and procedures. *Evaluation Review* 14:482-501.

Hammett, T.M., and S. Moini (1988) *AIDS in Correctional Facilities: Issues and Options*, 3rd ed. Washington, D.C.: National Institute of Justice.

Hammett, T.M., S. Moini, L. Harrold, and M. Weissberg (1989) *1988 Update: AIDS in Correctional Facilities*. Washington, D.C.: National Institute of Justice.

Horsburgh, C.R., Jr., J.Q. Jarvis, T. McArthur, T. Ignacio, and P. Stock (1990) Seroconversion to human immunodeficiency virus in prison inmates. *Journal of the American Public Health Association* 80:209-210.

Hoxie, N.J., J.M. Vergeront, H.R. Frisby, J.R. Pfister, R. Golubjatnikov, et al. (1990) HIV seroprevalence and the acceptance of voluntary HIV testing among newly incarcerated male prison inmates in Wisconsin. *American Journal of Public Health* 80:1129-1131.

Johnson, D. (1990) More prisons using iron hand to control inmates. *New York Times* November 1:A-10.

Kamerman, J. (1991) Corrections officers and acquired immune deficiency syndrome: balancing professional distance and personal involvement. *Death Studies* 15:375-384.

Kirp, D.L., S. Epstein, M.S. Franks, J. Simon, D. Conaway, et al. (1989) *Learning by Heart: AIDS and Schoolchildren in America's Communities*. New Brunswick, N.J.: Rutgers University Press.

Lambert, B. (1989) Learning to avoid AIDS: classes for former prisoners. *New York Times* July 8:25.

Lampinen, T.M., A.M. Brewer, and J.M. Raba (1991) HIV in prison: a counseling opportunity (letter). *Journal of the American Medical Association* 266:361.

Langan, P.A. (1991) America's soaring prison population. *Science* 251:1568-1573.

Lockwood, D. (1980) *Prison Sexual Violence*. New York: Elsevier.

Maisonet, G. (1990) Testimony before National Commission on AIDS. August 17, New York City.

Malcolm, A.H. (1991) More cells for prisoners, but to what end? *New York Times* January 18:B11.

Marini, J.L., C.I. Bridges, and M.H. Sheard (1978) Multiple drug abuse: examination of drug-abuse patterns in male prisoners. *International Journal of Addictions* 13:493-502.

Mauer, M. (1990) *Young Black Men and the Criminal Justice System: A Growing National Problem*. Washington, D.C.: The Sentencing Project.

Mauer, M. (1991) *Americans Behind Bars: A Comparison of International Rates of Incarceration.* Washington, D.C.: The Sentencing Project.

Mitford, J. (1973) *Kind and Usual Punishment: The Prison Business.* New York: Knopf.

Moini, S., and T.M. Hammett (1990) *1989 Update: AIDS in Correctional Facilities.* Washington, D.C.: National Institute of Justice.

Montefiore Medical Center (1990) Rikers Island health services. Photocopy. Montefiore Medical Center, New York.

National Commission on AIDS (1991) *Report: HIV Disease in Correctional Facilities.* Washington, D.C.: National Commission on AIDS.

Nelkin, D., and S. Hilgartner (1986) Disputed dimensions of risk: a public school controversy over AIDS. *Milbank Quarterly* 64:118-142.

Potler, C. (1988) *AIDS in Prison: A Crisis in New York State Corrections.* New York: Correctional Association of New York.

Pottenger, J.L., Jr. (1990) Testimony before the National Commission on AIDS. August 16, New York City.

Presidential Commission on the Human Immunodeficiency Virus Epidemic (1988) *Final Report of the Presidential Commission on Human Immunodeficiency Virus Epidemic.* Washington, D.C.: U.S. Government Printing Office.

Propper, A.M. (1981) *Prison Homosexuality: Myth and Reality.* Lexington, Mass.: Lexington Books.

Prout, C., and R.N. Ross (1988) *Care and Punishment: The Dilemmas of Prison Medicine.* Pittsburgh, Penn.: University of Pittsburgh Press.

Rooney, W. (1990) Testimony before National Commission on AIDS. August 16, New York City.

Schroeder, K. (1983) A recommendation to the FDA concerning drug research on prisoners. *Southern California Law Review* 56:969-1000.

Shenson, D., N. Dubler, and D. Michaels (1990) Jails and prisons: the new asylums. *American Journal of Public Health* 80:655-656.

Singleton, J.A., C.I. Perkins, A.I. Trachtenberg, M.J. Hughes, K.W. Kizer, et al. (1990) HIV antibody seroprevalence among prisoners entering the California correctional system. *Western Journal of Medicine* 153:394-399.

Smith, D. (1991) Facing AIDS in prison: an interview with physicians at Vacaville. *San Francisco Bay Times* June:29-31, 54.

Snider, D.E., Jr., and M.D. Hutton (1989) Tuberculosis in correctional institutions. *Journal of the American Medical Association* 261:436-437.

Starchild, A. (1988) How prisons punish AIDS victims. *New York Times* June 7:A-31.

Starchild, A. (1989) Mandatory testing for HIV in federal prisons (letter). *New England Journal of Medicine* 320:315-316.

U.S. Conference of Mayors (1989) AIDS/HIV in correctional settings: the Philadelphia experience. *AIDS Information Exchange* 6(4):1-12.

van Hoeven, K.H., W.C. Rooney, Jr., and S.C. Joseph (1990) Evidence for gonococcal transmission within a correctional system. *American Journal of Public Health* 80:1505-1506.

Viadro, C.I., and J.A. Earp (1991) AIDS education and incarcerated women: a neglected opportunity. *Women and Health* 17:105-117.

Vlahov, D., F. Brewer, A. Munoz, D. Hall, E. Taylor, et al. (1989) Temporal trends of human immunodeficiency virus type 1 (HIV-1) infection among inmates entering a statewide prison system, 1985-1987. *Journal of Acquired Immune Deficiency Syndromes* 2:283-290.

Vlahov, D., A. Munoz, F. Brewer, E. Taylor, C. Canner, et al. (1990) Seasonal and annual variation of antibody to HIV-1 among male inmates entering Maryland prisons: update. *AIDS* 4:345-350.

Vlahov, D., T.F. Brewer, K.G. Castro, J.P. Narkunas, M.E. Salive, et al. (1991) Prevalence of antibody to HIV-1 among entrants to U.S. correctional facilities. *Journal of the American Medical Association* 265:1129-1132.

Whitman, D. (1990) Inside an AIDS colony. *U.S. News and World Report* January 29:20-26.

Wiggs, J.W. (1989) Prison rape and suicide (letter). *Journal of the American Medical Association* 262:3403.

Wiseman, M. (1990) Testimony before the National Commission on AIDS. August 17, New York City.

8

Public Policies on Children and Families

The HIV/AIDS epidemic has touched American law at many points, both in legislation and litigation, in many jurisdictions. Most of the legislation has dealt with public health issues, which are discussed in Chapter 2. In litigation, a recent article states (Margolick, 1991:1): "A wave of AIDS-related lawsuits has swept over the courts. Most involve discrimination, the blood supply, and criminal prosecutions, but there are innumerable other permutations concerning everything from free speech to child custody to libel to will contests." Although the existence of litigation is unquestionable, the quantity is, in fact, unknown. Whether the "wave" is a tidal wave or a large surf is unclear. Nevertheless, U.S. law, at the legislative and judicial levels, has had to face difficult and sometimes unprecedented problems. The panel could have attempted an entire survey of the effect of AIDS on the legal system, but judged that the evidence, apart from public health legislation, was still too slim and scattered; we chose, instead, to focus on one area of legislation and litigation, namely, that which establishes public policy regarding families and children. This may be but a small corner in the world of law and public policy, but it is, in our judgment, of great importance in view of the populations most affected by the HIV/AIDS epidemic.

All societies have sets of norms that define what relationships count as *family* and dictate permissible forms of intimate interaction. In the United States and other industrialized nations, governments cast many of these norms into statutes and other formal rules that prescribe such matters as who can marry, who is financially responsible for the care of children, and what reproductive control methods are permissible. Governments also use less coercive policies to guide or reward family-related behavior. They use tax laws and welfare programs to recognize the needs and costs of those living in certain family configurations and to validate their acceptability. They use public health and school programs to encourage people to engage in behaviors considered socially desirable.

When the AIDS epidemic began, many U.S. policies bearing on families and other intimate relationships were in a period of transition, and AIDS raised difficult, often inconvenient, questions of family policy of at least three sorts. First, because AIDS is transmitted by sexual acts, governments had to come to grips with widely varying public attitudes about sexual behavior and about the appropriate role of government in influencing behavior. Everyone knew that many young people have sex (Hayes, 1987) and that many men have sex with other men (Fay et al., 1989). Some officials were not alarmed by these behaviors or, if they were, were willing to acknowledge they existed and urge precautions. Others, however, were unwilling to appear to condone the behaviors at all. School boards wrestled and are still wrestling with whether to distribute condoms to high school students (Galst, 1992), and states and the federal government responded variously to requests for support of programs that sought to eroticize safer sexual practices among gay men (Barnes, 1989). States have similarly wrestled with the degree to which they should rely on compulsory rules to induce desired sexual behaviors. Thus, many states considered and two states adopted and then repealed legislation requiring HIV-antibody testing before marriage (Joseph, 1989).[1] And many states adopted statutes making it a felony for persons who knew that they carried the virus to engage in sex without informing their partner (Hermann, 1990; see also Chapter 2).

Second, since AIDS is also transmitted perinatally, it necessarily involves the relationship between a woman and a fetus she is carrying. Government officials have thus struggled with the appropriate advice to give HIV-infected women regarding decisions about birth control and abortion (Bayer, 1990). Many women with HIV have been offered tortured advice wrapped in euphemisms to "postpone" having children (Centers for Disease Control, 1985). And, as described in Chapter 4, scientists who have wanted to administer AZT to HIV-infected pregnant women to learn whether they could prevent transmission of the virus to the fetus have encountered hostility from women's advocates seeking to ensure that the pregnant woman's health is in no way compromised in the name of trying to protect the unborn child.

Third, since AIDS is a protracted illness and invariably leads to death, family-related policy issues arise during the last stages of the disease and at the point of death. Disputes have erupted between gay men's lovers and parents over such issues as hospital visits or the authority to make decisions about life-prolonging medical procedures (Steinbrook et al., 1986). Women with HIV have wanted to keep their children with them as long as possible under welfare programs that provide little financial support and to control the placement of their children when they are no longer able to provide care.

This chapter presents case studies of the relationship between AIDS and two sets of family policies affected by AIDS; even more narrowly, it concentrates on these policies in a few selected cities and states. The first case study is that of public issues distinctly related to newborns and children with AIDS. In programs to keep children with their biological parents and in programs to respond to children who must be placed with others, New York and Florida have had to contend with familial issues under strained circumstances—issues of financial responsibility and parental control. The two states sometimes responded similarly and sometimes rather differently, but both of their responses reveal anomalies in public policies that bear on low-income families with children.

The second case study describes the efforts to gain legal recognition of nonmarital relationships, particularly the recognition of gay male and lesbian couples. We examine efforts in San Francisco to pass an ordinance to permit unmarried couples, including gay and lesbian couples, to register their relationship with the city and the quite different efforts in New York courts, legislatures, and agencies to expand the list of relatives entitled to remain in a rent-regulated apartment after the death of a tenant who had signed the lease. In each city, the issues had been debated before AIDS was a central feature of the city's life, but AIDS reshaped the debate in many ways.

NEWBORNS AND CHILDREN

Infants and children with AIDS pose different problems of social and family policy than adults with AIDS. Most of the differences stem from the necessarily dependent position of all young children. They must be cared for by others and decisions must be made for them. Policy makers have long debated how responsibilities for children and control over children should be divided between parents and the state (Mnookin and Weisberg, 1988).

In the context of AIDS, problems of social policy arise in painful, problematic, and revealing manners because AIDS persistently pushes to extremes the burdens and responsibilities of caretakers and the state. Every newborn who is HIV positive has a mother who is HIV positive, a woman who is probably poor and may already be ill herself, a woman who has probably been an intravenous drug user. Mothers of HIV-infected babies commonly feel both depression and anxiety due to their own illness and the illness of their children, and knowing that the child became infected through them, they frequently experience guilt and the need for denial (Seibert et al., 1989; Septimus, 1989).

All babies born to an HIV-infected mother carry passively acquired maternal antibodies to HIV. However, in only about one-third of such cases is the infant actually infected with HIV; those infants who are not infected will gradually lose maternal HIV antibodies, although they may persist until 15 months of age. Since standard tests for HIV detect HIV antibodies and not the virus itself, they cannot be used reliably to determine which infants born to HIV positive mothers have been infected until the child has lost the maternal antibodies. Even the use of less common and more expensive viral cultures is inappropriate in newborns because a negative culture is not sufficient to exclude HIV infection (Hardy, 1991). Therefore, the HIV status of infants born to HIV-infected mothers cannot be known by foster agencies or foster parents until well after birth.

All children who are actually HIV infected need extra attention from the point of birth (Hegarty et al., 1988). Unlike adults with HIV, roughly 20 percent of newborns with HIV become ill with AIDS-related infections within a year of their infection. Once ill, they tend to spend more days in the hospital than adults with AIDS. They typically have chronic growth problems, as well as developmental problems in both motor and language skills (Falloon et al., 1989). And all the required care will be delivered by someone who knows that it is highly probable that the child will die.

Pediatric AIDS thus provides an occasion to examine the impact of a new, chronic, and fatal illness on two strands of U.S. social policy relating to children and families. First, it raises the question of how much resources the nation is willing to devote to the care of children and their caretakers. AIDS tests the nation's commitment because the resources required for each child are large, and the children to whom the resources are devoted are among those who are most likely to be otherwise disenfranchised: babies with AIDS are overwhelmingly poor and African American or Hispanic. Yet, although they are the powerless offspring of powerless parents and pediatric AIDS cases (children under 13 years of age) represent less than 2 percent of all cases of AIDS (Centers for Disease Control, 1992), these children have received a substantial share of the public funds expended in response to the epidemic.

Second, pediatric AIDS permits an examination of the allocation of responsibility for children among parents, extended family, foster parents, and the state in regard to where a child will live, medical decisions, and financial costs. AIDS tests the strength of the state's traditional commitment to helping children remain with their biological parents and to affirming the authority of biological parents to control medical care decisions relating to their children (Gaylin and Macklin, 1982; for recent collections of essays on the responses to pediatric AIDS in the United States, see Schinazi and Nahmias, 1988; Seibert and Olson, 1989; and Anderson, 1990).

Resources and Special Programs

This section draws for illustrations on the responses to pediatric AIDS in New York City and Miami, Florida (and Dade County, of which Miami is a part), the two U.S. cities with the most cases of pediatric AIDS.[2] As of December 1991, 852 cases of pediatric AIDS had been reported in New York City and 198 cases in Miami.[3]

For half a century, the government's principal program of support for low-income families with children has been the program of Aid to Families with Dependent Children (AFDC). AFDC provides basic income support in the form of cash payments. Since the 1960s, Medicaid has been expected to meet the basic medical needs of AFDC families. Even with the social services that regularly accompany it, however, AFDC has never been sufficient in most states to meet the minimal requirements of poor families. In 1988, for example, two-thirds of states did not provide AFDC grants equal to the state's own determination of children's minimal needs. Even in states that did meet their own standard of need, the standards and grants were often very low.

In the early days of the HIV/AIDS epidemic, it became clear that the basic programs of AFDC and Medicaid would be so insufficient to meet the needs of infected parents and infants that additional governmental assistance was imperative. It was also apparent that traditional foster care programs and subsidies would be insufficient to attract foster families for HIV-infected children who could not live with their biological parents. Thus, states with growing numbers of pediatric AIDS cases began to develop new programs and, beginning in 1985, Congress began providing extra money to the states for services and foster care programs for children with AIDS.[4] With that money, New York City and Miami developed or expanded programs to provide added support to biological parents who were taking care of HIV-infected children and to provide noninstitutional settings for the children who could not live with their parents.

New York City

Special programs and resources created to respond to children with AIDS in New York City have been varied and substantial.[5] Nearly every public institution that regularly deals with families with children has developed task forces or programs for children with HIV disease. The state's Department of Health, for example, designated 10 hospitals in New York City as "AIDS centers." In those hospitals, every AIDS patient is assigned a caseworker, as case manager, who serves as the patient's advocate within the hospital and coordinates all eligible services; some workers are especially trained to work with mothers and children (AIDS Institute, 1990a). Other hospitals have created special units for HIV-infected mothers and their children. Harlem Hospital, for example, where, by early 1990, between 3 and 4 percent of all newborns had HIV antibodies, established a unit for women and children with HIV, which had a staff of 20.

To serve adults and children with AIDS during periods when they are not hospitalized, New York City's Human Resources Administration formed the Division of AIDS Services in 1985. By 1990, the division had a staff of 285. In turn, the division established a demonstration project, the Family and Children's AIDS Case Management Project, to coordinate all public services for any family with children in which one or more family members has been diagnosed with AIDS. Caseworkers in this unit carry much smaller caseloads than usual—1 caseworker for every 15 families rather than 1 worker for every 30 families. Most of the families in the program are under such stress from problems other than AIDS that they need the extra help wholly apart from AIDS. Thus, AIDS, which evoked a more sympathetic response than, for example, drug addiction, has opened services that other problems alone had not.

Since nearly all mothers of children with HIV antibodies served by the Division of AIDS Services are at risk of becoming disabled or dying from HIV while their children are young, caseworkers try to involve the mother's extended family, particularly grandparents or siblings of the mother, in helping while the mother is well enough to provide some care for the child and in providing care for the child when the mother is unable to continue. The New York project is particularly proud of these efforts. According to its director, in the first 3 years of operation, only four of the dozens of children the project had served had to be removed from the mother and placed in foster care with nonrelatives while the mother was still alive.

For the minority of children with HIV antibodies who could not remain with their parents or other family members, agencies in New York City have mobilized to find appropriate settings for them to live. Incarnation House, for example, was created to care for children so ill that they need to live in a setting in which they can have close medical supervision, but not so ill that they need to be in a hospital all the time. For the great majority of children with HIV antibodies who could not live at home, however, the goal was to find appropriate foster families. A crisis had arisen at several New York City hospitals in 1985 when a substantial number of babies medically ready for release became long-term hospital residents because their parents were unable or unwilling to take them home. The boarder babies, believed to be HIV infected, were initially even harder to find homes for than other children unable to live with their parents. They became the most visible manifestation of a foster care system already under severe stress due in substantial part to the growing number of parents with drug-addiction problems (Joseph, 1988).

Prodded by a lawsuit, New York City made two responses to the boarder baby situation. First, in 1987 it established a federally supported Hospital Baby Project to monitor all babies held at any hospital for more than 3 days after being medically ready for release. Once alerted to the presence of such a baby in a hospital, the project investigates the reasons for the delay and initiates the process for finding another placement. By 1989, according to the administrators of the project, almost no babies testing positive for HIV were being held as boarders in the city's hospitals.

Second, again supported by federal funds, the city's Human Resources Administration's Child Welfare Administration created a Pediatric AIDS Unit in 1988 to increase the number of qualified foster placements. The unit entered into contracts with 5 of the 74 private agencies through which foster children are placed in the city to create special programs for babies with HIV antibodies. By September 1990, the unit was overseeing the foster care placements of 426 children with HIV antibodies, about half of whom had been placed through the 5 specialized agencies and half through the other 69.

Under the special foster care program, foster parents receive much higher payments for caring for a child with HIV antibodies than they receive for caring for a healthy child without special problems (as of November 1990 $1,281 per child per month, compared with $400 to $500 a month for most other foster children). In addition, foster parents of children with HIV antibodies receive an annual clothing allowance of about $800, a modest additional amount to pay for respite care, and free equipment, such as carriages and cribs. A foster family caring for two children with HIV antibodies would thus be given about $32,000 a year, out of which they are expected to provide for all the children's needs apart from their medical care, which is paid for through Medicaid.

The largest AIDS foster care program in New York City is administered by Leake and Watts Children's Home, a private agency that began working with children with HIV antibodies in 1985 and, by 1990, had placed about 110 children into about 45 foster families.[6] A high proportion of the foster parents have worked as nurse's aides or have other nursing training. The foster parents receive high payments and attentive social services. To support its foster families, the agency employs a staff of social workers and nurses who make frequent home visits and are readily available for consultation. The agency is proud of the foster parents' record of taking care of the children: no child with HIV antibodies had been removed from a foster parent because of inadequate care by the foster parent and, of the 110 children with HIV antibodies placed through them since 1985, 104 were still alive in 1990.

The foster care relationships established through Leake and Watts have also been remarkably enduring and stable. Despite the traditional goal of foster care as a short-term intervention while efforts are made to reunite a child with the biological parents, only 4 of the 110 children placed with them had returned to their biological families. In fact, only a small proportion of the children are visited by their mothers or other biological family members. The agency attributes the small rate of reunions and visits primarily to the family situations of the newborns who come to them: the majority enter foster care directly from the hospital shortly after birth, and virtually all test positive not only for HIV, but also for heroin or cocaine. Thus, nearly all have mothers who are both drug users and HIV infected, and according to the agency, nearly all also have mothers who decided to leave their children at the hospital rather than take them home.

Because returning children with HIV antibodies to their biological parents is not often possible (or often is not in the infants' best interest), a further goal of New York City's program has been to arrange adoptions for as many of the foster children as possible. In the fall of 1990, roughly two-thirds of the children cared for through Leake and Watts were in some stage of the adoption process, nearly all of them proposed for adoption (or already adopted) by the foster parents with whom they had been living. In New York, for hard-to-place children like children with HIV antibodies, foster parents who adopt them continue to receive all the benefits and services they received as foster parents (except for the allowance for respite care).

Miami

Many of the same services provided for HIV-infected children in New York City have been developed in Miami.[7] Services there are provided through the state's Department of Health and Rehabilitative Services, the South Florida AIDS Network, Jackson Memorial Hospital, and private agencies. Jackson Memorial is a 1,250-bed public hospital; it provides care for more children with AIDS than any other hospital in the United States. As of the summer of 1990, it was providing inpatient and outpatient care to 198 HIV-infected children and to an additional large number of infants with HIV antibodies who were still too young to determine whether they actually carried the virus. Of the 198 children, 75 percent were living with one or both biological parents and another 14 percent were being cared for by grandparents or other family members.

Like Harlem Hospital in New York City, Jackson Memorial developed teams to provide coordinated services to women and children with HIV disease. To coordinate public services for families and children outside the hospital, the hospital undertook a demonstration project, similar to New York's, that was serving 160 families as of the summer of 1990. Project caseworkers carry smaller caseloads than usual, 30 families per worker (twice as high as New York's demonstration project but still substantially lower than the usual caseload in Miami). The project has been staffed to address the highly diverse cultural mix of Miami's population. As in New York, very few of the children in the demonstration project have been removed from a caretaking parent during the parents' lifetimes.

For the children who cannot remain with their biological parents, Miami has also established much the same range of foster care programs and support as New York City (Coppersmith, 1990). In Miami, nearly all children who have HIV antibodies and who require foster care are placed through a private agency, the Children's Home Society of Florida, which as of February 1991 was overseeing 36 children living in 21 foster homes; since January 1988 it had overseen the placement of 73 children.[8] As in New York, the substantial majority of the children in foster care are African Americans, were born with traces of heroin or cocaine in their systems, and were the children of women who were HIV infected and had at some point been drug users. Florida pays foster families that care for children with AIDS at an even higher rate than New York. The rate paid in the two states for an asymptomatic child is similar (about $1,300 per month), but because the Medicaid administrators in Florida have approved payments to foster parents for each day that a child is not in the hospital, foster parents caring for a child with AIDS receive a total of $2,621 per month ($31,452 annually).[9]

Adoption plays a much smaller role in policies for children with HIV antibodies in Florida than in New York. In Florida, the state has arranged adoption for only about 8 of the 73 children placed in foster homes through the Children's Home Society. Why so many more children have been adopted in New York is easy to explain: in New York foster parents adopting a hard-to-place child continue to receive nearly all the payments they received as foster parents; in Florida, on adoption, nearly all payments cease. Thus, in Florida, the only children in the HIV program who have been adopted have been a few of those who, on later testing, had seroconverted and were HIV negative. New York's principal goal in subsidizing adoptions has been to ensure continuity of care for hard-to-place children, but not one of the symptomatic children placed in foster care in Florida through the Children's Home Society has left the foster family even without an adoption subsidy program; thus, it is unclear whether New York's system of subsidized adoption has been needed to ensure continuity. The more significant value of New York's program, also unmeasured, may lie in helping children, through adoption, feel more a part of a family and in encouraging the foster and adoptive family to form as strong an emotional bond with the child as possible.

Anomalies in the Allocation of Resources

Miami and New York have developed impressive programs for responding to the needs of children with HIV infection. The projects just described are only part of the cities' extensive efforts. And yet, as ever, there are anomalies and inconsistencies in the public response. This section discusses some of the principal anomalies; although there are sometimes persuasive explanations for each of them, their cumulative effect remains troubling.

As a starting point, the very scale of the public commitment to infants with HIV infection may itself seem anomalous both as an absolute commitment of resources and in relation to expenditures for adults with HIV. The costs of caring for a baby with AIDS are very high. The medical costs alone often exceed $50,000 a year for children who spend many days in the hospital (Hegarty et al., 1988). If a child is in a foster home, the foster parents will be paid between $15,000 and $30,000 per year for the child's care. Whether or not the child is in foster care, social workers and other public employees who help oversee the child's care cost an additional several thousand dollars per child each year. The public commitment is also high when measured not in dollars but in people—specialized hospital staff, foster parents, social workers who serve biological and foster parents, and specially assigned agency staff. Some indication of the scale of such programs is the size of the Sixth Annual National Pediatric AIDS Conference, a five-day conference held in Washington, D.C., in February 1991, at which more than 200 papers were presented, a large proportion of which dealt with local programs of care around the country.

According to U.S. Department of Health and Human Services (1988), federal expenditures for children with AIDS in 1988 totalled $98 million, not including AFDC grants. State and local expenditures total several thousand more per child. In a nation frequently criticized for its uneven commitment to the well-being of children, and particularly to African American and Hispanic children, this expenditure of resources is substantial by any standard.

The commitment of high expenditures for HIV-infected children is in part easy to explain. As to hospital costs, for example, no special congressional appropriation was needed in the late 1980s to expend tens of millions of dollars each year on HIV-infected children. When the AIDS epidemic began, the Medicaid program was already in place to provide medical care for low-income adults and children; the critical public decision to respond to the medical care of the poor had been made in the mid-1960s. And even before Medicaid, public hospitals had been assigned the responsibility of treating the sick and dying who could not afford care.

More complex to explain are the new programs authorized by Congress that were specifically addressed to HIV-infected children—the programs, for example, that provided funds for the extra services in New York and Miami for HIV-positive children living with their biological parents and the funds for special foster care programs. The funds for these programs are not only substantial in themselves, but also in comparison with funds appropriated for extra services for adults with HIV. In the 1989 federal budget, for example, programs for out-of-hospital social services for children with HIV received $7.8 million; in comparison, such programs for adults received $14.7 million, even though there were over 40 adults with AIDS for every child with AIDS. In the 1990 budget, the support for such services for children nearly doubled to $15 million, but the budget for adult services increased only to $17.4 million, even though the number of pediatric cases had not increased as a proportion of all cases (Kirp, 1990). State budgets have also often been disproportional in their support of child-related HIV programs.

Because of their greater dependency, children may well require more expensive social services than adults, but that is hardly the total explanation for the proportionately greater commitment of resources to children. Part of the answer is simply that programs for poor children have always garnered more money than programs for poor adults. For example, neither the AFDC program nor any other federal program provides income support to nondisabled adults without children, no matter how poor they are. In one sense, the usual justification for higher public expenditures for children than adults does not apply in the context of AIDS: the usual justification, similar to the justification for public education, is that children are the nation's future, and income support and other programs are investments in that future, a way of providing opportunity. But sadly, of course, most children with HIV have very limited futures.

Thus, the better explanation for the higher expenditure for HIV-infected children is simply that as a nation, Americans are more sympathetic to their plight than to the plight of HIV-infected adults. Children with HIV may be viewed with more sympathy than adults because they are seen as morally blameless for the behavior that led to their illness. Moreover, to a degree vastly dwarfed by their number, the pediatric AIDS cases that have been brought to Congress's attention most forcefully have remained, even in 1990, the children with hemophilia or children who have received transfusions, not the children of heroin-injecting minority mothers. The major AIDS funding legislation of 1990 for both adults and children—the Ryan White Comprehensive AIDS Resources Emergency (CARE) Act—was, for example, named for a white, middle-class child with hemophilia.

A second anomaly in the deployment of resources is the differences in expenditures among the states. The AFDC program rests on federal legislation, but it is partially funded by the states, and the states are largely free to fix the grant levels. States are also free to vary the range of care provided through Medicaid. New York and Florida aptly illustrate the gross disparity of payments among the states. In New York, in early 1991, the basic AFDC grant for a parent and one child was $439 per month; in Florida, the same family would have received $211 per month. This difference cannot be explained by differences in the costs of living—Florida does not estimate that children need less to live on than New York estimates; rather, the difference lies in fundamental differences in the political environments of the two states. New York taxes its citizens at high rates (compared with almost all other states) and supports one of the nation's most extensive social welfare systems. Florida, without a state income tax, has chosen to spend much less on the needs of the poor and on services of all sorts. Florida ranks 48th among the states in expenditures per capita for health and social services, and it ranks 47th in Medicaid expenditures per capita for eligible poor people (Preston, Andrews, and Howell, 1989). In this light, Florida's unusually high payments to foster parents caring for HIV-symptomatic children is particularly anomalous.

AIDS arose in the context of a welfare system already widely divergent among states. In some respects, the federal response to AIDS has ameliorated the differences among states, for Congress has accepted the burdens of AIDS as so extraordinary that it has agreed that the federal government should bear nearly all the costs of special demonstration projects, such as those to provide extra services for HIV-infected children living at home. The Ryan White CARE Act similarly provides extra federal money to heavily affected cities, such as New York City and Miami, without regard to variations in the financial commitment that the particular cities and states have already made. Still, even with these extra infusions of money, a child with HIV who is eligible for AFDC in Florida and living with his or her mother has less income available and probably will be helped by a caseworker with a substantially larger caseload than a similar child in New York.

The disparities among states are matched by disparities within states. Even within Florida or New York, a child with HIV disease living in some settings receives much more support from the state than a child living in other settings. Some of these differences are the inevitable product of large bureaucracies and patchwork programs. In New York City, for example, some children with HIV disease are in the enriched, low-caseload demonstration programs for families operated by the Department of AIDS Services. Other children receive help from the division but not through a special program and have a caseworker with a larger caseload. Still others, particularly children who have HIV disease who live in a family in which no one is yet symptomatic, are not eligible to receive services from the division, and no special attention may be devoted to their HIV-related needs, such as prophylactic treatments that might delay progression of illness.

Some other within-state differences faced by HIV-infected children are more deliberate and more dramatic in their scale. As noted above, a child living with a foster family will receive vastly greater financial support from the state than a child living with a biological parent: in Florida, $2,621 each month to the foster mother, $211 in AFDC payments to the biological mother. The child living with his or her mother remains in poverty; the other child joins the middle class. Wide disparities exist even in the social services that these HIV-infected children receive. In New York, for example, a caseworker with Leake and Watts Children's Home will carry a caseload of only 9 to 12 HIV-infected foster children, even though the children are living with well-trained foster parents, while a caseworker for an HIV-infected child living with his or her mother will have a caseload of 15 to 30 children.

The gap in expenditures on HIV-infected children living with and living apart from their biological parents is, from one perspective, easy to explain, but it rests on assumptions about family responsibilities and the responsibilities of others that are rarely examined. In this country, states do not expect to have to pay biological parents to help them care for their children. When governments provide modest cash payments through AFDC and support for food through food stamps, most Americans think of the benefits not as compensation but as charity—the "dole"—or, at best, a social investment in the future of children (Marmor, Mashaw, and Harvey, 1990). In contrast, except in the context of adoption, government not only expects to have to pay strangers to take care of the children of others but also to pay them amply to take care of other people's children who are sick. The high payments for foster care for HIV-infected children have been based largely on an estimate of what it would take to attract a decent quality of care for a very needy group of babies. Foster care payments to third persons have always been higher, even for robustly healthy children, than AFDC payments to biological parents. With AIDS, the disparities are simply at their greatest. And the gap in the rate reveals a deep irony: a child is much better off when supported by the state to live with strangers than when supported by the state to live at home, although the latter is the setting governments claim to prefer. Legislators and policy makers extol the nuclear family, but in the context of AIDS they create a set of financial arrangements under which a mother who deeply loves her child might decide that she can show her love best by placing the child in foster care. Conversely, state officials, facing the huge difference between the payments to biological and foster parents, have an incentive to create policies that encourage leaving children with their biological parents even when a particular child seems at substantial risk of harm in that setting.

The disparity between payments for foster parents unrelated to a child and AFDC payments for biological parents provides the foundation for another nagging and more mundane problem of resource allocation that is also particularly visible in the context of AIDS. New York has repeatedly struggled with the appropriate foster payment scheme for children, with and without HIV disease, who are placed with a relative who has no legal obligation to care for the child but who nonetheless takes the child in. As described above, when a mother of a child with HIV disease becomes too ill to care for the child, the state tries to find another biological family member willing to provide the care. Biological relatives are preferred as caretakers when the parents are unable to provide care for some deeply rooted reasons of policy: to carry out the probable desires of the parents themselves, to preserve the child's emotional attachments with persons who have been significant to them, and to preserve cultural and blood ties for their own sake. Relatives are also preferred for a less flattering reason: they are expected to be willing to care for children for less money than strangers have to be paid to perform the same task. Thus, the goal in setting foster care payments for relatives, as it is for unrelated foster parents, seems simply to be to find the lowest rate that will induce enough relatives to become caretakers in a world in which many relatives will do so without special support and others will need an inducement.

In New York, a solution to the problem of foster payments for relatives was reached, after acrimonious litigation outside the context of AIDS (*Matter of Eugene F. v. Gross*, Sup.Ct., N.Y. County, Index No.1125/86), that reflects the ambivalence of both policy makers and relatives: if a parent places the child with a relative, such as a grandparent, without the intervention of the state, the grandparent is eligible for AFDC payments only, but if the state intervenes first, on the grounds that the child is without an appropriate caretaker, and arranges for the grandparent to take the child, then the grandparent (or aunt or other relative) is compensated at the higher foster parent rate. There is a rough logic to this compromise position: it distinguishes, it appears, between a relative who wants to take care of a child and a relative who has to be recruited. In practice, however, what often occurs is that families with relatives willing to help nonetheless contrive to get the state to intervene so that the relatives, often themselves living in poverty, can be eligible for the much higher foster parent payments.

In the context of AIDS (and other problems that make children especially hard to place), the disparity between foster care and AFDC payments is at its greatest, and thus the incentives are greatest for relatives to enlist the state's aid in arranging placements. Indeed, the incentive is such that it might enduce a biological mother to agree to the state's placing her child with a relative and then secretly continuing to live with the relative so that the child can receive the benefit of the most generous levels of payments and the care of her or his mother.

Anomalies in Policies Regarding
HIV Testing and Medical Decisions

The anomalies in the allocation of financial resources for HIV-infected children are matched by anomalies in the allocation of responsibilities for making decisions on behalf of children. The anomalies are particularly apparent in policies regarding testing children for HIV antibodies and the participation of HIV-infected children in clinical trials.

For testing, most clinicians now believe that it is important to identify in infancy children who may be infected in order to begin prophylactic treatment and to monitor them for signs of treatable infections (Cabat, 1990; Oleske, 1990). In March 1991, for example, the CDC issued guidelines for early prophylaxis for *Pneumocystis carinii* pneumonia (PCP) in HIV-infected children and called for testing of pregnant women and newborns (Centers for Disease Control, 1991). The Institute of Medicine also recently issued a report calling for a program of offering tests to all pregnant women in areas with a high prevalence of HIV (Hardy, 1991). Despite the wide agreement on the desirability of testing, hospitals in many states, even hospitals in areas of high incidence, do not routinely offer HIV antibody testing to all pregnant women. To some extent the problem is one of resources. Some hospital staffs would like to offer tests but lack the funds to hire the pre- and posttest counselors required by law and good medical practice. Recently, New York provided special funds to 23 hospitals as a part of a broad program of voluntary testing in the context of prenatal and postpartum care (AIDS Institute, 1990b), but many states, although providing care to children known to be ill with HIV disease, do not seek to identify all those who need care.

Even when hospitals do offer testing to pregnant women, however, many women decline to be tested and thus many infected newborns remain unidentified. In one study in a high-incidence area of New York City, for example, a hospital offered tests to 221 women who gave birth at a hospital without having previously received prenatal care. Of this group, a group thought likely to include an especially high level of HIV infection, only about one-half the women agreed to be tested (Hiranandani et al., 1991). Neither New York nor Florida imposes testing on pregnant women, and both refuse to test a child without parental consent. The Institute of Medicine, in its recent report, stressed the urgency of identifying infected children, but came out strongly against imposing testing on women and children (Hardy, 1991). The AIDS task force of the American Academy of

Pediatrics has concurred in this position, as has the Working Group on HIV Testing of Pregnant Women and Newborns (1990) at Johns Hopkins University. The reluctance to impose universal testing on pregnant women is generally justified by concern for the dignity and autonomy of women. If the motive for testing is for a woman's own sake, then the objections to doing so without her consent are the same as the objections to imposing other medical procedures on adults even when the state is confident that the procedure would be in the adult's best interest—a respect for individual choice and a skepticism about the motives of the state when it purports to act in such a paternalistic manner (Levine and Bayer, 1989). Thus, nearly all states impose testing on unwilling adults only in very narrow circumstances,[10] and the federal Ryan White CARE Act prohibits states' receiving funds under certain sections of the act from imposing testing on unconsenting adults except in a few instances (Section 2661(b)).

If the state's motive for testing a pregnant woman is solely to identify candidates for a program to reduce transmissions to children or for early medical intervention, then the objections are somewhat different. In these circumstances, the state is, in the view of many, using the woman simply as a vehicle for reaching her child. The hostility expressed toward testing for such purposes is similar to the objections that have been raised to clinical trials using zidovudine (AZT) on HIV-infected pregnant women solely to learn whether it is possible to prevent the transmission of the infection to their children (see Chapter 4).

Finally, if the state waits until after birth to test a newborn (but not her or his mother) without the mother's consent, it imposes two forms of intrusion on the mother. First, it compels her to learn her own status, which may be objectionable for the reasons just discussed. Second, even if it were possible to test a child without revealing the HIV status of the mother, imposing the test overrides the mother's control over her child in a society that leaves nearly all decisions about children to parents. States leave the control of children to parents in part because they believe that parents in general know better than anyone else what is good for their particular child. Even when the state believes it knows a child's needs better than the parents, it is reluctant across a very broad range to impose medical or other decisions over a parent's objections. They tend to do so only in circumstances, such as an emergency blood transfusion for a child of parents who are Jehovah's Witnesses, in which the child's life is at immediate risk (Bennett, 1976; Goldstein, 1977).[11]

The reasons that states do not impose such decisions reflect the most elemental views about parenting and the role of the state. Children are born to—come from the bodies of—particular parents, and most parents regard begetting and raising children as one of life's most fulfilling activities.

Affirming the responsibility of parents for making decisions on their children's behalf acknowledges this fundamental, socially useful drive. When the Supreme Court speaks of a constitutional presumption of biological parents' control over a child's life, it is speaking of rights that belong to the parent, not rights that belong to the child (*Smith* v. *Organization of Foster Families for Equality and Reform*, 431 U.S. 816 (1977)). Affirming the authority of parents also affirms, in general, the acceptability of diverse childrearing practices in a nation without a single orthodoxy about appropriate ways to raise children, and it helps preserve racial, ethnic, and religious identities in a nation of diverse cultures.

Yet empowering parents to refuse HIV testing for their newborn appears to pit the interests of parents against the interests of children since a child cannot be treated if her or his illness is not known. If early prophylaxis becomes increasingly effective for children, the tension between children's and parents' interests will become increasingly acute. At this time, the great reluctance to override parental choice is probably defensible. Arguments for state-imposed testing of newborns that rest on available treatments for the children who are identified have moral force only if the state actually makes such treatments available to all children who need them. But large numbers of children in the United States live in families ineligible for Medicaid and not covered by any type of private medical insurance: these children would be unlikely to receive appropriate care for HIV disease or AIDS. Even those children who are covered by Medicaid face obstacles to adequate care in many places (Hopkins, 1989).

Even if care were assured, there remain some child-centered reasons why a mother, especially a mother who does not know her own HIV status, might refuse testing for her child. The mother might justly worry about breaches of confidentiality and the stigma that would attach to her and to her child if others—neighbors, unsympathetic relations—learn that she and the baby have HIV. She might also worry about her own ability to cope with learning her status and the depression and anxiety that might then interfere with her capacity to parent. She and her child might both be better off if she could surmount those fears and learn her own status and the status of her child, but it cannot be claimed that a refusal to permit a child to be tested is always a selfish and unloving act. In addition, imposing testing on a woman who is poor may reinforce her own sense of powerlessness, while making testing within her control may not only give her some sense of power, but also encourage hospital staff to provide information about the values to the child of learning his or her status. A mother who has voluntarily consented to a child's testing, moreover, may be more likely to participate actively and enthusiastically in planning for meeting the medical needs of the child long after the test (Nolan, 1989).

The control that parents are accorded over HIV testing extends to other

decisions about the children's health care, including decisions to permit a
child to receive an experimental drug and decisions to authorize surgery and
other invasive procedures. All research on children poses difficult ethical
issues (Gray, 1989), and this section considers those issues in the context of
a final anomaly: Why is it that foster parents for HIV-infected children
(who are usually well trained and under less stress than the biological parents of the children) and other agents of the state are not permitted the same
authority as the biological parent regarding experimental drugs and surgery? For a child in foster care in New York, an agency that receives a
request for testing from a foster parent first tries to locate and obtain consent from the biological parent(s). Without a biological parent's consent,
the agency has to make a determination that testing will be in the child's
interests. In a few states the policies are so restrictive that no HIV testing
of a child in foster care is possible without consent of the biological parent(s),
and some parents cannot be found to give consent (Baughman et al., 1989).

The reasons that broad powers are accorded to parents were examined
above. To accord the same powers to foster parents might be seen as
undercutting or denigrating the authority of biological parents, even in circumstances in which the powers of the biological parent have largely been
suspended by placing the child in foster care.[12] The powers of foster parents are kept limited not only to recognize the authority of the biological
parents, but also because foster parents are, after all, paid agents or employees of the state, performing a job for the state. Although encouraged to
shower an HIV child with attention and affection—"Hugging and kissing
will help keep your [foster] child healthy," says one information sheet for
foster parents—they may inappropriately put their own interests ahead of
those of the child. Outside the context of AIDS, states have on several
recent occasions been sued by biological parents because of the abusive
treatment that a child suffered at the hands of foster parents (Oren, 1990).
Within the context of AIDS, however, it is questionable whether these reservations about foster parents have a reasonable foundation. At least in
New York and Florida, the child placement agencies believe that the highly
paid foster parents are exceptionally committed to their foster children's
well-being and exceptionally well informed about the children's medical
and other needs.

With regard to experimental drugs, even the state distrusts itself as
caretaker and seeks to protect children against any interests being taken into
account other than a specific child's. Thus, in New York, when a proposal
was made to permit children in foster care to participate in an experimental
drug trial, such as the initial proposals to give AZT to infants, the question
that the state agency put to itself was not whether all infants with HIV
would be benefited by the knowledge to be gained from the experiment,
but, rather, whether there was a sound basis for believing that the particular

children for whom the experimental drug was proposed would themselves receive a medical benefit from participating in the test. On that basis, foster children have not been permitted to participate in a clinical trial in which they might receive a placebo. Biological parents are not subject to such limits. For example, they might agree to a child's participation in an FDA-approved experimental protocol motivated not solely by concern for their child but also by altruistic concerns for other children, present and future, who might benefit from the treatment. It may seem paradoxical that biological parents are permitted to be less concerned for the welfare of their children than the state, but the state's self-imposed restraint is surely wise—at least in ordinary circumstances. It is wise because of the risk that the state will consider children for broader social goals without giving adequate weight to an individual child's needs.

There is, however, a problem with too much restraint in the context of AIDS. AIDS is a disease in which the current treatment of choice is often a drug still in the experimental stages. Restraint may prevent HIV-infected children in foster care from gaining access to drugs that will permit them longer lives. One study found that very few children in foster care have been among children included in clinical trials—no foster children in Florida, for example, had participated in clinical trials as of 1989—and concluded that many states needed new procedures to increase foster children's access to experimental medications (Martin and Sacks, 1990; see also U.S. Department of Health and Human Services, 1988).

LEGAL RECOGNITION OF
UNMARRIED COUPLE RELATIONSHIPS

San Francisco and New York, the two U.S. cities with the largest numbers of cases of AIDS among gay men, provide opportunities for examining family policies that primarily affect adults. They provide particularly rich opportunities to examine efforts to gain legal recognition for gay, lesbian, and other unmarried couples and the role of AIDS in the debates that accompanied those efforts. Although it is impossible to tell whether the changes in law that have occurred would have occurred anyway, it is at least certain that AIDS played a central role in framing the context for, and in shaping the public discourse that accompanied, those changes.

In both San Francisco and New York City, recent efforts to extend protections to people in unmarried relationships, heterosexual and homosexual, were an outgrowth of efforts that preceded the AIDS epidemic but were given new impetus by it. The 1970s and 1980s were a time of ferment in U.S. political and social history over the meaning of marriage (Bernard, 1972; Glendon, 1989) and the position of homosexual people in society (Altman, 1983). Until quite recently, in most states, most forms of sexual activity with another consenting adult of the same sex have been illegal, and only one sort of "couple" has been recognized by the law—the couple of a man and a woman married in a ceremony sanctioned by the state (Barnett, 1973).

Even today, in most states a couple, whether of the same or different sexes, who live together outside of marriage have no more rights or entitlements through their relationship than any two friends or roommates (Weitzman, 1981). They cannot file a joint tax return. If one dies without a will, the other will not inherit his or her property regardless of the nature of their relationship. And, even with a will, the survivor cannot obtain the benefit of state and federal estate tax laws that permit passing property to a spouse without payment of a tax. Nor can the survivor obtain Social Security survivor benefits.

In the two decades preceding the first reported cases of AIDS, changes had begun in some states' responses to unmarried couples in general and to gay and lesbian couples in particular. Those changes occurred largely in the courts, rather than the legislatures. A few courts began to provide relief to unmarried partners, heterosexual and homosexual, on the breakup of a relationship when they could prove some sort of explicit or implied agreement between the partners to share property or support each other (Blumberg, 1981). And some other state courts invalidated (and several state legislatures repealed) laws making voluntary sexual relations between persons of the same sex a crime (*Harvard Law Review*, 1989).

Efforts to gain more formal recognition of ongoing gay and lesbian relationships were more halting. The critical difference between the position of gay and lesbian couples and the position of heterosexual unmarried couples is that heterosexual couples, except in unusual circumstances, are free to marry if they choose but homosexual couples are not. Thus, some gay men and lesbians have fought for the recognition of homosexual marriage. In an effort to force recognition, some gay male couples have sought marriage licenses and, when a license was refused, have filed actions in court claiming that their state's statutes ought to be read to permit persons of the same sex to marry or, in the alternative, that denying same-sex couples a marriage license unconstitutionally deprived them of the equal protection of the laws. As of 1991, no courts had accepted the arguments. Nor had any state legislatures amended their marriage statutes to permit persons of the same sex to marry.

For many, the issue is highly symbolic. Marriage is a central public and communal ritual: if people of the same sex can marry, they can consider themselves brought within the community of respectable persons in the society (Stoddard, 1989). Other homosexual people, however, found aspects of the symbolism of marriage deeply troubling. Some lesbians, in particular, view marriage in its traditional terms as a state in which women are dependent, dominated, and systematically exploited (Ettelbrick, 1989).

Regardless of their views about marriage, however, nearly all gay and lesbian activists agreed that there were important pragmatic reasons for wanting to gain some sort of legal recognition for gay and lesbian partner relationships: the many benefits, such as access to health insurance and various government benefits, that one person can obtain through another or that two persons treated as a couple can obtain at lesser cost than two persons treated as individuals. Although in some sense, fighting for the right to obtain benefits through another person may reinforce images of dependency, most advocates viewed the issue as one of simple justice, of securing the advantages widely made available to heterosexual married couples.

In recent years, gay activists who work on issues relating to couples have largely focused their efforts on getting courts and legislatures either to recognize a special status for unmarried persons—often termed domestic partnership—or, more narrowly, to recognize the unmarried couple relationship for some particular purpose. For those who are uncomfortable with the social meaning of marriage, the term partnership conveys an attractive image of two persons as equals, not of two persons arrayed in a hierarchy. As described below, efforts to gain legal recognition for domestic partners have taken place in San Francisco and New York since the epidemic of AIDS began and seem to have been affected by the epidemic.[13]

San Francisco

In November 1990 voters in San Francisco approved an ordinance to permit unmarried persons to register with the city as domestic partners. The ordinance was adopted by a wide margin, and the gay community of San Francisco regarded the vote as a triumphant affirmation for all gay persons. The road to its passage, however, begun eight years earlier, had been strewn with potholes and detours.

The Early Years

The first effort in San Francisco for a domestic partnership ordinance occurred in 1982, after some cases of AIDS had been reported, but before AIDS had deeply imprinted itself on the minds of most San Franciscans. On that occasion, Harry Britt, at that time the only gay member of the city's Board of Supervisors, proposed legislation to permit unmarried couples to register with the city if they affirmed that they shared "the common necessaries of life" and that they were each other's "principal domestic partner." The bill prohibited the city from treating domestic partners and married persons differently.

The Board of Supervisors passed the bill, but the city's major newspapers and the Catholic church opposed it, and then Mayor Dianne Feinstein, who had supported many initiatives favored by gay men and lesbians, vetoed it. Mayor Feinstein objected to what she considered the broad potential reach of the bill and expressed fears about the impact of the bill on the institution of marriage. When Supervisor Britt introduced essentially the same bill the following year, the mayor announced that she would veto it again if it was passed, and the bill was withdrawn. AIDS played little role in the debate, although by 1983 many cases of AIDS had been identified, and some of those who opposed the bill argued that it would lead to medical insurance coverage for the partners of gay city employees and thus, eventually, to increased medical care costs for the city.

Six years passed before domestic partnership legislation was introduced again. In 1989 the effort was renewed, and an ordinance was initially adopted, rejected by the voters, proposed again, and finally adopted. Supervisor Britt continued to lead the efforts in a social and political context that had changed in the intervening years. A few smaller cities in California, including Berkeley, Santa Cruz, and West Hollywood, had by then adopted ordinances to provide health insurance coverage for domestic partners of city employees. Harry Britt was now president of the Board of Supervisors, and the city's new mayor, Art Agnos, had run on a platform supporting domestic partnership legislation. And AIDS had by then taken the lives of nearly 4,000 gay men in San Francisco alone and tens of thousands of others were HIV positive. By 1989, many believe, AIDS had substantially reshaped the meaning of nearly all political issues in San Francisco, including the issue of domestic partnership legislation, although it is, as ever, impossible to know what would have occurred over the 6 years in the absence of the HIV/AIDS epidemic.

Both proponents and opponents of the legislation believe that an initial broad way in which AIDS had altered the context by 1989 was that the epidemic had made gay and lesbian people more politically aware and active across a whole range of issues affecting their lives. Even in 1982 San Francisco had the most politically powerful gay and lesbian community among all large U.S. cities, and many lesbians had long been active in women's political forums. In the years after 1982, however, the number of gay men who became involved in political efforts grew substantially because of the large number whose lives were affected by AIDS and who believed that government needed to respond more forcefully to the epidemic (Altman, 1988). For many gay men through the early 1980s, if they were politically involved at all, their goal was to persuade the government to leave gay people alone to live their lives as they pleased. By the late 1980s, however, many gay men sought a far more active and responsive role from the state.

Just as AIDS made people more politically aware in general, so it also helped determine the particular political issues in which they became involved. Some issues were new and directly related to AIDS, such as efforts to persuade the California legislature and U.S. Congress to provide more funds for AIDS research and treatment programs and efforts to head off legislation that would have led to mandatory testing of people believed to be at high risk for infection. What was distinctive about Supervisor Britt's domestic partnership legislation was that it was an old issue infused with new content because of AIDS, in much the same way that efforts to provide legal protections for handicapped people have been enlarged by the inclusion of people with AIDS among those believed to deserve protection against discrimination.

For gay men and lesbians, AIDS altered the significance of the domestic partnership issue in two particular ways. In the widest sense, the large number of gay people who had cared for their ill partners made many homosexual people appreciate an aspect of their lives that had always been there but had never before seemed so salient. Jean Harris, a lesbian activist and assistant to Harry Britt, observed: "AIDS made us realize that our lovers are our support systems. It made us more aware of the importance of primary relationships. It made love and relationships even more important than they had seemed before" (interview, May 31, 1990). However, in some ways, especially for gay men, the very notions of domesticity and mutual dependence associated with long-term relationships seemed inconsistent with the spirit of liberation for which they had strived in the 1970s.

Much more specifically, AIDS also brought home the price that homosexual people had been paying for the social and legal nonrecognition of their relations. That price revealed itself when the biological families of gay men with AIDS tried to exclude their sons' partners from hospital visitation or from participating in decisions about life-prolonging medical treatment. It revealed itself, after death, in struggles over burial and property (Eisenberg, 1991). And, most urgently for many gay men, it revealed itself in access to medical insurance: many employers provided coverage to the spouses of their workers, but none provided coverage to a worker's unmarried partner. Many people with AIDS ceased to be able to work, lost their health insurance coverage, and could not obtain coverage through their partners (Padgug and Oppenheimer, 1990).

For people outside the gay and lesbian communities, AIDS had also altered the meaning of the domestic partnership issue. In San Francisco, many people knew and most had read about gay men who were providing care for a dying partner. They had heard about and seen pictures from the "Names Project," the quilt pieced from panels commemorating those who died of AIDS. For many, their image of the gay male community had expanded beyond hedonism to include tenderness, self-sacrifice, and suffering. With familiarity, they became more responsive to claims of a need to recognize gay partners than they had been in 1982.

For others, the association between AIDS and gay men remained different and negative. What came to mind when they thought about gay men's relationships was not the sympathetic image of bedside care but the sexual acts that were the means of HIV transmission. The public service ads posted all over San Francisco to encourage gay men to use condoms reminded some people not of lives that might be saved but of conduct they considered immoral. Some people who were unsympathetic also worried, more mundanely, about the financial costs of responding to the people with HIV disease. They rejected the idea of sharing the cost of providing benefits for people whose sexual behavior they abhorred.

During the campaign of 1989 (and 1990), the various conflicting images of AIDS helped shape the proponents' approach to drafting and promoting the domestic partnership legislation, as well as the response of the opponents. Thus, in the spring of 1989, when the domestic partnership bill was first reintroduced, it was framed slightly differently than the 1982 version. As before, the bill prohibited the city and county from drawing legal distinctions between married persons and persons who had registered as domestic partners. This time, however, to direct attention to the affective aspects of relationships, it defined domestic partners as "two people who have chosen to share one another's lives in an intimate and committed relationship of mutual caring." A new provision, clearly drawing on images from the epidemic, provided that, if a person was hospitalized and had made no designation of desired visitors, a person registered as a domestic partner would be permitted to visit.

The bill did not address medical insurance benefits for domestic partners because insurance matters were beyond the authority of the supervisors, even for city employees. Thus, even though the new bill prohibited discrimination on the basis of marital status, it would not, if passed, have imposed new health insurance costs on the city. By a separate action, the mayor, at the Board of Supervisors' direction, established a Task Force on Family Policy to study, among many issues, the feasibility of making insurance benefits available to domestic partners and other extended family members living with an employee and to make recommendations to the Health Services Systems Board, the agency with the authority over insurance benefits for city employees.

The Board of Supervisors unanimously passed the new domestic partnership bill in May 1989, and the mayor promptly signed it. Many conservatives were deeply dismayed. A group of Catholic and conservative Protestant clergy and laypersons banded together and gathered the signatures needed to place the ordinance on the ballot for the November election. A campaign then began to persuade voters to support or defeat the legislation. The HIV/AIDS epidemic affected the tactics of both sides. The proponents placed images from the epidemic at the center of their campaign. The principal flyer distributed by the Domestic Partnership Campaign Committee began as follows:

> Imagine having spent a lifetime with a partner, sharing a home, sharing responsibilities. Your partner becomes ill—and you don't even have the right to visit him or her in the hospital. Your partner dies—and you don't even have the right to leave work for the funeral. That's the cruel reality for many San Franciscans.

A few paragraphs later, the pamphlet subtly boosted the legislation as a tool to reduce the spread of AIDS. It asked, "Should the City of San Francisco encourage long-term, stable relationships, especially in the time of AIDS?" and then answered its own question, "Yes, of course." In much the same terms, a letter in campaign materials signed by a group of Republicans supporting the bill argued, "We believe it is good governmental policy to encourage the strengthening of stable, interdependent, caring and lasting relationships—particularly in the era of AIDS." The San Francisco Democratic Central Committee in its own campaign letter was more direct. The bill, it said, "helps in the fight against AIDS. It promotes long-term stable relationships."

Some people in the gay and lesbian communities were quite ambivalent about promoting the bill as a tool for encouraging gay men and lesbians to enter stable relationships. To be sure, they wanted to use whatever messages would attract voters, and there was something attractive about this appeal: it invited people by their vote to do their personal bit to halt the spread of AIDS, a civic gesture that had no cost in dollars. But many proponents resented the implication that gay men and lesbians needed legislation to learn to appreciate the values of loving relationships. Tens of thousands of lesbians and gay men in San Francisco were already in long-term relationships, and this group believed that most San Franciscans knew it. In their view, what gay people needed was recognition and equal treatment for relationships that already existed, not a public health gimmick to encourage monogamy.

The proponents also addressed AIDS in another way, by seeking to allay fears about the costs associated with the legislation. The pamphlet and other ads argued that the passage of the legislation would not, in itself, provide health or pension benefits to domestic partners. The point about costs would have been important to make even if AIDS had not existed, but it was especially important because it did.

At each stage of the political process, the proponents were thus responding to needs created by the epidemic and to the sympathies and fears that the epidemic had engendered. Although the legislation applied to un-married heterosexual couples as well as to homosexual couples, to lesbian couples as well as to gay male couples, to domestic partners who were well and domestic partners who were ill, the most frequent image conveyed by the proponents of the bill was of gay men and their partners in the context of AIDS. The proponents would have favored the legislation, just as they had in 1982, without regard to the epidemic, but AIDS had increased the urgency of recognition of partnership and affected the way they presented it to the public.

In mirror fashion, AIDS and the fear of AIDS did not provide the central motivation for those who organized the opposition to the ordinance—they would have opposed it without the existence of AIDS. But the oppo-nents also evoked their own images from the epidemic in their efforts to defeat the ordinance.

The Catholic and conservative Protestant clergy who were the principal opponents were not concerned about the prospects of higher health costs—the Catholic church had, for example, long favored generous social pro-grams to respond to health needs. What they disliked about the legislation was its central messages: that homosexual relationships and nonmarital relationships were socially acceptable. They believed that the traditional American family and traditional Christian values were under siege, and they viewed the legislation as encouraging their further disintegration. For them, calling a relationship a "domestic partnership" did not change the issue into an innocuous secular matter of shared finances. Whatever the relationship was called, it remained a direct affront to marriage. They were concerned about the high rate of divorce, the large number of children born outside marriage, and the temptations of homosexual life for children struggling with their sexual identity. They viewed the legislation as endorsing a style of life that they repudiated—wholly without regard to AIDS.

The campaign the opponents waged against the legislation was modest in scope. Several of the organizers refused to speak to the press. They did not purchase ads in the local papers or on local radio or television. They did, however, distribute two flyers widely. The Catholic archdiocese dis-tributed about 25,000 copies of one flyer through parish churches. The pamphlet never mentioned AIDS or homosexuality. It stressed instead that marriages deserve special treatment "in order to provide a secure and nur-turing environment for raising children," and it argued that the bill would give protection to transitory relationships and thus "cannot help but erode the commitment of marriage in the public mind."

The other flyer, supported by conservative Protestant groups, was mailed to 90,000 voters they hoped would be sympathetic. This flyer evoked im-ages from the epidemic, although it did so subtly. Its cover showed a silhouette of two men holding hands, with a caption reading "The Domestic

Partners Law. It isn't FREE . . . and it isn't FAIR." Except in two brief quotations, one from the Catholic archbishop, the other by the president of the Kong Chow Benevolent Association, the pamphlet made no explicit references to the traditional values that were the opponents' central concerns. Nowhere did it refer to homosexuality as immoral. Nor did it make unsympathetic references to people with AIDS. Instead, what it stressed repeatedly was the hidden dollar costs of the bill—that it would force an immediate increase in the medical insurance premiums that married city employees pay for insurance for their spouses and that it would serve as the opening wedge for forcing the city, and hence the taxpayers, to pay the premiums for unmarried partners. To bring AIDS to mind, the opponents claimed that the bill invited abuse. "City workers," the pamphlet warned, "might be pressured into claiming partnerships as a means of helping friends suffering from AIDS and other chronic diseases to obtain insurance." Echoing and reinforcing the cover of the pamphlet, the back showed a pyramid of silhouettes of men holding hands—2 men in the top row, 4 in the second row, 22 in the eighth row, each man with a dollar sign superimposed on his torso.

By election day, nearly all political organizations, newspapers, and television stations in San Francisco had announced themselves in favor of the legislation. Nevertheless, on election day, the bill went down to defeat—a narrow defeat by a margin of 1 percent, but defeat nonetheless. It had received overwhelming support in the Castro district, the predominately gay residential area, but it was roundly rejected by older voters in the western part of the city and narrowly rejected by the largely black community in Hunters Point.

The 1990 Election

Harry Britt would not give up. In the summer of 1990, he and three other members of the Board of Supervisors voted to again place the domestic partnership ordinance on the ballot in the November election. The ordinance they proposed was a variant of the one defeated the year before. It appeared to be the original bill stripped to its core. Gone were the provisions barring discrimination by the county between married couples and domestic partners. Gone was the special provision regarding hospital visitation. Retained was the central section defining a domestic partnership and setting up the mechanism for registering a partnership with the county clerk. Retained also was the section requiring partners to agree to be jointly responsible for basic living expenses for food and shelter, together with new language that permitted the agreement to be enforced by anyone to whom such expenses were owed. New also was an introductory section declaring that the purpose of the ordinance was "to create a way to recognize intimate committed relationships, including those who otherwise are denied the right to identify the partners with whom they share their lives." The idea was to invite a vote for the legitimacy of gay and lesbian relationships. One of the principal opponents viewed it more broadly—simply as "a referendum on homosexuality."

Each side geared up for another campaign. The opponents were somewhat more outspoken this time, and the proponents somewhat more muted, but in most respects the campaigns were the same. The proponents again emphasized the justness of treating all loving relationships equally and again claimed, as to costs, that there "was no bill to come due for tomorrow's taxpayers." Opponents warned again of the threat to family, but also continued to express their disbelief that there were no hidden costs to taxpayers. They widely distributed a similar pamphlet, using again the silhouettes of hand-holding men wearing dollar signs across their torsos. And, as before, all the city's newspapers and principal radio and television stations endorsed the proposal.

One of the few major differences between the 1989 and 1990 campaigns bore on the issue of AIDS. Shortly before the election, the wisdom of adopting the ordinance was strongly questioned by several groups the proponents had counted on as their allies. In early October, Clint Hockenberry, the director of the AIDS Legal Referral Panel of Bay Area Lawyers for Individual Freedom and a vocal advocate of gay rights, warned of potential adverse effects of the bill for people with AIDS. Pointing to the section in which partners had to agree to be responsible for each other's basic necessities, he worried that partners of people with AIDS would find themselves hounded by the creditors of their dying friend—and he labeled the bill "a creditor's bill of rights" (O'Loughlin, 1990). He also worried that the size of grants that a person with AIDS was eligible to obtain under various federal programs might be affected by the attributed income of the partner. Hockenberry did not object to unmarried partners accepting responsibility for each other. Rather, he was concerned that people with AIDS might not understand the possible consequences of registering and that the bill as drafted imposed responsibilities on domestic partners without providing any concrete benefits of the sorts accorded to married persons. Two weeks before the election, the city's Human Rights Commission, an agency responsible for protecting gay persons against discrimination, issued a staff memorandum entitled "Domestic Partnerships: Obligations without Benefits? Recognition without Equality?" that echoed many of Hockenberry's fears.

Hockenberry's attacks and the doubts of the commission staff left the proponents with little time before election day. Britt's staff regarded Hockenberry as a traitor. On the merits, they believed that, as a practical matter, very few people with AIDS would be hurt if the ordinance was adopted.[14] They also believed that Hockenberry was wrong in claiming that the bill gave no immediate benefits. One benefit was obvious—the symbolism of recognition. Another was more subtle but no less important. Although the bill did not in itself provide any financial benefits for domestic partners, the proponents believed that passage of the bill would goad San Francisco's Health Services Systems Board into arranging with insurance companies to permit city employees to obtain health insurance benefits for their partners. The language about joint financial responsibility had in fact been included to make providing insurance coverage more attractive to insurance companies.[15] Once the city provided access to insurance to domestic partners, private employers might be encouraged to follow.

Even though the proponents saw and believed in these benefits, they were nonetheless in an awkward position to respond. They could claim that the risks were not what Hockenberry forecast, but they were reluctant to advertise the bill as an opening wedge for insurance benefits for domestic partners of city employees, since they had been claiming, accurately if somewhat misleadingly, that nothing in the bill imposed any new costs on the taxpayers. The irony was that a provision in the bill that was intended to help pave the way for insurance coverage for the partners of city employees (some few of whom at any given time would have AIDS) had led to the condemnation of the bill as a whole by some other AIDS advocates who worried about a poorer group of people with AIDS, who were not partners of city employees—and that this condemnation might have jeopardized the entire bill.

The worries in the end proved groundless. For reasons that are not entirely clear, the city's newspapers gave little coverage to the dispute, and the coverage they gave made the matter seem technical and speculative. On election day, the ordinance carried by a wider margin—9 percentage points—than any other proposition on the ballot. A poll before the election had indicated that younger registered voters were overwhelmingly in favor of the ordinance and older voters overwhelmingly against it. In a survey conducted by the *San Francisco Chronicle*, of registered voters aged 18 to 34, 70 percent favored the bill and 24 percent opposed it; of voters aged 55 and over, 25 percent favored the bill and 65 percent opposed it. Voters aged 35 to 54 favored the bill 56 to 35 percent. Disparities that wide based on age are quite unusual—and one major difference between the 1989 and 1990 elections was that the 1989 elections had been in an "off year" when little else was on the ballot and fewer younger people eligible to vote actually did so.

The 1990 elections as a whole were regarded by San Francisco's gay political community as a triumph. In addition to the passage of the domestic partnership ordinance, two lesbians won positions on the Board of Supervisors, and a gay man was elected chair of the School Board. Some of the proponents of the domestic partnership bill believed that the popularity of the bill had helped secure the victory of the gay and lesbian candidates. In December 1990, as the proponents had quietly hoped during the campaign and the opponents had ominously forecast, the Health Services Systems Board voted to make health insurance available to domestic partners of city employees, an action that carried a $1.1 million initial cost to the county.[16] And, pushing one step further toward equality for domestic partners, the San Francisco Board of Supervisors, now with three gay or lesbian members, passed a unanimous resolution to recommend to the California legislature that it alter the marriage laws to permit same-sex persons to marry.[17]

New York City

The issue of domestic partnerships arose in New York in a quite different context, a context in which it was the judiciary, not the legislative or executive branches or the voters, that took the dominant role. In 1989, in the case of *Braschi* v. *Stahl Associates Co.*, New York's highest court, the New York Court of Appeals, decided that, for certain purposes, a same-sex companion counted as a member of his or her partner's "family" (74 N.Y.2d 201, 543 N.E.2d 48 (1989)). Here again, the particular issue might have arisen without regard to AIDS—in fact, had arisen often outside the context of AIDS—but AIDS made the problem seem more urgent and affected the tone of the debate and possibly even its resolution.

Succession Rights Before the Epidemic

The *Braschi* case arose in the context of New York's complicated schemes of rent control and rent stabilization and involved the problem often called succession rights. Succession questions arise on the death of a tenant in a rent-regulated apartment. For example, a tenant's spouse, partner, daughter, or mother has lived with the tenant for years but has never been a party to the lease and, after the tenant's death, wants to remain in what has become the family home. The person wants to remain in the apartment at the regulated rent, which is far below the rent for comparable unregulated apartments. The landlord in turn typically wants the person evicted because the rent regulation statutes provide that, once such an apartment becomes empty, the landlord is free to raise the rent for a new tenant to whatever the market will bear and to continue to raise rents annually at the percentage rate provided for rent-stabilized or, in certain cases, for free-market apartments. New York law provides different schemes of regulation for rent control and rent stabilization. Under both schemes, the regulations prohibit landlords from dispossessing some relatives on the death of a tenant. In the context of rent stabilization, landlords have persistently challenged the authority of the state's Division of Housing and Community Renewal to issue any regulations and have often been successful in the courts.

Over the years before the *Braschi* case, the Division of Housing and Community Renewal and the legislature had struggled with defining a group of family members who would be entitled to remain in a rent-stabilized apartment on the death of the tenant. At least six proposals had been adopted by the agency or passed by one house of the legislature over a period of a few years. None of the proposals, however, included a nonmarital partner among the protected survivors. The legislative and administrative efforts had centered on which persons related by blood or marriage would be covered and how long such a person would have to have lived in the apartment to be eligible for protection.

The struggle in the legislature over succession was less a public debate over the appropriate definition of *family* than simply one more skirmish in the unending political battles between tenants and landlords. In general, landlords detested rent control and rent stabilization and found a sympathetic ear in the state senate, which was controlled by Republicans and which typically supported landlords' positions. Landlords had no particular moral view to purvey about whether stepparents or siblings or even gay or lesbian partners deserved protection. They simply wanted a profit from their investments, and in that context any successor posed an impediment. Many tenants did care about protecting their family members, but succession rights were simply one of many matters about which tenant groups cared each time the legislature was considering rent regulation issues. In their lobbying, tenant groups had never given any special priority to protecting the interests of unmarried partners in general or gay and lesbian partners in particular. Tenants obtained their principal support from Democrats in the Democrat-controlled state assembly. On three occasions, the assembly voted for some form of succession rights for family members, and on each occasion, the senate refused to act on the proposal.

Succession Rights in the Context of AIDS

Between 1985 and 1989, while the legislature and the housing agency grappled fumblingly with a series of proposed solutions, the number of AIDS cases in New York City increased severalfold. The Legal Aid Society, which provides legal services for the poor, and the Gay Men's Health Crisis, a large HIV/AIDS service organization in New York City, began to receive frequent requests for help from men who had lost their partner (the tenant) to AIDS and wanted to remain in the apartment they had shared. In many cases, the surviving partner had taken care of the tenant over the course of a long illness and was now sick himself.

Thus, during this period, the lower courts in New York began to hear cases involving the gay partners of persons who had died of AIDS. The great majority dealt with rent-stabilized apartments, not rent-controlled apartments, because vastly more units in New York City are covered by the rent stabilization program. Facing cases of a surviving gay partner in a rent-stabilized apartment, a few judges started providing relief. One court, for example, held that, so long as a state agency continued to give protection to a list of relatives such as stepchildren or fathers-in-law, the equal protection clause of the Constitution required that a long-term gay domestic partner be given the same protection (*Two Associates* v. *Brown*, 502 NYS 2d 604 (Sup. Ct. 1986)). The court reasoned that there was simply no rational basis for giving relief to a stepchild or father-in-law, who may have depended little on the deceased, while denying it to a life-long gay companion, who was much more likely to have been emotionally tied to the deceased. Some lower courts agreed, but others did not.

During this same period, the only legislative proposal that would have provided succession rights to an unmarried partner came from Governor Cuomo. In January 1989 he proposed that succession rights be made available to any person (partner or otherwise) who had lived in the tenant's apartment for 5 years or more. The governor's proposal was never introduced into the legislature. By the summer of 1989, the agency's powers to issue protective regulations of any sort were still in doubt and the legislature, caught in the usual crossfire, enacted no legislation. In fact, some politicians and agency and other officials were by this time looking to the New York Court of Appeals in hopes of a resolution.

The *Braschi* case, the case that everyone watched when it came before the Court of Appeals, arose under the rent control program, the smaller, older, and more rigorous rent regulation scheme, a program that was in disfavor with the legislature and that was slowly being phased out. Since the 1940s that program had included a specific regulation that dealt with succession. In the mid-1980s, the succession section provided that, on the death of a tenant in a rent-controlled apartment, the landlord could not dispossess "either the surviving spouse or some other member of the deceased tenant's family who had been living with the tenant" (New York City Rent and Eviction Regulations). An unresolved question the state agency and courts faced was whether a domestic partner counted as part of the tenant's "family." The agency had consistently interpreted the term to include only a list of people related by blood or marriage.

The particular case that came before the Court of Appeals involved a gay man, Miguel Braschi, who had lived with his partner, the tenant, for 10 years and had cared for him through a long illness. At Braschi's request, the papers filed with the court were silent about his partner's illness, but anyone reading the record would have inferred that the partner had died of

AIDS. In preparing to bring the case before the Court of Appeals, Braschi's lawyers believed that the many accounts in newspapers and on television of gay partners taking care of a partner with AIDS were likely to have made sympathetic impressions on the judges, impressions that could be helpful as the court decided how expansively to interpret the term "family." Thus, in their brief, Braschi's lawyers emphasized the close and loving relationship between the partners and the "painstaking care" that Braschi had provided during his partner's illness and hospitalizations (*Braschi* v. *Stahl Assoc. & Co.*, Brief of Plaintiff-Appellant, p. 2). They urged the court to reject a narrow and technical view of family based on blood or marriage and to accept instead a functional definition more in keeping, in their view, with twentieth century living patterns. In oral argument before the court, the lawyers drew on examples from the HIV/AIDS epidemic to remind the judges of the many partners who faced eviction, and the judges in turn responded with questions that drew on the epidemic.

To drive home the AIDS-related concerns in this case, a group of AIDS care providers, including organizations from several boroughs of the city, filed a brief with the court that stated that, while exact numbers were impossible to calculate, there were surely thousands of gay men with AIDS living in New York with partners much like Braschi (*Braschi* v. *Stahl Assoc. & Co.*, Brief of Gay Men's Health Crisis, pp. 15-19). They also brought in materials on the growing problem of homelessness among people with AIDS. They referred the court, by name, to 16 other cases involving succession rights then pending or recently decided in the lower New York courts, all of which involved an unmarried partner, nearly all of which involved a tenant with AIDS, and some of which involved a surviving partner who was himself ill and desperate to remain in the joint apartment (pp. 23-24). The City of New York filed a similar brief emphasizing the problem of homelessness for HIV-infected people (*Braschi* v. *Stahl Assoc. & Co.*, Brief of City of New York, pp. 2-3).

The record before the court also included a submission from Russell Pearce, general counsel of the city's Commission on Human Rights, who reported an increasing number of complaints of discrimination against people with AIDS—414 complaints in the first six months of 1988, nearly as many as in the entire preceding year. Pearce argued that if the court did not rule for Braschi, "thousands of people affected by AIDS who live in non-traditional family units will face eviction at a most difficult time in their lives" (*Braschi* v. *Stahl Assoc. & Co.*, Affirmation of Russell Pearce).

The apartment Braschi wanted to retain was owned by a real estate company. The company's lawyers, in their briefs and arguments to the court, tried to stay away from AIDS (*Braschi* v. *Stahl Assoc. & Co.*, Brief of Defendant-Respondent). They mentioned the disease only once in their brief, in a footnote that seemed to try to deflect sympathy based on AIDS by pointing out that there was no evidence in the record that Braschi's partner had AIDS. They also sought to undercut sympathy for Braschi in particular by pointing out that his partner was a rich man and that, as his heir, Braschi could afford other housing at prevailing market rates. On the legal issues, they urged the court to accept a traditional definition of family, one that would be more consistent with the agency's practices and more certain of application. Unlike the opponents of the domestic partnership ordinance in San Francisco, they were not motivated in their opposition by moral concerns about family values or about homosexuality, and they did not make such appeals to the court. Nor did the Roman Catholic archdiocese or other religious groups appear before the court to make such arguments.

The court, in its decision, accepted Braschi's position. Cutting through all that the legislature had been unable to resolve, the court began by observing that the term "family" in the rent control statute was neither defined elsewhere in the statute nor discussed in any legislative materials over the years. With such a vacuum, the court believed that it would be most consistent with the legislature's purpose of protecting "a narrow class of occupants other than the tenant of record" to look not to "fictitious legal distinctions or genetic history" but rather to the "reality of family life" (*Braschi* v. *Stahl Assoc. & Co.*, p. 53). Accordingly, the court decided that the proper definition of family should include, among others, "two adult life-time partners whose relationship is long-term and characterized by an emotional and financial commitment and interdependence" (*Braschi*, p. 54). The court prescribed a list of factors for the lower courts to consider in deciding individual cases—factors such as the longevity and exclusivity of the partners' relationship, their level of emotional and financial commitment, and the reliance the couple placed on one another for daily services.

The court ended its decision by sending Braschi's case back to the trial court to permit the trial judge to determine whether Mr. Braschi met the new criteria, but in summarizing the facts alleged by Braschi, the court left little doubt about the appropriate outcome. If Braschi could prove what he had alleged—a relationship of 10 years, with the partners regarding each other as "spouses," holding themselves out as a couple to friends and relatives, and sharing finances, and with Braschi the primary heir of his partner's estate—he should be considered a member of the tenant's family and assured succession. The court never mentioned AIDS, but almost everyone with any connection to the case believed that AIDS had been on the judges' minds.

By any standard the decision of the New York Court of Appeals was adventurous. As a dissenting judge pointed out, the decision seemed inconsistent with the legislature's overarching goal of phasing out the rent control program as original tenants of apartments died, inconsistent with the traditional definition of family, and inconsistent with the practice of the agency administering the rent control statute, which had always limited its interpretation of family to a small group of relations by blood or marriage. Worse yet, the dissenting judge complained, while the narrower view of family merely requires a simple determination of a blood tie or a link by marriage, the new interpretation placed an already overworked agency in the unfortunate position of having to make inquiries, on a case-by-case basis, into a number of highly personal, subjective factors, such as two persons' level of emotional commitment to each other (*Braschi*, pp. 55-57).

The decision, when announced in July 1989, received a great deal of attention in the press. Legislators had predictably opposing reactions. Many in the Assembly praised the decision. In contrast, conservative State Senator Marchi proposed an amendment to New York's constitution that would have limited the meaning of "family" in all statutes and regulations to spouses, their children, their parents, and their in-laws. No legislation was ever seriously considered in either house. In the succeeding months, nearly all official activity shifted once again to the rules relating to rent stabilization, the larger rent regulation program, for nothing in the *Braschi* case, a rent control case, dealt directly with rent stabilization, and the legislature remained as paralyzed as ever in deciding between the conflicting demands of tenants and landlords.

Impact of the Braschi Decision

After months of delay and intense lobbying from a variety of groups, including gay rights organizations, the Division of Housing and Community Renewal in 1990 issued new regulations to cover rent-controlled and rent-stabilized apartments (Title 9, New York City Rent Regulations, Subtitle S, Subchapters A and B (1990)). Despite intense resistance from representatives of the landlords, *Braschi* carried the day for rent control and rent stabilization. The new regulations began with findings of fact to support the regulations. In its findings, the agency emphasized the general problems of homelessness and the HIV/AIDS epidemic, which, by the estimates on which it relied, had infected between 124,000 and 235,000 New Yorkers. Of this group, the great majority, the agency stated, were gay men or members of "low-income groups . . . two groups most likely to live in nontraditional households" and were thus most in peril of losing their homes. In the new rules themselves, the agency expanded its old list of people related by blood, marriage, or adoption and provided succession rights to other persons "who can prove emotional and financial commitment and interdependence" with the tenant. The regulations went somewhat further than *Braschi* and made clear that a sexual relationship between the parties was irrelevant; thus, a long-term resident who had a relationship with the tenant much like that of a child or a sibling would also be protected. Finally, in a provision reminiscent of San Francisco's domestic partner registration, the new regulations provided that people who wished to be in a position to claim succession rights could file with the landlord a form provided by the agency informing the landlord of the familial relationship.

At the time the new rules were issued, William Rubenstein, Braschi's attorney in the Court of Appeals, exulted that they were "the most far-reaching recognition of lesbian and gay relationships ever granted by any government agency in the United States." After extended litigation, the new regulations have been upheld (*Rent Stabilization Association of New York* v. *Higgins*, 562 NYS 2d 962 (App. Div. 1990)).

Braschi may have already exerted some effects in New York beyond rent regulations. Immediately after *Braschi* was decided, then Mayor Edward Koch announced another form of recognition of the domestic partnership relationship. By executive order, he expanded the policy on "bereavement leave" available to city employees to cover bereavement leave for a domestic partner (or a domestic partner's child or parent) in the same manner as bereavement leave for a spouse (Executive Order No. 123 (1989)). City employees who might want to take such leave under the policy were to register their partnerships with the city's Department of Personnel. The changes in bereavement policies were already being drafted in the mayor's office when *Braschi* was announced, but the generally positive public response to *Braschi* may have encouraged the mayor's office to proceed with releasing them and helped to create a positive climate at the time they were released.

CONCLUSIONS

Newborns and Children

The most significant effect of AIDS on social policies bearing on newborns and children has been to force a response by social service systems that are already under stress to families who are similarly already under stress. The responses have often revealed basic tensions, inconsistencies, and anomalies in governmental policies that relate to children and their families.

Children with HIV arrive into a world of social services and legal doctrines formed before they were born and shaped without children like them in mind, shaped by compromises among many conflicting social goals. It should thus hardly be surprising that high points and gaps appear in the public response to them: model programs, generously funded and of which cities can be proud, reach only some of the affected children, while large numbers of other children have needs that are not met at all or are met much less well. Funding for children with HIV disease is more generous in many regards than funding for adults with HIV disease, but it is uneven in ways that reflect society's ambivalence about the parents of these vulnerable children.

Children with HIV disease or AIDS might be better off if most of the policies discussed in this chapter were different—if there were not wide disparities among states in support programs for families, if within states the payments to biological parents caring for a child were closer to the payments to foster parents, if all pregnant women were tested for HIV infection whether they wanted to be tested or not, if foster parents for HIV-infected children had as wide authority as biological parents to make decisions on behalf of the children in their care. Yet each of these policies is supported by deeply held beliefs about the roles of government and parents in an individualistic democracy, and thus far, the HIV/AIDS epidemic has not led to any fundamental reappraisal of those beliefs. What the long-term effect of the epidemic will be on these policies is as yet impossible to say. At this time, it seems likely that the epidemic will simply serve as another example of the durability and resilience of long-held public values in the United States regarding families and the state.

Recognition of Unmarried Couple Relationships

Looking back, what role did AIDS play in shaping the political and judicial struggles that led to the new, broad housing rules to protect domestic partners and other nontraditional family members in New York City and to the domestic partnership ordinance in San Francisco? That question cannot be confidently answered. It can at least be said, however, that it is highly unlikely that the state agency in New York would have acted when it did to protect such families if it had not been for the *Braschi* decision and for the lobbying of the agency by gay rights and AIDS groups, who were outside the usual political fights between tenant and landlord groups.

The question that is harder to answer is whether *Braschi* itself would have been decided the way it was but for the epidemic of AIDS. The case that came before the New York Court of Appeals, the case of Miguel Braschi, not only evoked some sympathy in itself—a loving partner who had cared for his dying companion—but also surely evoked images of many other similar companions and of yet other homeless persons dying of AIDS in city shelters. In their briefs, the supporters of Braschi had certainly gone out of their way to evoke such images in the belief that they would affect the judges. More globally, in the years that immediately preceded *Braschi*, what AIDS had also done, as it had done in San Francisco, was to raise the political consciousness of many gay men and lesbians and lead to the creation of organizations that urged the courts and legislatures to adopt an enlarged view of families.

It thus seems quite possible that AIDS contributed in New York and in San Francisco to the recognition of domestic partnerships and to the recognition of other nontraditional family relationships for which no lobbying voice exists. In both New York City and San Francisco, the recognition of domestic partnerships would have been important to gay and lesbian couples even if AIDS had never happened, but AIDS, for all its tragic effects, may have led the larger community in both cities to confront and accept, at least for certain purposes, families who had once been unseen or, if seen, rejected as different. If this has been the role of AIDS, it is in some sense an amiable paradox: a fatal disease, associated in the public mind with promiscuous sexual acts, a disease so stigmatizing that Miguel Braschi had not wished its name to be mentioned, nonetheless contributed to the recognition and acceptance of a variety of emotionally intimate and interdependent family ties that were once outside the law.

NOTES

1. Illinois and Louisiana passed and later repealed statutes mandating premarital HIV antibody screening, largely because of their lack of cost effectiveness (Childress, 1991).

2. Northern New Jersey is the geographic area with the third largest number of pediatric AIDS cases; for a brief description of the response to AIDS in Newark, see Williams (1989).

3. Pediatric AIDS cases constitute about 1.7 percent of the cumulative U.S. total through December 31, 1991 (Centers for Disease Control, 1992); in December 1991, they constituted about 3.2 percent of the cumulative cases in Miami and 2.3 percent of cumulative cases in New York City.

4. For example, see the provisions for pediatric AIDS health care demonstration projects in P.L. 100-202 administered by the Office of Maternal and Child Health of the Health Resources and Services Administration.

5. The information in this section is based on the materials cited and interviews with staff members of state and city agencies and private foster care agencies.

6. The description is based on interviews with staff members of the Leake and Watts Children's Home and on Gurdin (1990).

7. The information in this section is based on the materials cited, presentations made at hearings by the panel in Miami on July 1, 1990, and interviews with the staff of Jackson Memorial Hospital and other agencies in Miami.

8. Some of the children left the program when, after initially testing positive for the HIV antibodies, they later seroreverted to HIV negative.

9. A few years ago, payments for foster parents caring for a child with AIDS were even higher. Florida's pattern of high payment rates was set at a time when Jackson Memorial had many boarder babies. Payments of even $3,000 per month per child seemed a bargain to many public officials in comparison with the even higher costs—$800 to $1,000 per day per child by some estimates—and the negative publicity they received when housing children in the hospital.

10. To protect mothers, Jackson Memorial Hospital in Miami generally will not permit a biological father to give consent to test a child in circumstances in which the hospital is not certain whether the father knows the HIV status of the mother (interview with Dr. Terry Mastrucci, October 1990).

11. Some people and groups object to state-imposed testing over a mother's objections on broader grounds. They oppose mandatory testing of any group—babies, prisoners, health care providers, air traffic controllers, etc.—on the grounds that the arguments for it are tenuous and that the risks are great that approval of it will lead to even less justified mandatory testing of other groups and, ultimately, to greater discrimination against HIV-infected people.

12. Obtaining the consent of the biological parent(s) consent also protects the state from a lawsuit by the only people likely to sue if the test is performed.

13. This section is based on interviews with proponents, opponents, and observers in both cities and on examinations of legal materials, newspaper accounts, and political campaign literature.

14. Julia Lopez, head of San Francisco's Department of Social Services, issued a memorandum stating that "passage of the domestic partners initiative would not have any effect on the eligibility for benefit programs administered by the department." The Human Rights Commission staff thought Lopez might have been hasty in her conclusions.

15. Some insurance companies insist that dependents of an employee to whom they provide coverage be a person to whom the employee has some legal obligation.

16. San Francisco's health plan for its employees does not provide coverage even for spouses; rather, it allows employees to purchase coverage for their spouses (and dependent children) at group rates. The board's action in December 1990 permitted employees with domestic partners to purchase insurance for their partners at the same rates. The extra $1.1 million in costs to the county was due to the fact that the insurance companies demanded a higher premium for all dependents if domestic partners were to be covered, and the city wanted to make certain that adding domestic partners did not force employees with spouses to pay higher premiums than they already were.

17. A ballot initiative seeking to repeal San Francisco's domestic partnership ordinance failed in November 1991 (Chung, 1991).

REFERENCES

AIDS Institute (1990a) Intensive Case Management Services for HIV Infected Women and Children: A Report for the Committee on the Care of Women and Children with HIV Infection. New York State Department of Health, New York.

AIDS Institute (1990b) Obstetrical HIV/Counseling/Testing Care Initiative: Program Status Report. New York State Department of Health, New York.

Altman, D. (1983) *The Homosexualization of America*. Boston: Beacon.

Altman, D. (1988) Legitimation through disaster: AIDS and the gay movement. In E. Fee and D.M. Fox, eds., *AIDS: The Burdens of History*. Berkeley, Calif.: University of California Press.

Anderson, G.R., ed. (1990) *Courage to Care: Responding to the Crisis of Children with AIDS*. Washington, D.C.: Child Welfare League of America.

Barnes, M. (1989) Toward ghastly death: the censorship of AIDS education. *Columbia Law Review* 89:698-724.

Barnett, W. (1973) *Sexual Freedom and the Constitution: An Inquiry into the Constitutionality of Repressive Sex Laws*. Albuquerque, N.M.: University of New Mexico Press.

Baughman, L.N., C.H. Morgan, S. Margolis, and M. Kotler (1989) *Infants and Children with HIV Infection in Foster Care*. Washington, D.C.: U.S. Department of Health and Human Services.

Bayer, R. (1990) AIDS and the future of reproductive freedom. *Milbank Quarterly* 68:179-204.

Bennett, R. (1976) Allocation of child medical care decision-making authority: a suggested interest analysis. *Virginia Law Review* 62:285-330.

Bernard, J. (1972) *The Future of Marriage*. New York: World Publishing.

Blumberg, G.G. (1981) Cohabitation without marriage: a different perspective. *University of California at Los Angeles Law Review* 28:1125-1180.

Cabat, T. (1990) The development of an early intervention model for HIV-infected women and their infants. In G.R. Anderson, ed., *Courage to Care: Responding to the Crisis of Children with AIDS*. Washington, D.C.: Child Welfare League of America.

Centers for Disease Control (CDC) (1985) Recommendations for assisting in the prevention of perinatal transmission of human T-lymphotropic virus type III/lymphadenopathy syndrome. *Morbidity and Mortality Weekly Report* 34:721-726, 731-732.

Centers for Disease Control (CDC) (1991) Guidelines for prophylaxis against *Pneumocystis carinii* pneumonia for children infected with human immunodeficiency virus. *Morbidity and Mortality Weekly Report* 40(RR-2):1-13.

Centers for Disease Control (1992) *HIV/AIDS Surveillance Report*. Atlanta, Ga.: Centers for Disease Control.

Childress, J.F. (1991) Mandatory HIV screening and testing. In F.G. Reamen, ed., *AIDS & Ethics*. New York: Columbia University Press.

Chung, L.A. (1991) SF apartment vacancy control proposition defeated; domestic partner repeal fails. *San Francisco Chronicle* November 6:A-5.

Coppersmith, S. (1990) Foster care for children with HIV infection: special mission in a loving environment. In G.R. Anderson, ed., *Courage to Care: Responding to the Crisis of Children with AIDS*. Washington, D.C.: Child Welfare League of America.

Eisenberg, R. (1991) Personal and estate planning. In P. Albert, R. Eisenberg, D.A. Hansell, and J.K. Marcus, eds., *AIDS Practice Manual: A Legal and Educational Guide*, 3rd ed. San Francisco: National Lawyers Guild.

Ettelbrick, P.L. (1989) Since when is marriage a path to liberation? *Outlook* 2(6):9, 14-17.

Falloon, J., J. Eddy, L. Wiener, and P.A. Pizzo (1989) Human immunodeficiency virus infection in children. *Journal of Pediatrics* 114:1-30.

Fay, R.E., C.F. Turner, A.D. Klassen, and J.H. Gagnon (1989) Prevalence and patterns of same-gender sexual contact among men. *Science* 243:338-348.

Galst, L. (1992) The right to a safe education: American's teens and AIDS activists push for condom availability in high schools nationwide. *The Advocate* February 11:46-48.

Gaylin, W., and R. Macklin, eds. (1982) *Who Speaks for the Child?: The Problems of Proxy Consent*. New York: Plenum.

Glendon, M.A. (1989) *The Transformation of Family Law: State Law and Family in the United States and Western Europe*. Chicago: University of Chicago Press.

Goldstein, J. (1977) Medical care for the child at risk: on state supervention of parental autonomy. *Yale Law Journal* 86:645-670.

Gray, J. (1989) Pediatric AIDS research: legal, ethical, and policy influences. In J.M. Seibert and R.A. Olson, eds., *Children, Adolescents and AIDS*. Lincoln, Neb.: University of Nebraska Press.

Gurdin, P. (1990) Quality care for children: a specialized foster care program. In G. Anderson, ed., *Courage to Care: Responding to the Crisis of Children with AIDS*. Washington, D.C.: Child Welfare League of America.

Hardy, L.M., ed. (1991) *HIV Screening of Pregnant Women and Newborns*. Committee on Prenatal and Newborn Screening for HIV Infection, Institute of Medicine. Washington, D.C.: National Academy Press.

Harvard Law Review (1989) Developments in the law—sexual orientation and the law. *Harvard Law Review* 102:1508, 1519-1537.

Hayes, C.D., ed. (1987) *Risking the Future: Adolescent Sexuality, Pregnancy, and Childbearing*. Panel on Adolescent Pregnancy and Childbearing, National Research Council. Washington, D.C.: National Academy Press.

Hegarty, J.D., E.J. Abrams, V.E. Hutchinson, S.W. Nicholas, M.S. Suarez, et al. (1988) The medical care costs of the human immunodeficiency virus-infected children in Harlem. *Journal of the American Medical Association* 260:1901-1905.

Hermann, D.J. (1990) Criminalizing conduct relating to HIV transmission. *St. Louis University Public Law Review* 9:351-378.

Hiranandani, R. et al. (1991) HIV counseling and testing in a high-risk post-partum population. Paper presented at the Sixth Annual National Pediatric AIDS Conference, Washington, D.C., February 2-12.

Hopkins, K.M. (1989) Emerging patterns of services and case finding for children with HIV infection. *Mental Retardation* 27:219-222.

Joseph, S. (1988) Adoption, foster care and day care issues in New York. In R. Schinazi and A. Nahmias, eds., *AIDS in Children, Adolescents and Heterosexual Adults: An Interdisciplinary Approach to Prevention.* New York: Elsevier.

Joseph, S.C. (1989) Premarital AIDS testing: public policy abandoned at the altar (editorial). *Journal of the American Medical Association* 261:3456.

Kirp, D. (1990) The politics of pediatric AIDS. *The Nation* May 14:666-668.

Levine, C., and R. Bayer (1989) The ethics of screening for early intervention in HIV disease. *American Journal of Public Health* 79:1661-1667.

Margolick, D. (1991) Tide of lawsuits portrays society ravaged by AIDS. *New York Times* August 23:1.

Marmor, T.R., J.L. Mashaw, and P.L. Harvey (1990) *America's Misunderstood Welfare System.* New York: Basic Books.

Martin, J.M., and H.S. Sacks (1990) Do HIV-infected children in foster care have access to clinical trials of new treatments? *AIDS and Public Policy Journal* 5:3-8.

Mnookin, R.H., and D.K. Weisberg (1988) *Child, Family and State.* Boston: Little, Brown.

Nolan, K. (1989) Ethical issues in caring for pregnant women and newborns at risk for human immunodeficiency virus infection. *Seminars in Perinatology* 13:55-65.

Oleske, J. (1990) The medical management of pediatric AIDS: intervening in behalf of children and families. In G.R. Anderson, ed., *Courage to Care: Responding to the Crisis of Children with AIDS.* Washington, D.C.: Child Welfare League of America.

O'Loughlin, R. (1990) Liability question makes Prop. K more controversial. *Bay Area Reporter* October 11:21.

Oren, L. (1990) *Deshaney's* unfinished business: the foster child's due process right to safety. *North Carolina Law Review* 69:113-158.

Padgug, R.A., and G.M. Oppenheimer (1990) AIDS health insurance and the crisis of community. *Notre Dame Journal of Law, Ethics & Public Policy* 5:35-51.

Preston, B., R. Andrews, and E. Howell (1989) *Case Study of Miami AIDS Service Demonstration Project.* Final report submitted to the Health Resources and Services Administration. Washington, D.C.: McGraw-Hill/Systemetrics.

Schinazi, R., and A. Nahmias, eds. (1988) *AIDS in Children, Adolescents and Heterosexual Adults: An Interdisciplinary Approach to Prevention.* New York: Elsevier.

Seibert, J.M., and R.A. Olson, eds. (1989) *Children, Adolescents and AIDS.* Lincoln, Neb.: University of Nebraska Press.

Seibert, J.M., A. Garcia, M. Kaplan, and A. Septimus (1989) Three model pediatric AIDS programs: meeting the needs of children, families and communities. In J.M. Seibert and R.A. Olson, eds., *Children, Adolescents and AIDS.* Lincoln, Neb.: University of Nebraska Press.

Septimus, A. (1989) Psycho-social aspects of caring for families of infants infected with human immunodeficiency virus. *Seminars in Perinatology* 13:49-54.

Steinbrook, R., B. Lo, J. Moulton, G. Saika, H. Hollander, et al. (1986) Preferences of homosexual men with AIDS for life-sustaining treatment. *New England Journal of Medicine* 314:457-460.

Stoddard, T.B. (1989) Gay marriages: make them legal. *New York Times* March 4:27

U.S. Department of Health and Human Services (1988) *Final Report: Secretary's Work Group on Pediatric HIV Infection and Disease.* Washington, D.C.: U.S. Government Printing Office.

Weitzman, L. (1981) *The Marriage Contract.* New York: Free Press.

Williams, L. (1989) Inner city under siege: fighting AIDS in Newark. (Second of a four-part series, "The Changing Face of AIDS.") *New York Times* 2/6/89:A-1.

Working Group on HIV Testing of Pregnant Women and Newborns (1990) HIV infection, pregnant women, and newborns: a policy proposal for information and testing. *Journal of the American Medical Association* 264:2416-2420.

9

The HIV/AIDS Epidemic
in New York City

The panel planned to study in some detail the impact of the HIV/AIDS epidemic in several locales as part of an effort to understand the localized dimensions of the epidemic. Our plan had been to focus on three cities, New York, Miami, and Sacramento, to determine the epidemic's impacts in places with quite different social, cultural, and demographic characteristics. Unfortunately, it proved logistically and financially difficult to carry out this plan. Fortunately, however, since several members of the panel lived or worked in New York and had convened for regular discussions over the several years of the panel's life a group of experienced observers of the epidemic, the panel was able to complete one of its planned empirical studies, that of New York City.

"Completed" is not quite accurate: many aspects of the epidemic in New York City are not included in this chapter and much more needs to be done before a picture that is in any way complete can be presented. We refrain from calling this chapter a case study in the proper sense, since such a study, being only one and thus lacking comparisons with similar studies, would require much more detail and depth before either causal connections between the complex phenomena can be discerned or even tentative generalizations can be suggested. Still, the panel believes that the New York City study, as it stands, offers a vivid portrait of the epidemic in a particular place and illustrates with particular force the principal conclusions of this report: namely, the epidemic is not spreading uniformly throughout the population but is highly localized, and the epidemic is now progressing in such a way that a convergence of social ills creates a nidus in which it can flourish. It is our belief that New York City, special though it may be, exemplifies these conclusions. In New York City, as in the United States, the epidemic is highly localized and is flourishing in social settings where there is a "synergism of plagues" (Wallace, 1988).

Much of the attention given to the epidemic has focused on national estimates and national needs. Although these are perfectly appropriate concerns, it must be understood that ultimately the epidemic, its impacts, and the responses to the impacts are experienced in specific locales. The United States, unlike many European countries, is composed of states and other political subunits that can and do pursue quasi-independent policies in many aspects of social life. For instance, all states, counties, and most large cities have their own public health agencies, which have differing traditions and varying levels of quality. In addition, these subnational, geopolitical units often have different political, economic, welfare, and crime control practices, all of which are involved in dealing with HIV/AIDS.

Although these subnational jurisdictions are smaller in size and population than the country, they are not homogeneous social and cultural units. Affluent people live in some parts of a city, and poor people live in others; individuals of European descent live in some communities, and African Americans and persons of Latin descent live in others. In some cities there are residential communities of gay men and lesbians, but in many there are not. Because HIV is not spread through casual contact, the structure of social networks in different localities and the geographical mobility of persons engaging in risky behavior shape the transmission of the virus. Sexual relationships and the sharing of drug injection paraphernalia are not random activities, but are embedded in other patterns of social interaction. HIV/ AIDS is thus a disease of neighborhoods and communities, of high-prevalence localities and low-prevalence localities. Even a cursory look at the patterns of CDC-defined AIDS cases suggests distinct patterns in different cities. For example, many cities have few intravenous drug users who are infected and hence few women and infants who are HIV positive, while others have many intravenous drug users and so many infected women and infants.

New York has always been described as "special," meaning that it is unlike any other city in the United States. This view has considerable truth in it: New York City is an unruly, chaotic urban place, which regularly seems to verge on being economically and politically unmanageable. Its residents are the children of old immigrants who came by boat and new arrivals just off an airliner. New York City is actually a large number of collaborating and competing communities with disparate levels of power and resources. Many of these communities have no direct contact with other communities and compete with each other over resources and entitlements in distant arenas, while others directly confront each other on the streets of the city over specific pieces of turf.

This study only partly confronts the complexity of the city and its response to the HIV/AIDS epidemic. It does not, as it might, list all of the people who took leadership positions and made the limited institutional reforms that characterized the city's best efforts. It is therefore a somewhat gloomy and admittedly partial vision. There is little discussion about the local media and its responses and nonresponses to the epidemic. We have used articles in the local press to track various controversies. A number of commissions and committees have attempted to analyze the epidemic in New York and plan for the future. We have read and quoted from their studies, even though we do not describe their special efforts (e.g., Citizens Commission on AIDS for New York City and Northern New Jersey, 1991).

Other local studies of the epidemic are needed (see Andrews et al., 1989). We hope there are researchers who will attempt to find out what happened in Los Angeles, San Francisco, Miami, Houston, Dallas, and Atlanta, as well as in Chicago, Detroit, and Denver. We believe the research community needs to discover the stories of the epidemic from the perspectives of the streets of the South Bronx and the apartments of Chelsea, the emergency rooms and pediatric units of Harlem, Bronx Lebanon, Woodhull, and St. Vincent's Hospitals, and the offices of the Gay Men's Health Crisis (GMHC), AIDS Coalition to Unleash Power (ACT-UP), Association for Drug Abuse Prevention and Treatment (ADAPT), and God's Love We Deliver, as well as providing the epidemiological models and health cost estimates that are the accounting frames that are only mere summaries of the realities of human action.

COURSE OF THE EPIDEMIC

Current Situation

By March 1992, 37,952 cases of AIDS had been reported to the Centers for Disease Control (CDC) for the New York City metropolitan statistical area (MSA)—the five boroughs of New York City and the immediate suburban counties of Putnam, Rockland, and Westchester (Centers for Disease Control, 1992); the five boroughs account for more than 95 percent of the cases. Those cases comprised 37,062 adults and 890 children less than 13 years old: 17.6 percent of all adult and 24.7 percent of all child cases of AIDS reported to the CDC by health departments in the United States. The proportion of the national epidemic represented by the New York City MSA has declined somewhat over the course of the epidemic. For cases reported from March 1990 to February 1991, the proportion from the New York City

MAS was 15.6 percent; from March 1991 to February 1992, it was 14.8 percent.

All these figures, however, are an underestimation of the numbers of actual AIDS cases. There are four sources of this underestimation, which mirror the undercount problems on a national level. The first is the lag in the reporting of cases from the local site in which the disease is diagnosed to the local health department; the next lag is from then until the cases are reported to CDC and entered into the AIDS Case Registry. In New York City, one-third of AIDS cases are reported to the city health department within 1 month of diagnosis, about 85 percent are reported by 6 months, and the count is as nearly complete as it is likely to be after about 15 months (New York City Department of Health, 1989a). According to the U.S. General Accounting Office (1989), the lag time between diagnosis and reporting is growing longer rather than shorter.

A second source of underestimation is the extent of undercounting, that is, the number of cases that, if diagnosed and reported, would meet the current CDC case definition. These are cases that are lost to the system by inadvertence and overwork, failures of paperwork, deliberate decision, or by death from other causes among individuals whose AIDS was not diagnosed because they were not in contact with the health care system. The proportion of undercounted cases varies by geographical location and by risk group (U.S. General Accounting Office, 1989; Buehler, Berkelman, and Stehr-Green, 1992).

A third source of underestimation of the dimensions of the epidemic is HIV-infected people who die from complications of the disease prior to a diagnosis of AIDS. This may be a very significant factor in New York City.

The final source of underestimation is the occurrence of either new opportunistic infections that are the result of HIV infection or infections specific to particular populations that do not conform to the CDC case definitions. These are viewed by some as indications of the changing natural history of the disease or as symptoms of HIV/AIDS among less studied populations.

Of the 26,336 cases of AIDS reported in the state by December 1989, 87 percent were from the five boroughs of New York City, and an additional 7.8 percent were from the four counties with the most intimate social and economic connections with the city (Nassau, Suffolk, Westchester, and Rockland)—in all, 95 percent of all cases reported in New York State (AIDS in New York State, 1989).

Whatever the precise number of cases of AIDS, deaths from the opportunistic infections that are associated with end-stage HIV disease accounted for a very large proportion of the total mortality among young men and women in New York City in 1989. Among men aged 25 to 44, AIDS was the leading cause of death: 31.6 percent of deaths of men aged 25 to 34 and

35.2 percent of deaths of men aged 35 to 44. Among women aged 25 to 34, AIDS accounted for 26.1 percent of all deaths; in addition, 10 percent of the mortality among women aged 15 to 24 and 17 percent of the mortality among women aged 35 to 44 was also directly attributable to AIDS.

Localization of the Epidemic

One of the most striking features of the HIV/AIDS epidemic is its concentration in and within large urban centers. This is manifested across the United States, and New York is no exception. As noted above, 87 percent of all cases in New York State are concentrated in the five boroughs of the city. But that is only the first level of concentration of the epidemic. Within the city itself, AIDS cases are concentrated both in individual boroughs and in neighborhoods within the boroughs. Data on various characteristics of AIDS cases by 41 neighborhoods in the five boroughs have been published by the New York City Department of Health (1990a,b,c,d,e). Although there are other ways to define neighborhoods, these 41 areas—10 each in Manhattan, Queens, and Brooklyn, 7 in the Bronx, and 4 in Staten Island—have the virtue of being used for a wide variety of other epidemiologic, health care, and planning purposes.

The incidence rates vary as much within New York City as they do across the counties of New York State. Table 9-1 presents data on the number of adult persons with AIDS by selected demographic characteristic or risk categories and ethnic groups, reflecting the intense concentration of the epidemic in certain city neighborhoods. The variation in Manhattan, which is the hardest hit of the boroughs, remains quite large (from 341 to 1,802 per 100,000 persons). A more precise pattern is evident when the cumulative AIDS case data for the city are plotted using zip codes; see Figure 9-1. Within the larger geographical units, as defined by the United Hospital Fund's community health areas, one can observe the zip code areas with the highest concentrations of cumulative AIDS cases. In vast areas of the city, cumulative AIDS cases are fewer than 175 per 100,000, but in a small set of zip code areas, the rates are more than 700 per 100,000.

A similar geographical pattern can be found in the data on rates of HIV antibody seropositivity among women bearing children in New York City. Since 1987 all infants born in New York State have been tested for antibodies to HIV in anonymous serologic surveys of blood routinely taken (from the heel) for testing for inherited metabolic disorders. Such surveys are indirect measures of the rate of HIV infection among newborns, since only a fraction of babies born to HIV-infected mothers are themselves infected and since an infant may carry antibodies from its mother but not in fact be infected. They are, however, accurate indicators of the serostatus of the mother. Of 359,470 babies tested in New York City between November 1987 and September 1990, 4,453 women were determined to be infected

TABLE 9-1 AIDS Cases by Neighborhoods in New York City, Cumulative Incidence from 1981 to June 1990

Borough and Neighborhood	Number of Cases	Rate per 100,000	Percentage[a]				
			Women	Gay Men[b]	IVDU	African American	Hispanic American
Manhattan	10,523	—	9	67	29	25	21
Washington Heights/Inwood	487	348	10	59	32	39	36
Central Harlem/Morningside Heights	1,107	722	22	32	59	81	11
East Harlem	873	1,125	21	26	65	50	41
Upper West Side	1,807	925	6	78	20	18	21
Upper East Side	597	341	5	86	10	9	14
Chelsea/Clinton	1,986	1,802	3	84	14	11	15
Gramercy Park/Murray Hill	979	852	4	79	18	13	16
Greenwich Village/Soho	1,175	1,524	2	81	17	10	13
Union Square/Lower East Side	1,434	960	12	57	39	16	32
Lower Manhattan	96	748	16	58	36	23	25
Bronx	3,855	—	22	23	64	37	53
Kingsbridge/Riverside Dr.	114	163	14	44	39	26	36
Northeast Bronx	269	174	16	34	47	53	28
Fordham/Bronx Park	699	420	22	25	61	29	56
Pelham/Throgs Neck	611	268	22	22	62	32	50
Crotona/Tremont	748	730	24	21	64	41	55
Highbridge/Morrisania	866	795	24	21	68	48	49
Hunts Point/Mott Haven	548	1,047	22	16	73	27	70

249

Brooklyn	5,297	—	20	31	51	50	26
Greenpoint/Williamsburg	700	450	22	19	67	32	56
Bensonhurst/Bay Ridge	207	128	14	39	50	9	16
Downtown, Heights, Park Slope	907	523	12	56	37	33	25
Bedford Stuyvesant/Crown Heights	1,516	523	24	24	57	78	14
East New York	406	361	22	20	65	57	33
Sunset Park	207	296	19	27	57	10	64
Borough Park	218	140	19	35	49	15	27
East Flatbush/Flatbush	716	293	23	28	34^c	73	14
Canarsie/Flatlands	147	110	24	35	41	31	14
Coney Island/Sheepshead Bay	273	120	21	34	51	25	23
Queens	2,916	—	15	41	45	39	26
Long Island City/Astoria	279	158	12	51	41	25	24
West Queens	852	309	8	52	40	19	47
Flushing/Clearview	160	88	14	50	32	20	25
Bayside/Littleneck	42	65	14	29	33^d	14	17
Bridgewood/Forest Hills	206	110	7	48	40	6	23
Fresh Meadows	65	82	13	46	42	22	18
Southwest Queens	257	147	14	45	44	25	25
Jamaica	665	334	21	26	58	81	10
Southeast Queens	252	172	22	36	41	62	12
Rockaway	138	177	30	20	65	63	16

Continued on next page

TABLE 9-1 *continued*

Borough and Neighborhood	Number of Cases	Percentage[a]					
		Rate per 100,000	Women	Gay Men[b]	IVDU	African American	Hispanic American
Staten Island	357	—	17	33	52	22	16
Port Richmond	70	153	24	16	57	31	11
Stapleton/St. George	188	188	19	40	45	24	19
Willowbrook	38	47	8	39	45	3	13
South Beach/Tottenville	61	43	8	18	71	18	15
Total Borough	25,260[e]						
Total Neighborhood	22,948[f]						

[a] Does not equal 100 percent because a person can be counted in more than one category.
[b] More broadly, men who have sex with men.
[c] Thirty-two percent of cases defined as other.
[d] Twenty-six percent of cases defined as other.
[e] 186 unknown addresses.
[f] 2,126 cases without zip code.

SOURCE: Data from New York City Department of Health (1990a,b,c,d,e).

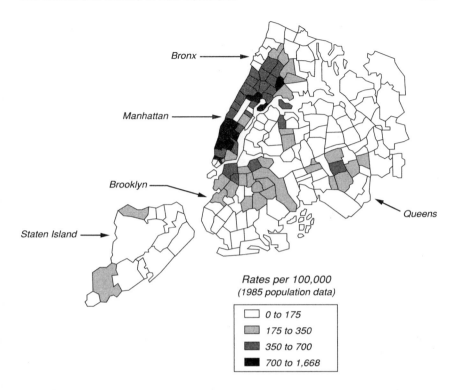

FIGURE 9-1 AIDS case rates in New York City, by zip code, as of April 1989. SOURCE: Data from New York City Department of Health (1990a,b,c,d,e).

with HIV—a citywide seropositivity rate of 1.24 percent (Novick et al., 1991); see Table 9-2. This proportion has not changed substantially since testing of infants began, indicating there have not been rapid increases in seropositivity among women who are having children. This seroprevalence measure does not estimate the rates of HIV infection among all women of childbearing age: it excludes women who are not having children because of contraceptive use, infertility, celibacy, or spontaneous or induced abortion.

These data for childbearing women show a pattern similar to the AIDS data for women. Rates are high among African American (2.21 percent positive) and Hispanic women (1.41 percent positive) and particularly high for women aged 25 to 34. However, the rates vary substantially for both African American and Hispanic women by borough of the city; again, the highest rates are found in Manhattan and the Bronx. Since there is evidence of higher rates of sexually transmitted diseases among African American women than other women, there may be some consequent reduction in

TABLE 9-2 Seroprevalence Among Mothers of Newborns in New York
City, November 1987-September 1990, by Borough and Neighborhood

Borough and Neighborhood	Number Tested	Number Positive	Percent Positive
Manhattan Total	44,141	697	1.58
Washington Heights/Inwood	8,808	57	0.65
Central Harlem/Morningside Heights	7,907	213	2.69
East Harlem	5,057	163	3.22
Upper West Side	5,239	39	0.74
Upper East Side	4,352	16	0.37
Chelsea/Clinton	2,894	61	2.11
Gramercy Park/Murray Hill	2,461	36	1.46
Greenwich Village/Soho	1,500	4	0.27
Union Square/Lower East Side	5,071	95	1.87
Lower Manhattan	852	13	1.53
Bronx Total	50,512	853	1.69
Kingsbridge/Riverside Dr.	2,091	7	0.33
Northeast Bronx	5,165	63	1.22
Fordham/Bronx Park	10,128	125	1.23
Pelham/Throgs Neck	8,655	95	1.10
Crotona/Tremont	9,805	183	1.87
Highbridge/Morrisania	9,093	225	2.47
Hunts Point/Mott Haven	5,575	155	2.78
Brooklyn Total	89,240	1,169	1.31
Greenpoint/Williamsburg	10,782	148	1.37
Bensonhurst/Bay Ridge	4,343	16	0.37
Downtown, Heights, Park Slope	7,509	127	1.69
Bedford Stuyvesant/Crown Heights	21,134	452	2.14
East New York	7,838	119	1.52
Sunset Park	4,670	46	0.99
Borough Park	7,677	29	0.38
East Flatbush/Flatbush	13,710	155	1.13
Canarsie/Flatlands	4,367	24	0.55
Coney Island/Sheepshead Bay	7,210	53	0.74
Queens Total	59,550	376	0.63
Long Island City/Astoria	5,337	42	0.79
West Queens	13,010	70	0.54
Flushing/Clearview	6,441	15	0.23
Bayside/Littleneck	1,828	1	0.05
Bridgewood/Forest Hills	5,269	20	0.38
Fresh Meadows	2,239	4	0.18
Jamaica	9,468	113	1.19

TABLE 9-2 *continued*

Borough and Neighborhood	Number Tested	Number Positive	Percent Positive
Southwest Queens	6,953	36	0.52
Southeast Queens	5,212	36	0.69
Rockaway	3,793	39	1.03
Staten Island Total	11,835	68	0.57
Port Richmond	1,881	25	1.33
Stapleton/St. George	3,200	27	0.84
Willowbrook	2,306	6	0.26
South Beach/Tottenville	4,448	10	0.22
New York City Total	255,278	3,163	1.24

SOURCE: Data from New York City Department of Health (1990a,b,c,d,e).

childbearing capacity that would result in an underestimation of the seropositivity rate among this group (Aral and Holmes, 1990).

HIV seropositivity for women of childbearing age follows the general geographical pattern of AIDS cases for women and intravenous drug users in the city. The rates of highest seropositivity can be seen in the band extending from the northern edge of Manhattan into the central Bronx, across Manhattan below midtown, and in a solid band across the northern edge of Brooklyn. The scattered nature of the areas of high seropositivity suggests the decentralized and local nature of the epidemic in large portions of the city.

Predicting the Future of the Epidemic

As the AIDS epidemic evolves, the proportion of persons at various stages of the disease has also been changing. If a major surge in infections in New York City occurred in the late 1970s and early 1980s, the early to mid-1990s should be the period, in the absence of effective therapies, when a majority of those who were infected will begin to show the symptoms of "frank" AIDS. Although the distributions in Figure 9-2 reflect substantial errors of measurement, they offer some numerical guidance as to what the future has in store for the city. The number at the apex of each pyramid is an indicator of the impact on the acute-care components of the health care system. The numbers in the two lower strata of each pyramid indicate people in the early stages of disease who could benefit from prophylactic measures to prevent or delay the onset of opportunistic infections. Those in the middle strata of the pyramid will require increased levels of outpatient care.

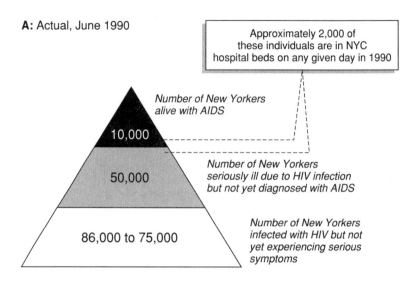

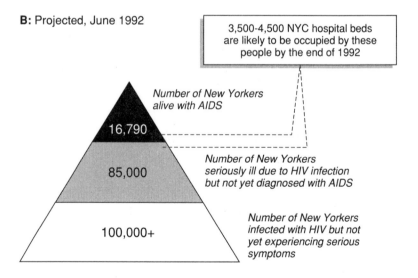

FIGURE 9-2   Estimate of numbers of New York City residents in various stages of HIV-related illness and infection. NOTE: Total estimated number of HIV-infected people in New York City, 126,000-235,000. SOURCE: Data from New York City Department of Health (1989a,b; 1990); Carey (1990:10).

The New York City Department of Health estimates that the incidence of new HIV infections is about 2 percent per year, which would add about 4,000 new cases to the total each year at the present time (Carey, 1990). If this incidence figure remains stable and there is substantial future mortality (which would reduce the numbers of persons with HIV/AIDS), the prevalence of persons with HIV/AIDS in the city should decline substantially by the end of the 1990s.

Estimating the size of a present or future epidemic is not, however, as it might seem superficially, a neutral scientific act. It is a complex calculation that works with uncertain numbers, and they can be manipulated for many purposes. The results often have political reverberations. A July 1988 report by former health commissioner Dr. Stephen Joseph reduced by one-half the estimated number of HIV-infected individuals (Bayer, 1991; Lambert, 1988a,b); the original estimate of 400,000-500,000 was revised to a range of 149,000 to 225,000, provoking a confrontation with AIDS organizations. The suddenness of the change created an outcry within the larger AIDS community that garnered considerable press attention (Lambert, 1988a,b,c,d; Trafford, 1988; Loomis, 1989a,b,). The revised estimate was part of a general rethinking of the dimensions of the epidemic (Centers for Disease Control, 1990), but in New York City it seemed to presage a decline of interest in those who were ill or would become ill in the near future. Despite this initial reaction, however, the reduced numbers have become the accepted figures.

In the most recent report of the New York State Department of Health (1990), three different modeling methods were used to estimate the future course of the statewide epidemic by risk group, producing three substantially different estimates. All are included in the report to show the significant difficulties in generating "precise" estimates of the future course of the epidemic. Indeed the estimates in 1990 vary considerably from those made in 1989. Of particular interest are the differences in the estimates of the future course of the epidemic among women. Modifications in the program used to estimate the logistic growth curve, which assumed very high rates of sexual partnering of intravenous drug users with nonuser partners, resulted in estimates of women infected through sexual contacts with men that are about three times higher by 1996 than are estimates produced by other methods. Studies of the actual sexual partnering patterns of women in New York City do not support such a high estimate (Fordyce et al., 1991). In the absence of additional systematic studies of sexual partnering and sexual behaviors in the general population, estimates will inevitably be very imprecise (see below).

If the projected decline in expected number of AIDS cases among all groups at risk is correct, it may be explained by a number of possible factors, including:

• overestimation of the size of risk groups. There may have been fewer people in the identified risk groups (men who have sex with men or intravenous drug users) than was originally estimated in the mid-1980s.

• overestimation of the proportion of people who are HIV positive. There may have been fewer persons in the identified risk groups who were infected because those who fell into the seroprevalence studies were not a representative sample of the social groups to which they belonged. This would mean that fewer persons have HIV/AIDS than expected.

• reductions in high-risk behaviors early in the epidemic. Changes in sexual practices among gay men may have occurred sufficiently early in the epidemic so that the number of men who might have been expected to become infected in the period between 1982 and 1986 was dramatically reduced. This argument is supported by the rapid decline in rectal gonorrhea rates observed in New York City by Fordyce and Stoneburner (1990) during this period and by other studies of rectal gonorrhea reported by CDC for other cities (Centers for Disease Control, 1990:16). Similar changes in risk behaviors may have also occurred among intravenous drug users, although these changes are less well substantiated.

• impact of the use of prophylactic medications on the onset of HIV-associated infections. The decline in the diagnoses of new AIDS cases may reflect the longer period between HIV infection and the appearance of opportunistic infections of those persons who are being treated with antiviral drugs and the early prophylactic treatment of *Pneumocystis carinii* pneumonia.

• increase in outpatient treatment of persons with HIV before and after the onset of opportunistic infections with delays in reporting. Anecdotal evidence and a few studies suggest that many physicians do not report AIDS diagnoses among outpatients in a timely fashion (indeed, the majority of AIDS case reports come from hospitals). This produces an unmeasured delay in reporting as well as the loss of some cases to the record-keeping system (Greenberg et al., 1990). This is more likely to occur among those populations with access to private health care, and it interacts with the effects of prophylactic care.

• undercounting of the morbidity and mortality that is associated with HIV infection as well as the failure to count persons who would have met the criteria for an AIDS diagnosis. This factor is of particular importance in New York City, where intravenous drug users make up a large proportion of the infected population. Using a variety of data sources, Stoneburner and his colleagues estimated that instead of the 2,440 narcotics-related AIDS deaths that were expected (on the basis of historical experience in the period studied) (Stoneburner et al., 1988:918):

[there was] a cumulative number of 6,157 narcotics-related deaths, 1,197 of which were reported as AIDS cases. Subtracting the expected 2,440 deaths and the 1,197 deaths reported as AIDS cases from the 6,157 actual deaths leaves 2,520 excess deaths that we suggest are HIV-related, but not yet recognized as AIDS.

Adding those deaths to the total number of deaths among intravenous drug users officially attributed to AIDS would increase the total number of HIV-related deaths of intravenous drug users in the official case registry by 35 percent. Such an undercount has dramatic consequences for public- and private-sector responses to the epidemic in New York City, where intravenous drug users comprise one-half of the recognized AIDS cases.

The number of women with HIV/AIDS, their rates of morbidity and mortality, the misfit between their symptoms and CDC-defined AIDS, and their access to health and welfare entitlements associated with an AIDS diagnosis are also deeply controversial issues and are especially important in New York City, where women represent approximately one-fifth of new AIDS cases. In 1988-1990, women accounted for nearly 20 percent of new AIDS cases in the Northeast as a whole (Miller, Turner, and Moses, 1990). Using data from New York State, the Newborn HIV Seroprevalence Study (Lessner, 1991) reports that an estimated 25,196 women aged 15 to 44 were infected with HIV during the period of 1981-1988. From these data, Lessner estimates that there will be 8,295 new cases of AIDS among women in that age group between 1989 and 1993 and about 2,000 new cases in 1993. Using sexual behavior data from a probability sample survey of women in New York City, Fordyce et al. (1991) modeled the number of women in New York City infected with HIV as the result of sexual contact with intravenous drug users. According to their model, new infections for women aged 15 to 44 in 1988 ranged between 867 and 1,668, and the total number of women infected by this mode of transmission for the 1977-1988 period ranges from 5,390 to 10,230 (the midpoint is 7,810). These data suggest that there will be substantial growth in the number of HIV-infected women in the 1990s and, as a consequence, an increase in the number of children born with HIV.

THE TWO EPIDEMICS

From the beginning, New York has had at least two socially, and therefore epidemiologically, separate epidemics. The first involves two linked, but not overlapping, populations of men who have sex with men. One comprises the gay community, which is primarily white but includes men from all ethnic groups. The other includes men of African or Hispanic descent whose sexual contracts are in semi-independent, ethnically homogeneous sexual communities that are only somewhat identified as gay.

The second HIV/AIDS epidemic is composed of intravenous drug users, their sexual partners, and their children, who largely reside in the impoverished, ethnically segregated communities of the inner city. In recent years, the ratio of AIDS cases between men who have sex with men and male intravenous drug users has reached parity, and there has been a significant increase in HIV/AIDS among women and children.

For the period from 1982 to 1985, the proportion of women diagnosed with AIDS in New York City hovered around 10 percent. Since 1985 it has increased steadily each year: 12.4 percent in 1986, 15.8 percent in 1987, 16.4 percent in 1988, and 21.7 percent in 1989 (based on incomplete data for the year) (AIDS in New York State, 1989:60). Of the total number of female AIDS cases reported in New York State by December 31, 1989, approximately 57 percent were reported to have been infected through their own drug use and about 23 percent were infected through sexual contact with a drug user. There is no difference by ethnicity in these proportions (New York State Department of Health, 1989).

Epidemic #1: Men Who Have Sex with Men

In June 1981 the Centers for Disease Control reported that between October 1980 and May 1981, five young gay men had been diagnosed with *Pneumocystis carinii* pneumonia, an illness that would soon be so common that it would become known by its initials, PCP. The next month CDC reported that 26 cases of the formerly very rare Kaposi's sarcoma (KS) had been diagnosed among gay men in the prior 30 months. These reports provided the first intimations of an epidemic that would infect very large numbers of men who had sex with men. A decade later, the HIV/AIDS epidemic has passed through the stage of being regarded as the "gay plague" or being referred to as a "gay-related immune disorder."

Today, the epidemic has manifested itself in other populations, and the rapid spread in new infections in the gay community has slowed somewhat. However, it must be noted that of the approximately 1 million persons infected with HIV in the United States by the end of 1989, between one-half and two-thirds are men who had sex with men. Although gay men responded rapidly with preventive education, patterns of safer sex are not constant across groups and regions, and there is still concern that micro-epidemics may flare up again in the gay community (Stall et al., 1990).

In the period between 1981 and 1991, large numbers of gay men became ill and many died. Many others can be expected to become ill over the next 4 years. This is nowhere more true than in New York State, where it is estimated that by 1996 between 36,000 and 47,000 men will have been diagnosed with AIDS (using the current case definition) (New York State Department of Health, 1990). Between 75 and 80 percent of those men will have died at the end of 1996 if there is no substantial advance in available treatments.

Scholars have noted that plagues and natural disasters have similar psychological consequences (Erikson, 1976). Both shatter the sociocultural order of a community and cause massive emotional reactions among the survivors, which typically appear in the form of collective and individual traumas. *Collective trauma* denotes the loss of communality—the loss of a network of relationships and shared meanings that provide intimacy, support, and a sense of self that ties individuals to the social order. *Individual trauma* refers to the emotional responses to death or devastation, which are shock, numbness, disorientation, guilt, and emotional depletion.

The HIV/AIDS epidemic has had many of these consequences for the gay community and the individuals who are part of it. Of particular importance is the epidemic's impact on a youthful cohort among gay men (those between 25 and 45 in 1980). Death in the United States is usually the province of the elderly, and its incursion into a youthful community means that social and psychological issues that are normally allocated to the end of the life course have to be dealt with at an early age.

An appreciation of the impact of the epidemic in the gay communities requires more than calculation of the numbers of persons infected, ill, or dead. The HIV virus and the emerging gay and lesbian community cultures in New York interacted in ways that profoundly influenced the course of the epidemic, the general public response to it, and the institutional structures and social identity of the gay community.

Evolution of the Gay and Lesbian Community

The pre-HIV/AIDS gay and lesbian community in New York City developed out of the stigmatized social conditions that existed prior to mid-1960s. From World War II until the end of the 1960s, persons identified as "homosexuals" by the medical profession and "dykes," "queens," "fags," and "degenerates" by the public (Levine, 1979) sought to establish identities free of social marginalization and stigma and the harsh social sanctions they fostered (Weinberg and Williams, 1974). New York State criminalized same-sex contact and solicitation, which exposed lesbians and gay men to police harassment, imprisonment, and blackmail. Most mental health professionals considered both female and male homosexuality as a curable form of mental illness, which left these individuals open to mandatory psychotherapy and psychiatric hospitalization. Ridicule, ostracism, and even physical violence from family, friends, and strangers were common (Weinberg and Williams, 1974). Stigmatization thus shaped the structure of New York's lesbian and gay community. The threat of sanctions led to the formation of isolated social networks that functioned as surrogate kin structures and included friendship cliques providing companionship, emotional support, and material aid (Helmer, 1963).

During the 1950s the homosexual community was discreetly clustered within several Manhattan and Brooklyn neighborhoods and entertainment zones (Weinberg and Williams, 1974). Middle- or upper-class lesbians and gay men filled the apartment buildings and townhouses of the East Side, Greenwich Village, and Brooklyn Heights (Helmer, 1963). Most of these men and women were white; only a handful were black or Puerto Rican. Working-class lesbians and gay men, who were predominantly white except for a sizable Puerto Rican contingent on the West Side, lived in tenements and rooming houses of Times Square, the seedy parts of Greenwich Village, and the Upper West Side. These neighborhoods also contained clandestine concentrations of lesbian and gay gathering places (Weinberg and Williams, 1974).

Stigma and oppression were the most important features of the pre-1960s homosexual community and the individuals who constituted its membership. The constant dangers associated with same-gender erotic desire produced a secret world that has been called the "closet culture." The belief that same-sex desires constituted immorality or pathology blocked some lesbians and gay men from having erotic contacts. The threat of exposure, entrapment, or involvement with police raids forced some lesbians and gay men to shun the opportunities for sexual or emotional relations. Thus, the homosexual community in New York City prior to the 1950s and 1960s was relatively fragmented, secretive, and constantly under threat. Some individuals were entirely socially isolated from the community, others used it only as a sexual marketplace, and still others lived in small friendship cliques. Most concealed their sexual desires to family, friends, coworkers, as well as their religious counselors.

The lesbian and gay liberation movement of the 1960s and early 1970s significantly reduced the stigma placed on female and male homosexuality (Marotta, 1981). The decision to embrace the names "lesbian" and "gay" was similar to the decision by "Negroes" to rename themselves "blacks," to claim a name that was formerly an epithet. The gay liberation movement partook in the same spirit that energized the feminist, countercultural, antiwar, and civil rights movements. Its activists strove to eradicate the stigma attached to same-gender sex and, within the sphere of sexual preference, to promote personal autonomy and the right to live within the larger society in accord with one's own values and choices (Adam, 1987). In addition, activists promoted values of self-expression and personal liberation, especially in regard to the use of drugs and to sexual behavior (Marotta, 1981). Political and legal protests were used to counter antigay and antilesbian discrimination in New York City. In response to these activities and general cultural changes, the New York State sodomy statute was declared unconstitutional, and mental health professionals officially ceased treating same-sex love as a psychological disorder (Bayer, 1981). Destigmatization of same-sex desires within the gay and lesbian and gay community during the 1970s allowed many gay men and lesbians to regard themselves as normal, healthy, and sexual. The parallel increase in social tolerance and modest decline in discrimination from the larger community allowed lesbians and gay men to "come out" before a wide range of audiences. Thousands of white, middle-class New Yorkers stopped passing as heterosexual and publicly expressed their gay identity. This identity took on the tones of an "ethnic" self-conception and fostered a massive expansion of the community's territorial, institutional, and cultural base.

The creation of a visible community with a wide range of services had wealth-creating consequences. Businesses that were owned by and that employed gay men and lesbians gained patronage. The community acquired many features of traditional ethnic groups that trade preferentially within their community group. Such practices enabled gay men to buy housing in the local community, and it increased discretionary funds for community service and political activities.

Gay liberation involved both changes and continuities in the sexual styles of gay men and lesbians. The visibility of the community and its members meant that gay sexuality did not necessarily involve personal secrecy. Changes in gender codes meant that many gay men began to adopt entirely masculine styles of personal presentation.

Some elements of prior practice continued for men whose sexual lives had been heavily secretive and repressed by social conditions of the past. This was particularly so in the maintenance of the tradition of "tricking" (having casual sex) with large numbers of partners. The increased visibility, size, and density of the gay community and the public emergence of institutions that were designed to promote easy congregation (baths, bars, discos) made meeting other men in anonymous and erotic circumstances far easier than it had been. There is limited evidence from interviews conducted by Kinsey in the 1940s that even under historically restricted conditions men who were part of the "homosexual" community accumulated large numbers of partners. Under the more open circumstances of the 1970s there were substantial increases in numbers of sexual partners by men in the community (Blumstein and Schwartz, 1983).

Levine has identified the visible world that emerged in these circumstances as dominated by the "clone culture" (Levine, 1989). The term clone emerged from the similarity in look and life-style among a large number of men that set them apart from other groups in the gay world. Levine's point is that not all gay men were clones, but that this culture represented the gay world in popular culture (in the same way that "queen" culture, "drag," and "camp" had done so in earlier eras). Four features distinguished clones:

(1) strongly masculine dress and deportment; (2) uninhibited recreational sex with multiple partners, often in sex clubs and baths; (3) the use of alcohol and other recreational drugs; and (4) frequent attendance at discotheques and other gay meeting places. Clone culture with its pattern of sexual availability, erotic apparel, multiple partners, and reciprocity in sexual technique became an important organizing feature of gay male life during the 1970s. It also became a seedbed for high rates of sexually transmitted diseases as well as frequent transmission of the hepatitis B virus. Many treated sexually transmitted diseases as a price that had to be paid for a life style of erotic liberation.

Initial Response to the Epidemic

The response of the gay community to the beginning intimations of an epidemic were complex. The historical evidence is that the first response of afflicted communities and individuals to epidemics is denial and minimization. Gay men and the communities in which they lived were no exception. The accumulating evidence that the new disease (which was not yet called AIDS) was probably transmitted by sexual contact and that people with many sexual partners who were living in "the fast lane" were either already infected or likely to become infected was met with some disbelief. Some of the disbelief was in the form of "not me," but other responses were more ideological. In the minds of some, the liberation of gay life was identical with the expression of open and free sexuality: gay identity was focused on sexual freedom, and the denial of sexual expression seemed to be a denial of much that the gay movement had struggled for.

Those whose life-styles were not centered around the sexual aspects of gay life were more receptive to the first messages of changing behavior. Some were in the health professions, others were in conventional paired relationships, others had work that took them outside of the recreational life of the gay community, and still others who simply disapproved of what they saw as the sexual excess of some gay male life. Nevertheless, all gay groups urged voluntary behavior changes rather than public health intrusions into the civil rights of those at risk.

The early days of the epidemic in New York saw deep conflicts in the gay community. On one side were those who did not see the small number of cases as evidence for the need to change their sexual conduct and those who felt that the urging to change was coming from the medical profession that so recently condemned them as perverse and neurotic. The message and the messenger seemed untrustworthy. However, as early as mid-1982, community members were beginning to respond to the epidemic in an organizational way by the formation of Gay Men's Health Crisis (GMHC) (officially founded in November 1981) with planning meetings and fund raisers that occurred earlier that summer (Chambre, 1991). As the number of ill and dying rose, it was clear that the community could not, by itself, care for them and that there was a serious need for governmental intervention. From 1981 to 1983 there was increasing community pressure on local and state governments to respond to what was beginning to be recognized as a profound health crisis.

In comparison with the rapid mobilization of public resources in San Francisco, where the gay community was a powerful political voice, the New York public health system moved slowly in response to the epidemic. In contrast to San Francisco, the New York gay community was a much smaller political constituency (San Francisco has a population of approximately 750,000, New York City, approximately 11 million) and had a much more complex political structure. GMHC and other volunteer agencies helped fill an institutional vacuum, focusing on the epidemic among gay men that was happening in their own community. The openly active gay community was willing to recognize it as their own. This contrasted with other similarly afflicted communities. As late as 1987 the major institutions of the African American and Hispanic communities had made only minimal formal responses and there was little evidence of AIDS-related organizations.

Substantial behavioral changes in sexual practices were documented in the gay community—the reduction of unsafe sex, particularly anal intercourse, and numbers of sexual partners. These changes antedated the initiation of formal educational programs to promote behavior change. Studies both in San Francisco and New York indicated that changes in behavior had begun by 1982-1983. By 1986 there had been dramatic declines in risky behavior in all age groups among gay white men (Hansfield, 1986). In New York, studies of the rectal gonorrhea rate (a proxy for risk of HIV transmission) showed about a 10 percent drop between 1981 and 1983 and a drop of close to 80 percent between 1983 and 1986. Similar declines are believed to have occurred among African American and Hispanic men, although lagging behind changes among white men). Martin, Garcia, and Beatrice (1989) reported that the gay-identified men in a nonrandom sample of 745 individuals had reduced their numbers of partners and incidents of anal intercourse by three-quarters (see also Siegel and Glassman). This change appears to have occurred as a result of informal feedback into the community from community-based organizations rather than from formal education programs sponsored by specific health agencies.

Evolution and Role of Volunteer Organizations

By the late 1980s the rate of new HIV infections among gay-identified men began to fall—partly because those at highest risk had already been infected, but also because those still at risk had modified their behaviors. Young gay men were not getting infected at the rates that characterized the age cohort that came of age between 1975 and 1985. This period marked a major transition in the New York gay community. The volunteer agencies had emerged as a potent political force. Voluntary efforts had been the primary force in staying the epidemic of transmissions within the gay community and had also supplied most of the social support resources of those who were ill. The reduction in new infections and steady increase in the numbers of persons needing health care and other services caused the major volunteer agencies to turn their attention to issues of treatment and care. This attention extended to both the delivery of care and attempts to mobilize the governmental sector.

The Gay Men's Health Crisis (GMHC) is probably the largest central volunteer agency in New York providing supportive care to the gay community in New York City. Their activities included buddies; crisis intervention; support in securing and preventing discrimination in housing, health care, and employment; and providing educational services. By June of 1991, it had served 11,362 clients and had a current caseload of 3,266 persons. GMHC has taken stands on most of the major issues facing the gay community and attempted to extend its outreach to nongay-identified and other men who had sex with men throughout the city.

Although recognizing GMHC achievements, some within the gay community thought its political strategies were too moderate. The perceived need for a more radical political effort gave birth to ACT-UP (AIDS Coalition to Unleash Power). ACT-UP was created as a nonhierarchical direct action organization that made decisions concerning demonstrations ("actions" or "zaps") or policies on the basis of an open democratic forum. Although a committee structure developed around specific issues, the town meeting format has sustained itself in the face of substantial increases in membership. There are now ACT-UP groups in many cities across the country, and there is still no central office.

ACT-UP/New York has been an important player in conflicts within the city in a variety of areas and has extended its interests well beyond the gay-identified community. ACT-UP has been visible in a number of New York City conflicts, including those over the reduction in estimates of numbers of persons with HIV in New York City (Bayer, 1991); the appointment of Woodrow Meyers as Health Commissioner (Purdum, 1990; Bayer, 1991); the dispute about condoms in the schools; a continuing conflict with Cardinal John O'Connor about various positions of the Roman Catholic Archdiocese of New York related to AIDS and gay life; and attempts to improve police practices in dealing with the gay and lesbian community (ACT-UP/New York, 1991). On the national scene, ACT-UP/New York has played both an insider's and outsider's role in putting pressure on the National

Institutes of Health, the Food and Drug Administration, and the major pharmaceutical houses to speed the development and release of new drugs (Bryant, 1991; Taylor, 1990). The tactics of ACT-UP, while often compelling and sometimes effective, have also generated strong criticism, and some gay activists believe them to be counterproductive. Events such as the disruption of U.S. Health and Human Services Secretary Louis Sullivan's speech at the International AIDS conference in 1991 and the zaps at St. Patrick's and Holy Cross cathedrals aroused considerable criticism, leading observers to wonder whether they were, on balance, more harmful than helpful.

Volunteer efforts on AIDS have been critical elements in delivering services and reducing the financial impact of the disease, and they have characterized New York's response from the very first moments of the epidemic. Volunteering in a systematic way, however, has been primarily a characteristic of the gay community (Chambre, 1991). This is not to say all volunteers are AIDS-infected gay men. They include the uninfected, women, persons who are not themselves gay, as well as a large number of professionals from a variety of fields.

Agencies and organizations that serve the gay community have attempted to reach other groups of men who have sex with men, intravenous drug users, and women, with mixed results. Of particular importance has been outreach to men who have sex with men in communities that have limited links to the organized gay community. Many African American, Hispanic, and Asian American men have strong contacts with the largely white gay community that is centered in Manhattan. However, these men find themselves caught between their identities as gay men and their bonds with their own ethnic communities that have negative attitudes toward men who have sex with men in general and toward gay men in particular. In addition, the white gay community also exhibits racism, which limits outreach efforts.

Men Outside Identified Gay Communities

Men who have sex with men are found not only in the predominantly white gay community, but also among men of African and Hispanic descent who are only somewhat identified as gay. At the onset of the epidemic little was known about men who had sex with men in various communities of the city. What has been learned about African American men and Hispanic men has largely emerged from research concerning the rates of HIV infection in these groups and ways of preventing further infection. Of all African American men who have been reported with AIDS in New York State, 33 percent are reported to be men who had sex with men; 49 percent are intravenous drug users; and 5 percent have both risk factors. Of all Hispanic men who have been diagnosed with AIDS, 33 percent are reported to be men who have sex with men; 55 percent are intravenous drug users; and 5 percent have both risk factors (New York State Department of Health, 1990). Nationally, the majority of racial and ethnic minority men diagnosed with AIDS have contacted the disease as a result of having sex with men. However, because of the stigma of being known as someone who has sex with men, it is believed that there have been some false reports by African American men that their risk behavior is intravenous drug use.

A number of social networks in the African American community of men who have sex with men are epidemiologically separate from the gay community and show markedly different patterns of infection. A study of 57 African American gay men (who did not self-identify with the predominantly white gay community), raised in stable middle- or working-class, two-parent families showed that this discrete population was not HIV infected. They did not observe safe sex (at the time of the interviews in 1988, none was using condoms), and sexual encounters often followed drinking in bars, at parties, and in private homes, but they selected partners from a neighborhood pool that was as yet uninfected (Hawkeswood, 1991). Other subgroups of men who have sex with men in the African American community appear to be at very high risk for infection because of involvement in street prostitution and "hustling." What little is known about these groups through anecdotes and informal reports suggests relatively high rates of unprotected sex as well as a considerable risk of arrest and imprisonment.

The Hispanic communities in New York City are enormously complex, and many have not been studied at all. An estimated 400,000 Dominican immigrants live in New York City, and Cubans and others from the Caribbean and Central America are also represented, but the major Hispanic community in New York City is Puerto Rican. All share a common cultural perspective on sexuality that is vastly different from prevalent American beliefs. Researchers have found that men who have sex with men in these cultures are divided roughly into two groups, "passivos" and "activos." Activos insert their penis into another man, either orally or anally, and the passivos receive a penis: these are usually, though not always, exclusive roles. Activos are defined as men since they insert, which is what men do to women, and passivos are defined as women since they receive the penis. The inserter is not viewed as homosexual: thus, the distinction between "heterosexuality" and "homosexuality" as commonly understood does not fit this group. (Similar distinctions are found among prisoners and other groups of men who do not view the inserter as homosexual.)

The strength of this pattern depends on the level of acculturation of Hispanic populations into the culture of the United States. Carrier (1989) reports that the active/passive pattern is common among men in Mexico and among recent Mexican immigrants to the United States. Acculturation produces sexual styles more equivalent to those of white gay-identified men.

The pattern appears similar among New York Hispanic men. The continuing belief that the passive homosexual male is a woman has consequences for "coming out" in this community. There remains a tendency for some young men to offer an effeminate self-presentation; cross dressing is common, and some engage in prostitution as women. Such belief structures have important implications for public health practices directed to these communities.

There are few volunteer organizations that work solely with minority men who have sex with men. A general denial of the existence of HIV/AIDS characterizes many Hispanic communities in the city, accompanied by specific denials regarding men who have sex with men who have HIV/AIDS. In part this is a denial by the larger community that there are such men, but another element is the denial by the men themselves. Men who do not self-identify as gay may have some difficulty accepting services directed at those who are identified as gay or homosexual (Russell, 1990). The higher rates of morbidity and mortality in these populations and their lack of access to medical services may result in part from these cultural norms.

Individual Impacts: Discrimination and Impoverishment

For the reasons noted above—recognized rates of infection, a willingness to accept the reality of the epidemic, and active community-based groups monitoring its evolution—the impact of the epidemic has been best recorded in the gay-identified community. The impact on other infected communities is not well documented, and when their histories are better understood they may differ in important respects from the New York gay community. Nonetheless, many features of the experience are common.

HIV/AIDS is a disease that increases the likelihood of discrimination and reduces the economic prospects of individuals even if they do not lose their jobs. It is impoverishing, eliminating opportunities and destroying social networks. The new social networks it creates are often linked to dealing with illness and death.

A major portion of the work of various community-based organizations is providing assistance for gay men with HIV who have encountered discrimination. For example, GMHC provides free legal service to all persons in the New York City area diagnosed as HIV positive. In 6 years they have served 4,000 clients with problems in housing, insurance, health care, and employment. A survey of 60 persons with AIDS and of AIDS service organizations by the New York City Commission on Human Rights (1989) reported cases of discrimination, noting the social impact of discrimination on costs of and access to health care, social services, education, and prevention must be factored into all programs and policy planning.

As previously noted, one of the results of the gay liberation movement was an increase in income and assets of the gay community. Much of the wealth consists of salary and wages, rather than savings. A prolonged illness of any type can impoverish even the solidly middle-class and professional segments of the population (Hansell, 1990); AIDS, however, can be particularly quick in producing financial ruin. Many gay men have been fired when their HIV disease was discovered. Most find it difficult to continue working full time as the disease progresses, yet they hesitate to stop work because of the almost inevitable loss of health insurance coverage. Many who are able to continue working discover that they are occupationally immobile because of health insurance considerations.

Those who are ill find themselves caught in a cycle of high treatment costs and inadequate insurance coverage. To avoid workplace discrimination, men sometimes pay for their own health care rather than submit bills to health care insurers (Oppenheimer and Padgug, 1991). An important share of the costs of HIV/AIDS treatment is the expense of drugs, and typical insurance restrictions on the coverage of prescription drugs (including exclusion of experimental drugs) results in high, out-of-pocket costs. The decline in the costs of AZT, the primary drug of treatment, from $10,000 to between $2,000 and $3,000 a year has been a help, but the costs of other drugs remain high.

The declining ability to work and the daunting costs of health care for HIV disease results in the phenomena of individuals' "spending down" into Medicaid. While only 10 percent of GMHC clients are Medicaid eligible when they first contact GMHC, within 1 year nearly 60 percent have become eligible. GMHC staff estimates that it takes 1 year, on average, for a middle-class, self-supporting individual with HIV to become at least partly dependent on public resources (Hansell, 1990).

Limited public resources have been supplemented by the volunteer community, both in terms of money and services. Productive working people who might have spent more time earning money are now instead involved in volunteer caretaking. Money that would have been saved or invested is spent on charity. Some have described the gay community as an economic colony of the health-care professions, the hospitals, and the pharmaceutical houses (Oppenheimer and Padgug, 1991).

Epidemic #2: Drug Users

In the opening stages of the epidemic it became apparent that sharing of drug injection paraphernalia among heroin addicts was a critical element in HIV transmission (Drucker, 1986). New York City, which had experienced an epidemic of heroin use from the late 1960s into the middle 1970s, is thought to have an aging population (people aged 30 to 40) of some 200,000 heroin users. Experts believe the actual numbers could vary by as much as 50 percent, but 200,000 remains the best estimate possible given the illegal status of drug use and the limitations of any drug-user surveillance system (Turner et al., 1989). However, it was clear that a very large community existed at high risk for infections with a blood-borne viral disease. Indeed, early studies of HIV seropositivity among intravenous drug users showed a rapidly increasing rate. By 1985 it was estimated that intravenous drug users had a seropositivity rate that exceeded 50 percent (Des Jarlais, 1985; Drucker, 1986). Annual incidence rates for the same period were estimated to be between 1 and 11 percent.

Estimating the effect of the HIV/AIDS epidemic on the already existing population of older heroin addicts was complicated by the emergence of cocaine as a readily available street drug. Researchers reported that the majority of methadone patients reported injecting cocaine in the period from 1978 to 1985 (Selwyn and Schoenbaum, personal communication reported in Drucker, 1986). The short-acting effects of cocaine, when injected, increased the frequency of injections and the likelihood of contact with an infected needle.

The dynamic potential for rapid change in the social ecology of drug use was demonstrated by the introduction of crack cocaine in the mid-1980s in response to interruptions in previously plentiful supplies of marijuana. Retrospective analyses suggest that smokeable cocaine in the form now called crack was becoming available on the street in a number of cities (principally, Los Angeles, Miami, and New York) as early as mid-1984 (Hamid, 1990). Beginning in 1987 it became clear that crack added a variety of new complications. In its smokeable form, a nearly immediate, but extremely transitory "high" is experienced, leading to relatively frequent use. The drug was cheap in comparison with either high-quality cocaine or heroin, and the price fell as markets expanded. Since polydrug use has always been common—for example, many, if not most, users of heroin also used other drugs, including alcohol and marijuana—the addition of crack to the drug-use repertoire was not surprising.

Crack was inexpensive enough to be used by young people without much money, and it requires little preparation, creating a new class of youthful users and dealers. The drug was attractive to women, in part because its route of administration did not require injection. Ethnographic research among crack users in Harlem in 1989 found, in addition, that women with a chronic dependency felt crack changed the nature of their relations with men, making them feel powerful and in control of sexual interactions (Clatts, 1992). Unlike heroin or alcohol, which are sedatives, crack cocaine is a stimulant. Because it appears to act as a defense against feelings of low self-esteem and depression, crack became the drug of choice among homeless youths and women who traded sex for drugs (Clatts et al., 1990a,b).

The explosion in crack use during the late 1980s deepened social problems in the areas of New York City that were already most affected by HIV/AIDS. In the opening phase of the crack epidemic, individuals who first began to use the drug exhibited acute signs of personal and social disorganization. Some individuals reported a nearly immediate loss of control and rapid escalations in use and an equally rapid collapse in the stability of personal relations. During this period, the behavior of crack users was thought to be entirely a function of the power of the drug and its impact on the brain, and a number of clinicians thought that such users were not amendable to treatment. The mass media struggled with how to interpret the problem, reporting in early 1989 that crack was "a disaster of historic proportions" (New York Times, 1989:E14). The police responded with concentrated surveillance and arrests in areas overrun by crack dealers, but dealers and buyers simply moved to other sites. Surges in arrests clogged the court dockets and the jails, but they did not appear to produce significant reductions in drug use. Indeed, the police commented that they could arrest four to five times more offenders if there were greater capacity to process them.

A variety of extremely serious second-order problems followed. Crack increased the likelihood of high-risk sexual behavior among female users of all ages. The emergence of "crack prostitutes" was widely reported—a pattern of sexual conduct that involved the exchange of sex by crack-addicted women for money or drugs (Tierney, 1990; Inciardi, 1991). In the most extreme cases, women were reported to be staying in crack houses and exchanging sex for drugs on an indiscriminate basis with many sexual partners, at least some of whom were infected with HIV (Williams et al., 1988).

Exchanges of sex for drugs also involved an increased risk of sexually transmitted diseases that might act as cofactors for HIV transmission. Crack use was identified in one New York City study as a significant behavioral cofactor reported by HIV-positive women visiting a municipal sexually transmitted diseases clinic (Chaisson et al., 1990). Three factors were thought to increase risk of transmission: (1) an increase in sexual partners; (2) the fact that men on cocaine maintain erections for longer, thereby increasing risk of vaginal dryness, leading to abrasions that provide access for the virus; and (3) oral lesions due to blisters caused by hot crack pipes, which increase the likelihood of transmission during oral sex.

In addition to increased risks of transmission, crack use significantly modified patterns of personal and social behavior. Although there is a strongly skewed sex ratio in traditional drug-use patterns (many more men than women), reports confirm that many more women than men have become addicted to crack (see e.g., Hamid, 1990). A variety of experts in New York City commented on the disordering effects that crack use had on women, noting that women had become violent property offenders to an unprecedented degree (Hamid, 1990). A substantial increase in child neglect, abuse, and abandonment affected the workings of the family court and foster care systems, which were already under severe stress. In addition, there was a rise in the number of babies born in the city who showed evidence of maternal cocaine use, and some of those babies required many days of intensive care at very high cost. The "crack babies" added to the problems caused by the number of babies born who were HIV positive. The impact of crack on women was especially serious in minority communities, where women are often the only stable caretakers for children.

PUBLIC HEALTH AND HEALTH CARE

The concentration of the epidemic, both socially and geographically, has differentially affected the component agencies and services of the health care and social welfare systems of New York City. For example, municipal hospitals serving areas with large numbers of people with HIV/AIDS who do not have health care insurance usually have a very large number of patients in various stages of HIV disease. These municipal hospitals are already underfunded, understaffed, and threatened with further budgetary cuts, all of which affect their ability to provide care (Gage et al., 1991).

The lack of private care physicians in the inner-city communities enhances the importance of municipal hospitals. For instance, in the Mott Haven/Hunts Point section of the Bronx there are only 34 office-based primary care physicians for every 100,000 people, in contrast to 1,451 per 100,000 in the Upper East Side of Manhattan (Carey, 1990). Moreover, the few community-based physicians who are available have limited practices. In a recent study of 701 primary care providers in nine low-income communities, only 28 (3.9 percent) were able to provide "accessible, comprehensive and coordinated primary care," and only a quarter had admitting privileges to hospitals to which the poor have access. Those without such privileges must refer patients to the closest emergency room for hospital-level care (Carey, 1990). In such areas of the city, the emergency rooms of the municipal hospitals often serve as the health care providers of the first resort.

Of the 72 hospitals in New York City, 13 serve over one-half of the AIDS patients in the city: 3 are operated by the Roman Catholic Archdiocese and 10 by the New York City Health and Hospitals Corporation. The United Hospital Fund estimates that by 1993, 15 to 25 percent of beds in university hospitals and 50 percent of beds in municipal hospitals will be occupied by persons with diseases related to HIV/AIDS. This will be in a hospital system with close to 90 percent occupancy rates and for which no expansion in beds is expected (Carey, 1990). The concentration of people with HIV/AIDS in certain facilities results from a variety of factors, including: the disease prevalence in community areas served by those hospitals; the expertise developed by institutions with significant concentrations of HIV/AIDS patients; reimbursements available for AIDS care; and resistance of some hospitals to caring for people with HIV disease or people without health insurance. This phenomenon is not restricted to New York City: national data indicate that in 1987, 20 percent of the hospitals in the nation provided 77 percent of the care for persons with HIV/AIDS, and 4 percent of the hospitals provided 32 percent of the care (Rothman et al., 1990).

Within the service areas of the hospitals that provide the largest amount of health care for persons with HIV/AIDS, there is evidence that some specific local areas (as defined by zip code) have a disproportionate number of AIDS cases. Of 542 recent AIDS-related discharges by Bronx Lebanon Hospital, for example, more than one-half had addresses in only two zip code areas. Bronx Lebanon provides a dramatic example of the way in which the HIV/AIDS epidemic can dominate a hospital's health care activities. In 1991 the hospital's average daily census of inpatients with HIV/AIDS ranged from 100 to 120, about four-fifths of whom were housed outside the specialized AIDS unit of 22 beds. Overall, the hospital estimates that one-third of its inpatients are HIV infected. And during 1990, approximately 10,000 visits were made by persons with HIV/AIDS to the outpatient AIDS unit.

The high concentrations of HIV disease in New York City can be documented to the level of clusters of city blocks. HIV/AIDS in impoverished populations in the inner city is transmitted by behaviors that imply a common residential pattern. For example, intravenous drugs users appear to be a relatively immobile population that depends on a strong network of neighborhood residential and social ties to maintain contacts with "running buddies" and drug suppliers. This population's sexual partners are also relatively immobile, and often they and their children share common households with the drug users. Such factors increase the concentration of persons with HIV/AIDS within narrow boundaries and focus the impact of the epidemic in those communities.

A similar process of geographical concentration had occurred with gay men, but for quite different reasons. The areas in New York City with the highest concentrations of people with HIV/AIDS are those that are home to large numbers of gay men (United Hospital Fund areas Chelsea-Clinton and Greenwich Village-Soho), and within those two areas, the majority of persons living with HIV/AIDS reside in two (of nine) zip code areas. The construction of these quasi-ethnic communities, which provide a wide range of social and cultural services, also created an environment in which there were high rates of sexual interaction, which resulted in transmission of HIV and other sexually transmitted diseases among some men. These residential communities now contain substantial numbers of men who are living with HIV/AIDS and who are users of the services provided by local hospitals and physicians (often gay themselves), as well as by the voluntary organizations that have been created in response to the AIDS epidemic. The everyday fact of living with the epidemic is thus concentrated in a small number of communities, which are in large measure insulated from the rest of the city.

The social concentration of the epidemic in some neighborhoods also has limiting effects on the proportion of health care professionals and facilities that come in contact with persons living with HIV/AIDS. Patients with HIV disease are concentrated within the catchment areas of specific hospitals. In addition, African Americans and Hispanics with HIV/AIDS (as well as those white gay men who are impoverished by HIV/AIDS) are more likely to be treated in municipal rather than private hospitals. During the week of January 21, 1990, for example, municipal hospitals in New York City had 16 percent of the beds but 37 percent of the AIDS patients (Carey, 1990).

Within some hospitals in New York State, specialized facilities have been developed to handle persons with HIV/AIDS, and a number of hospitals in the city have been designated AIDS centers by the state. (To be so designated hospitals must meet 14 standards of care; in return, they receive a higher level of reimbursement.) As of October 12, 1990, 13 hospitals in New York City were designated as AIDS centers. As of the same date, no municipal hospital had met the standards for center status, even though municipal hospitals have the largest proportions of HIV/AIDS patients in the city (except for three voluntary hospitals administered by the Archdiocese of New York and Bronx Lebanon).

The concentration of persons with HIV/AIDS in various locations does not necessarily mean that only physicians who maintain practices in those areas, either community- or hospital-based, are likely to see patients in any stage of HIV disease. In a 1988 telephone survey in New York City of a probability sample of 473 primary care physicians (internists, family care practitioners, general practitioners, and obstetricians-gynecologists), 61 percent said that they had "ever" had a person with HIV in their practice, and those physicians had accumulated an average of six patients who had AIDS. About one-third of the physicians said that they were currently treating patients who were HIV positive, and on average, those physicians had 15 such patients in their practice. Another one-third, however, said they would refer an asymptomatic HIV-positive patient elsewhere rather than treat the patient (Gemson et al., 1989). The data in this survey suggest that many primary care physicians in New York City have had some contact with persons with HIV/AIDS. The physicians who reported having such patients were more often younger, better trained, less averse to or fearful of homosexuality, and more likely to know someone other than a patient who has AIDS. These findings suggest that some experience with persons with HIV/ AIDS is relatively widely distributed among physicians.

The survey data do not necessarily conflict with data on concentrations of patients in hospitals, data on the neighborhood concentrations of AIDS cases, or the evidence from AIDS voluntary organizations that many physicians do not treat patients with HIV/AIDS. Although many physicians in private practice may have a small number of patients with HIV/AIDS (particularly middle-class men), the majority of persons with HIV are treated by a smaller number of health care professionals and agencies. The Gay Men's Health Crisis has a referral list of only 45 AIDS specialists in Manhattan (Lambert, 1990b). Even though there is evidence for some contact between many physicians and persons with HIV/AIDS, there is other evidence, even in New York City, that only a modest number of medical professionals in private or hospital practice regularly come into contact with persons with HIV/AIDS. Given the concentration of HIV/AIDS in specific neighborhoods and social communities, a substantial proportion of that number are professionals working in public-sector hospitals and physicians in private practice in gay areas of the city.

Despite the recommendations of various AIDS commissions and task forces that the burden of HIV/AIDS be dealt with on a citywide basis (New York City Department of Health, 1989a,b; Rothman et al., 1990), the epidemic is disproportionately felt in limited areas of the city. Indeed, although there are no single-disease hospitals for HIV, some hospitals and medical practices are in fact dominated by HIV/AIDS (Navarro, 1991). This is, in some measure, a result of the geographical concentration of the epidemic, which limits which health care providers and hospitals will be in the neighborhoods of AIDS patients. Another factor that has considerable influence is the limited health care resources that exist in the areas in which economically impoverished members of ethnic minorities live—poverty reduces physician availability and concentrates patients in the municipal hospitals. HIV/AIDS in this sense is not a citywide disease.

Public Health Effects of HIV/AIDS Concentration

The concentration of HIV/AIDS in particular neighborhoods of New York City reveals a chilling epidemiological fact: HIV/AIDS is but one in an overlapping cluster of epidemics. The affected neighborhoods, marked by poverty, poor access to health care, drug addiction, and social disintegration are beset with co-epidemics of disease. The most striking lesson to be learned from the concentration of AIDS in particular neighborhoods is that

AIDS cannot be viewed in isolation. The map of HIV disease in New York City is also a map of the epidemic spread of other diseases, including sexually transmitted viral and bacterial diseases, as well as some nonsexually transmitted diseases, particularly tuberculosis. AIDS cases are also concentrated in zones of urban poverty, poor health care, drug addiction, and social disintegration.

Gonorrhea, syphilis, and chancroid—the three classic venereal diseases that had nearly disappeared except for momentary and treatable recurrences—are increasing at epidemic rates among urban minority populations in the United States (Aral and Holmes, 1991). Syphilis and herpes have been associated with HIV infection in heterosexual men and women and homosexual men in the United States. HIV infection leads to altered manifestations of sexually transmitted diseases (STDs) and is thought to promote their spread. Thus, it has been suggested that HIV and other STDs interact to facilitate the sexual transmission of HIV (Aral and Holmes, 1991:66).

The recent spread of nonsexually transmitted infectious diseases is also occurring in neighborhoods already suffering from a high concentration of AIDS and other STDs. Certain parts of urban centers of the United States have become "islands of illness" (Rosenthal, 1990:1) as their residents experience a resurgence of measles, mumps, rubella, and whooping cough—all of which are diseases that can be prevented with vaccines. In addition, during the 1980s (following almost two decades of decline), New York City experienced a 132 percent increase in the incidence of tuberculosis (New York City Department of Health, 1991). New cases rose by more than 38 percent in the city in 1989-1990, almost four times the rate of increase in the previous year. The highest rate was found in central Harlem, where there were 233.4 cases per 100,000, more than 23 times the national average. Although African Americans made up 28.7 percent of the city's population in the 1990 census, they accounted for 58 percent of the tuberculosis cases. The association between tuberculosis and HIV disease has been documented in a number of studies (see, e.g., Barnes et al., 1991).

The rise of tuberculosis in impoverished communities is in part linked to the movement of people in and out of prison and jail systems in which crowded conditions, inadequate health care, and the presence of HIV/AIDS facilitate the transmission of the bacillus. The annual incidence of tuberculosis in the New York State correctional system increased from 15.4 cases per 100,000 in 1976-1978 to 132.2 cases in 1988. African Americans and Hispanics aged 30 to 39 who had used intravenous drugs were those usually infected, as one might expect. There is no evidence for a common source of the epidemic within the institutions, a finding that would confirm the view that the epidemics in New York City and in the prisons are part of a common epidemiologic community (Hammett et al., 1989).

The increase of tuberculosis in New York City was accompanied by an epidemic of homelessness during the same period. In the late 1960s, homelessness in New York City meant "skid row,"—large numbers of predominantly white men (often employed) living in an area called the Bowery. In marked contrast, today's homeless are more likely to be young (late 20s and early 30s), minorities, and, increasingly, mothers and children who are members of single-parent families (Hopper, 1990). By 1989, 69 percent of men living in the streets were African American, 17 percent were white, and 12 percent were Hispanic; of those regularly using city shelters, 72 percent were African American, 7 percent white, and 16 percent Hispanic (Hopper, 1990).

Recent research suggests that homelessness and the social disorder associated with it are critical factors in the increase of tuberculosis (Brudney and Dobkin, 1991). In research conducted at Harlem Hospital, which serves the area of the city with the highest tuberculosis rate, 224 consecutive patients with tuberculosis were studied during the first 9 months of 1988: 50 percent of those patients had HIV/AIDS, 68 percent were homeless, 64 percent used crack cocaine or injected drugs, and 50 percent had high rates of alcohol use. Of the 178 who were discharged, 89 percent were lost to follow-up and did not complete treatment. The situation of many people with tuberculosis is so compromised by unemployment, poverty, and drug and alcohol use that even when they are diagnosed and prescribed a treatment regimen, they often fail to comply.

According to the same study, there has been a substantial disinvestment in tuberculosis control in both New York City and New York State. Traditional programs of inpatient tuberculosis care had been eliminated in the 1970s, but there was also a dramatic decline in funding outpatient treatment of tuberculosis. The fiscal crisis of the city in the 1970s led to reduced funds for tuberculosis control, and the state terminated its support for all city tuberculosis control activities in 1979. At the same time, the Public Health Service was also decreasing its support for tuberculosis control (Brudney and Dobkin, 1991). Yet even before the HIV/AIDS epidemic began, tuberculosis was resurgent. The dramatic increases in homelessness and in the use of shelters have created the seedbed for transmission and for noncompliance with treatment routines.

More recently, there has been a major surge of interest in the dangers of a tuberculosis outbreak as the dire predictions of the tuberculosis control workers have come true. A disturbing aspect of the resurgence of tuberculosis involves small outbreaks of a strain of the bacillus that is resistant to conventional treatments, representing a particular danger to individuals whose immune systems are compromised by HIV infection. Multiple drug-resistant tuberculosis (MDR-TB) is both more expensive and more complex to treat than non-drug-resistant varieties of tuberculosis. Following a November 1991 outbreak of MDR-TB in which 12 HIV-infected inmates and a guard died, the Department of Corrections announced it will put in place programs of screening inmates and employees and isolating those inmates with tuberculosis in quarantine units in remodeled infirmaries (McFadden, 1992).

The problem of adherence to tuberculosis treatment routines has become especially important as the disease has become common among those with the most disorderly lives in the society: the homeless, the drug addicted, and those in these groups who have lost hope as a result of their infection with HIV. Inadequate support for the machinery of tuberculosis control compounds these problems. A recent request for $13 million from the federal government (to add to the $8 million budget for the city's Tuberculosis Bureau's) resulted in two grants totaling only $1.4 million (Belkin, 1991). In December 1991 an allocation of $8 million was promised from city, state, and federal funds to invest in "sweeping health measures to limit the spread of TB" (Altman, 1991), although there was no specification of how much of these funds was new money. The new program involved increased personnel and incentives for compliance, as well as the requirement that hospital rooms have better ventilation and ultraviolet lamps. In recent months there have been anecdotal reports that persons with HIV/AIDS may be avoiding hospitals because they are afraid of being infected with tuberculosis (Navarro, 1992).

Ethnicity and Residence:
Data Collection and Other Public Health Issues

There is some evidence to suggest that the impact of HIV/AIDS differs among ethnic groups in New York City, although the way in which AIDS data are currently collected provides only limited insight into the situation. The CDC method of data collection (identifying only black/white/Hispanic and, more recently, Asian-Pacific) does not allow researchers or health care practitioners to trace the impact of the epidemic in particular ethnic communities, reducing opportunities to devise culturally appropriate prevention and treatment programs. The absence of data on income, education, or occupation invites the fallacy of attributing to *skin color* effects that are in fact the result of poverty and racism and of further stigmatizing disadvantaged communities.

Puerto Ricans are the ethnic group most severely affected by the HIV/AIDS epidemic in New York City. This fact has been determined despite the absence of incidence data for those born in Puerto Rico and the difficulty of determining ethnicity among those classified as Hispanic in AIDS mortality data (Menendez-Bergad et al., 1990). Between 1982 and 1987, AIDS accounted for a steadily increasing proportion of deaths among Puerto Rican born males, reaching 12 percent among Hispanics, compared with 6 percent for African American, and 2 percent for whites in 1987 (Menendez-Bergad et al., 1990).

The Puerto Rican incidence data provide important insights into the epidemic, suggesting that culturally distinctive patterns of behavior and residential segregation play a role in the spread of HIV disease. For example, all Puerto Ricans have U.S. citizenship and thus have no need to marry U.S. citizens to ensure continued residence (unlike other Hispanics born outside the United States). Indeed, Puerto Ricans marry each other in greater proportions than other Hispanic-origin groups in New York City, and they are also more likely to have sexual contact with other Puerto Ricans than with individuals from any other groups. In addition, needle-sharing networks among intravenous drug users are often racially or ethnically homogeneous (Schoenbaum et al., 1989), which further concentrates the virus. Puerto Ricans also maintain close links with family and friends, and many Puerto Ricans diagnosed with HIV disease in New York City return to Puerto Rico following diagnosis, underlining the idea that the Puerto Rican communities in New York City and San Juan can be thought of as a single social and epidemiologic "neighborhood" (Lambert, 1990a).

Women's ability to observe safe sex practices—specifically to persuade their partners to use condoms—is heavily influenced by cultural expectations. A study of 304 African American and Hispanic women of childbearing age at two inner-city health facilities showed that Hispanic women were more likely than African American women to believe that there was nothing they could do if their partners did not want to use condoms. Moreover, foreign-born women were more likely than native-born women to hold that view and also to know less about AIDS and safer sex practices (Worth, 1989; Ricardo, 1990). Thus, significant differences of epidemiologic relevance stem from distinctive cultural patterns of social and sexual contact, differences in national origin, in migration history, and in the prevalence of HIV in particular communities (Menendez-Bergad et al., 1990).

Very little is currently known about these important cultural and social differences for the many ethnic groups in New York City. Knowledge is particularly wanting for Hispanics. Prior to 1965, for example, Puerto Ricans accounted for the largest proportion of Hispanic immigrants to New York City. Since that time, immigration from Puerto Rico has declined and that from other locations has increased, especially from the Dominican Republic. Dominicans are now the second largest Hispanic group in New York City, approximately 50 percent of whom are thought to be illegal residents (Wasserman et al., 1990). The implications for health behavior and health care remain largely unexplored.

The Crisis of Infant Health

The impact of the AIDS epidemic among children in the city is now well known, but the epidemic is only one indication of the problematic status of child health among the minority poor in the city. Data from as early as 1985 suggested a growing health crisis for infants and children in the most impoverished sections of the city, including a leveling off in the previous long-term decline in infant mortality rates.

Data on low birthweight infants (less that 2,500 grams), a phenomenon highly associated with infant mortality as well as a precursor of a variety of problems for a child who survives the first year of life, are highly variable across the city. Gager (1988) have identified health center districts in the city with much higher than average rates of low birthweight infants. The four areas characterized by the largest proportion of low birthweight infants in 1985 (1 infant in 8 in contrast to 1 in 12 in the city at large) in Upper Manhattan and the South Central Bronx (Central Harlem, Morrisania, Mott Haven, and Tremont) had nearly 70 percent of all births paid for by Medicaid, 40 percent with late or no prenatal care, and 20 percent of all births to teenage mothers. The districts with a high prevalence of low birthweight infants have a familiar ring when compared with the neighborhoods that have been the sites for the highest rates of reported AIDS cases among poor adults and children. They are again those areas in the city where HIV/AIDS is interactive with other social and health crises.

The low-weight births are also concentrated in the same hospitals that serve the largest number of AIDS cases among minority adults and children. The largest number of low-weight births in Central Harlem occurred at Harlem Hospital: 50 percent of those births were to women who had late or no prenatal care and 80 percent were paid for by Medicaid. In East Harlem, most low-weight births occur at Metropolitan Hospital, and they too are largely paid for by Medicaid, although there is evidence of more prenatal care: only one in four mothers had late or no prenatal care. The data are similar for some hospitals in the Bronx, such as Lincoln (two-thirds late or no prenatal care and two-thirds supported by Medicaid). Similar patterns occur for the remainder of the city, with the voluntary hospitals reporting lower proportions of women who have late or no prenatal care.

The complex association among infant health, drugs, HIV seropositivity, and measures of socioeconomic status remains. Data that present the ecological correlation among HIV-seropositive births, low birthweight infants, drug-related discharges from hospitals, and proportion of births to mothers with less than 12 years of education show a remarkable overlap by city area (Morse et al., 1991).

CORRECTIONAL SYSTEMS

The concentration of intravenous drug users in the impoverished inner-city communities of New York and the intimate association between drug use and criminality have led to a steady flow of drugs users in and out of the criminal justice system. The criminalized status of drug use and the crimes that are often committed by drug users involve a cycle of addiction, arrest, imprisonment, release, and relapse to addiction. This revolving-door pattern has been characteristic of the life of the users of illegal drugs in the United States—particularly those using opiates and opiate derivatives—since the late 1920s (Musto, 1987). Since World War II, the cycle of addiction and criminalization has been disproportionately centered in minority communities, even though there is evidence of widespread illegal drug use in other communities.

When the federal war on drugs was declared in the 1980s, increased numbers of low-level drug users and sellers (who are often users themselves) were arrested, resulting in larger numbers of people at high risk for HIV infection being processed by criminal justice institutions. Of all correctional institutions, prisons are probably the most severely affected since they hold people for the longest periods of time and have responsibility for the health of their inmates.

Of the 130,000 people who are processed through New York City's correctional system each year (daily censuses are about 20,000 people), it is estimated that more than one-half have histories of drug use (though not all are intravenous drug users). Of the 50,000 or more intravenous drug users, it is estimated that between 20 and 25 percent are HIV positive. Thus, between 10,000 and 15,000 people with HIV disease were in the city's correctional system during 1988 alone (Association of the Bar of the City of New York, 1989). Approximately 54,000 people are held in state prisons, 60 to 70 percent of whom have histories of drug use (although not all are intravenous drug users); about 75 percent of the total are from New York City.

Women with HIV/AIDS are a particularly serious problem for the city (and state) correctional systems. About 5 percent of the prisoners in the state system are women; the midyear 1990 count was 2,721 prisoners. About 19 percent of female prisoners are HIV positive, and 57 women have died in prison from AIDS (Smith et al., 1991). Women are more likely to be committed to the state prison system for drug offenses than for crimes of violence, and many have been recently imprisoned as the result of crack cocaine use. In the city system, about 10 percent of the prisoners are women, and about one in five is HIV positive. Female inmates with HIV/AIDS require special services including drug treatment, frequent medical attention to the gynecological needs, pregnancy testing, and access to information about infection control between mother and child (New York State Department of Health/New York AIDS Institute, 1989).

The inmates who flow through the correctional institutions of the city and the state are not drawn equally from every community in the city. The city is itself residentially segregated along ethnic lines, and although data do not exist on the residential distribution of those who enter the criminal justice system, it is not unreasonable to argue, given their ethnic distribution, that they are drawn from the areas that house the poor of the city. Currently, on any given day, 23 percent of all African American men in New York State aged 20 to 29 are in some form of control by criminal justice authorities—prison, jail, probation, or parole (see Table 9-3). Of those young men, 48 percent are in jail or prison. It is important to note that these are lower-bound numbers because they represent the count on a single day. Across an entire year, the proportions are somewhat higher. The proportion under the control of the criminal justice system is smaller for Hispanic men of the same age (14 percent), but the proportion of those in custody who are in prison or jail is the same—48 percent. In contrast, only 3 percent of whites in the same age range are in custody of any kind (Gangi and Murphy, 1990). More than 80 percent of all of the Department of Corrections Services prisoners in New York State are African American or Hispanic. The proportions in the jails of the city of New York are similar.

HIV/AIDS makes a special contribution to the bleak situation of many of these men and the women. The number of minority men in New York City who will die from HIV/AIDS (largely in their 30s and early 40s) will be substantial; estimates range between 50,000 and 100,000 (although the actual number will never be known precisely). Many of these men will pass through the criminal justice system, challenging its ability and willingness to deal humanely with HIV-infected inmates. The system's success in meeting that challenge will be felt not only by the inmates, but by the poor and minority communities from which they come and to which they may return.

Currently, 41 states plus the District of Columbia, Puerto Rico, and the Virgin Islands are under a court order or consent decree to improve conditions of confinement or limit the prison populations either for their entire prison systems or for specific institutions (Cade, 1990). Neither the New York City nor the New York State correctional systems are under such court orders or consent decrees, but both have had to expand rapidly to accommodate the rapid rise in prisoners over the past decades. In 1973, New York State had 12,500 persons in the state prison system; by September 1990, that number was more than 54,000 (Gangi and Murphy, 1990). In December 1991 it was reported that this number had reached 57,000 and that the state would add from 3,000 to 6,000 new beds through double bunking in the medium-security prisons (Raab, 1991). Similarly, the num-

TABLE 9-3 Criminal Justice Custody Rates for Males Aged 20-29, by Ethnicity or Race, New York State

Group	State Prisons	County Jails	Misdemeanor Probation	Felony Probation	Parole	Total Population	Under Custody Number	Under Custody Percent
White	3,613	2,092	15,459	10,944	2,000	1,243,189	34,108	2.7
Black	13,123	8,354	7,186	11,004	5,092	193,222	44,759	23.2
Hispanic	5,641	3,813	2,052	5,511	2,704	164,575	19,721	12.0
Total	22,377	14,259	24,697	27,459	9,796	1,600,986	98,588	6.2

SOURCE: Adapted from Gangi and Murphy (1990).

ber of prisoners in the New York City correctional system has increased—from 7,000 per day in 1980 to 20,000 per day in 1990 (Gangi and Murphy, 1990).

The state was expected to spend $3 billion in 1990 to cover the cost of operations and construction of the prison system. It costs approximately $58,000 a year to keep an inmate in a city jail; the cost of constructing a new jail cell is close to $200,000 (Gangi and Murphy, 1990). Not only are these costs high, resources used for prisons become unavailable for alternatives to imprisonment, for drug treatment, or for the health care system at large. This trade-off has raised questions about the wisdom of incarcerating drug offenders (Gangi and Murphy, 1990).

The focus on law enforcement solutions to drug problems, particularly in the visible communities of drug users in minority populations where the epidemic of HIV disease has centered, has created a major crisis in the criminal justice system, especially in prisons and jails (Association of the Bar of the City of New York, 1989). People with HIV disease, including those with AIDS, come in contact with the full gamut of the agencies of the criminal justice system—police, court officers, correctional officers, and probation and parole officers, as well as lawyers and judges. They find themselves at the double disadvantage of being accused or convicted offenders and ill with a disease that creates fear in many of the officials with whom they come in contact. Recent reports suggest that although some workers in the system have been particularly helpful to people with HIV/AIDS, there are many incidents of prejudice and discrimination that are harmful to the health and legal cause of persons with HIV/AIDS (Association of the Bar of the City of New York, 1989). There is evidence of trial delays and limitations on court access because of HIV status, problems with the behavior of court officers (e.g., wearing gloves and protective masks), problems with the transportation of HIV-infected accused and convicted people, and failures of confidentiality of HIV status (Association of the Bar of the City of New York, 1989).

Correctional System's Response to Inmates with AIDS

The New York City Department of Corrections has tried to be responsive to the AIDS crisis. In 1987, for example, a 40-bed infirmary unit was established on Rikers Island, a New York City jail, to house inmates who were diagnosed with AIDS. (The unit replaced the very inadequate facilities that had existed since 1984.) In 1989 prisoners with AIDS were moved to an expanded 66-bed annex to the infirmary. These improvements were taken under threat of court action by inmates with HIV/AIDS and concerned nongovernmental organizations. The new facility at Rikers Island is considered to be a model of efficient and humane care, but it is a segregated unit, and all of the men in the unit know they have a fatal disease. The extended report on the situation in Rikers Island by Dobie (1990) indicates that the fear of dying in prison is widespread among the men in the unit and that there are difficulties in arranging compassionate release even for seriously ill men.

The policy of segregating inmates with "recognizable" AIDS (most inmates with "unrecognized" HIV disease are in the general prison population) was justified on a number of bases, including the risks to those infected if their status were known to other inmates. However, the segregation appears to be based on management considerations relating to institutional efficiency and movement in the institution and to and from court, as well as for health care and public health considerations. Actual medical care in the institution is now provided under contract by Montefiore Hospital (located in the Bronx), and acute care takes place in a number of municipal hospitals with secure units when beds are available; in 1989 there were a total of 66 such beds in two hospitals, Bellevue and Kings County. When beds are not available or specialized care is needed, prisoners, including those with HIV disease, are placed in wards meant for the general population. The prisoners are usually shackled 24 hours a day, although there are some circumstances in which manacles are not used. (For a detailed discussion of the use of manacles, see Association of the Bar of the City of New York, 1989:201.)

The New York State Department of Corrections Services has, for a variety of reasons, been less responsive to the issue of HIV/AIDS. In part this has been the result of a policy decision at the highest administrative levels. In 1988, Thomas A. Coughlin III, the commissioner of the department, stressed that their primary mission is not one of health care (quoted in Association of the Bar of the City of New York, 1989:207):

> As Commissioner I would resist any attempts to redefine our mission to include primary responsibility for health care. Our system is predicated on the use of community health resources . . . AIDS is a devastating personal and societal problem; prison should not be the place to treat that problem. Any attempt to replicate in prison services that should be provided in the community to treat this problem is, in my opinion, bad public policy.

Although this position is understandable given the limited resources of the Department of Corrections Services, some 3,500 persons with HIV/AIDS are estimated to be in the state prison system. The sentences of state offenders are longer than those of inmates in the city correctional system. As a consequence, state inmates are more likely to find themselves in the end stages of their disease while imprisoned. State prison facilities are far flung, often in rural counties, far from the concentrated health care resources of the urban regions. Prior to the epidemic the state prison system

depended on limited-care infirmaries within the institutions, a few dedicated acute care beds in outside hospitals, and a case-by-case arrangement
with community hospitals. Since the epidemic, problems have increased,
but the response of the department has been modest—special needs units
have been established in three institutions and a dormitory in a fourth.
According to various external reports, the department's health-care facilities are currently inadequate for the needs of the inmates with HIV/AIDS
(see New York State Department of Health, 1988). Furthermore, although
the department has "mainstreamed" many of its prisoners with HIV/AIDS,
it has also attempted to create specialized segregated facilities, which was
halted by court order (Association of the Bar of the City of New York,
1989:219).[1]

There is evidence that the survival rate for prisoners in state custody
who have histories of intravenous drug use and who have HIV/AIDS is far
shorter than for people with similar characteristics in New York City who
are not incarcerated: the latter survive 318 days from diagnosis to death;
the former survive 159 days. There is also evidence that 25 percent of
inmates who die in prison of HIV/AIDS are diagnosed only after autopsy;
this percentage appears to be lower than that for people who die undiag-
nosed in the community (Potler, 1988; Stoneburner et al., 1988).) The
differential in survival time may have a number of causes, including delays
in identifying those who are infected and show signs of illness, inadequate
care as a result of limited staff training, and understaffing (Potler, 1988).
One might add to these causes the relative lack of treatment drugs available
to prisoners (especially to those who are asymptomatic) and the stressful
conditions of life for prisoners.

The failure of attempts to remediate the current health care crisis in
state institutions is signaled by the fact that this most recent report of the
Correctional Association now focuses on early release and clemency for the
terminally ill while treating a major improvement in the health care facilities of the prison system as desirable goal. Medical parole for terminally ill
inmates has been urged by a number of legislators, inmate groups, citizen
groups, and correctional officials. According to recent press reports, there
are now between 8,000 (the correctional systems estimate) and 12,000 inmates (citizens' groups estimate) with HIV/AIDS in the state prison system,
and 2,600 prisoners are now being treated for HIV disease (Dao, 1992). A
clemency program might increase contacts between terminally ill inmates
and their families and would prevent prisoners from dying alone. In addition, it would save the prison system money by transferring the costs of
treating terminally ill prisoners to the budgets of nonprison institutions.

IMPACT OF HIV/AIDS ON
WOMEN, CHILDREN, AND FAMILIES

Women make up a growing proportion of persons with HIV/AIDS, particularly in New York City and northern New Jersey, which already lead the nation in the cumulative number of CDC-defined AIDS cases among women. They are nearly almost all poor and from African American or Hispanic communities. The highest rates of HIV-infected women occur in the South Bronx, Chelsea-Clinton, and Central and East Harlem in Manhattan and in Bedford Stuyvesant in Brooklyn (see Table 9-1 above). As noted above, researchers modeling HIV/AIDS among women in New York predict as many as 2,000 new cases in 1993 and a related increase in the number of babies born with HIV/AIDS.

A number of investigators have noted the importance of distinguishing between women with HIV/AIDS, children with HIV/AIDS as a result of perinatal transmission, and the interactive relationship between women and children, one or both of whom may have HIV/AIDS. Women are often viewed only in terms of their "reproductive function," and an invidious distinction is drawn between "guilty" women infected by drug use or sex and "innocent" children (Chavkin, 1990).

The distinction between innocent and guilty sufferers has serious consequences for resource allocation. Funds are more readily devoted to babies and children with AIDS than to women who need drug treatment, housing, or other social resources. In addition, such a distinction between guilty and innocent affects interactions between women with HIV/AIDS and the traditional systems of care and caretakers. Ethnographic studies document numerous negative experiences on the part of poor African American and Hispanic women in their interactions with the health care system. These have the effect of disempowering women, reducing their sense of control over their own lives, and preventing them from seeking health care or complying with instructions given to them (Kenny et al., 1990).

Finally, the division of the world into guilty mothers and innocent children focuses the health care debate for women around the issues of childbearing, the prevention of reproduction, and decisions that women "ought to make" about whether to have children. Such debates generally do not result in the practical programs that are required to give women the resources with which to manage their own choices about sexuality and reproduction.

Research activity is also skewed toward women in their relation to their children or to children rather than to women themselves. The scientific reasons offered for the exclusion of women from clinical trials for drugs for HIV disease are complex. A number of feminists have pointed out, however, that women were previously excluded from other trials (e.g., those related to heart disease), for which the specific complexities of HIV/AIDS did not obtain.

There has been widespread support for specialized health training and facilities for the care of women with HIV/AIDS; Bronx Lebanon Hospital has such a clinic for women (Citizens Commission on AIDS for New York City and Northern New Jersey, 1991). Such clinics, as planned, would focus on the social, economic, political, and psychological situation of women, factors that are often at the center of dealing with the nonmedical cofactors that affect the transmission and management of HIV disease.

As rates of HIV infection among women have increased, a number of medical investigators have begun to question earlier findings about the effects of HIV infection on the outcome of pregnancies. Asymptomatic HIV-infected female intravenous drug users in a New York City methadone program were not found to have decreased pregnancy rates or increased risk of adverse pregnancy outcomes. Moreover, acceleration in HIV disease during pregnancy was not found to be common (Selwyn et al., 1989b).

Data suggest that HIV-positive women are giving birth at rates normal for their age. Knowledge of their own HIV infection does not necessarily deter women from bearing children. Medical investigators associated with Montefiore Medical Center in the Bronx found that knowledge of HIV antibody status was not the overriding factor in decisions to terminate pregnancies; matters related to pregnancy—such as experience with a prior elective abortion, a negative emotional reaction to pregnancy, and whether the pregnancy had been unplanned—were more important (Selwyn et al., 1989a). Research conducted by anthropologist Anitra Pivnick among the same community of women explored the notion of reproductive choice in a broader context of family and social relations, economic circumstances, and cultural influences (see Pivnick et al., 1991). The 120 women in the study population—62 percent Hispanic (predominantly Puerto Rican), 30 percent African American, and 8 percent white—had a mean age of 34.9 years. Three factors distinguished HIV-positive women who chose to bear children from those who chose to terminate their pregnancy: prior abortion experience, the duration of knowledge of serostatus, and history of the mother's residence with existing children. Women who elected to continue with their pregnancies had a significantly lower lifetime abortion rate than women who chose abortions. They had also known of their serostatus for a significantly longer period of time, which presumably enabled them to consider decisions about childbearing without the pressures of pregnancy. Finally, women who had not lived with any child for 100 percent of the child's life were more likely to choose to bear a child than women who had that experience. (Many women in the study had themselves been "given away" by their own mothers and had confessed to life-long feelings of sadness and reproach.) Women who had managed to keep at least one of their own children felt a profound sense of accomplishment. The study suggests that drug treatment options and family services, the first steps in keeping families together, could relieve many women of the need to replace lost offspring by giving birth to infants who face an unpromising future (Pivnick et al., 1991).

HIV positive women have difficulty obtaining abortions. In one study, test calls were placed to 25 abortion clinics. After the appointment was made, the caller revealed that she was HIV positive: 16 clinics (64 percent) canceled the appointment and refused to perform the procedure; others charged higher rates (Franke, 1989).

Data from a national, population-based survey to measure the prevalence of HIV infection in women giving birth to infants indicate that an estimated 1.5 of every 1,000 women giving birth to infants in 1989 were infected. The highest HIV seroprevalence rates were observed in New York (5.8 per 1,000) the District of Columbia (5.5 per 1,000), New Jersey (4.9 per 1,000), and Florida (4.5 per 1,000). Assuming a perinatal transmission rate of 30 percent, the authors estimate that approximately 1,800 newborns acquired HIV infection during one 12-month period (Gwinn et al., 1991). In another study, blood specimens collected from parturients in a recent New York City study indicate that as many as 2 percent of live births occur among women with HIV infection (Barbacci et al., 1990).

Further evidence of the high rates of HIV infection in childbearing women in New York is provided by the New York State Department of Health's newborn seroprevalence study. On the basis of the testing of blood specimens obtained from all infants born in the state between November 30, 1987, and March 31, 1990, the study found an overall seropositivity rate of 0.66 percent for childbearing women. The magnitude of the health problem was most striking in New York City, where in some zip code areas as many as 1 of every 22 childbearing women were found to be HIV infected (Novick et al., 1991). The rates were highest in the Bronx, followed by Manhattan and then Brooklyn. The rates for Queens and Staten Island were more than twice the rates for the two New York State regions adjacent to New York City (New York City Suburban and Mid-Hudson Valley) (Novick et al., 1991). The lower overall seropositivity rate for New York State exclusive of New York City (0.17 percent) is deceptive, however, since zip code analyses revealed small areas with rates approaching those in New York City. This underscores the need for small-area information in assessing large geographic areas: apparently low seropositivity may mask communities with rates that are a serious public health concern (Novick et al., 1991).

The New York State study also showed the mothers of black and Hispanic newborns with the highest (0.87 percent) seropositivity rate. The rate of 0.12 percent for whites and for other racial and ethnic groups, however, confirms a significant incursion of HIV infection in these populations as well (Novick et al., 1991). Moreover, newborn seropositivity increased with maternal age: an especially sharp rise in the infection rate was seen for women in New York City—from 1 in 624 at age 14 to 1 in 71 at age 24. Although racial/ethnic and maternal age patterns are needed for projections and resource allocation, race and age are not as such risk factors. Identifying the patterns offers insight into the environmental factors that determine prevalence and that allow for the targeting of preventive measures. Furthermore, as the rate of HIV infection among heterosexuals increases, current policies of offering HIV testing only to women with currently acknowledged risk factors will become even more inadequate (Barbacci et al., 1990).

Women with HIV/AIDS in poor urban neighborhoods also have special needs. Women in single-parent households must deal not only with the impact of their illness, but with their concerns about the children they will be leaving behind when they die (Indyk et al., 1990). It is expected that 20,000 children will be orphaned by AIDS in New York City by 1993 and that over the next few years 60,000-70,000 children will lose one parent to AIDS (Citizens Commission on AIDS for New York City and Northern New Jersey, 1991). Children of a mother who has died of AIDS are likely to confront stigma in school and in the community). Ignorance and prejudice about AIDS still undermine the intervention efforts of community-based health organizations attempting to deal with the special educational needs of those children.

Caring for Infected Children: Examples in Harlem

Pediatric HIV infection is a family disease: more than 80 percent of pediatric AIDS cases reported to the CDC identify perinatal exposure as the mode of transmission. Thus, a child with HIV disease is often the index case that leads to the identification of infected parents and siblings previously considered healthy. Extended kin often assist in the care of these children, providing support or acting as foster parents, and uninfected siblings are left to witness the deterioration and destruction of their family. Few diseases of childhood affect an entire family with such clarity (Abrams and Nicholas, 1990).

The situation at Harlem Hospital was described for the panel by pediatrician Elaine Abrams. The Pediatric AIDS Unit at Harlem aims to provide high-quality care for HIV-infected children largely in the context of highly disenfranchised families. Only one-half of the children are accompanied by their natural parents; many are in alternative or foster care settings. Extended kin—aunts, uncles, and especially grandmothers—often provide care for the children. The grandmothers, who may be suffering from the loss of their natural children, also face the burdens of failing health, limited financial resources, and multiple responsibilities, which further complicate the medical management of a sick child (Abrams and Nicholas, 1990). The care program at Harlem Hospital is supported to a significant degree with research funds. Although supporting clinical care through research grants is a strategy born of necessity, participation in a research protocol can enhance overall care. A research protocol enforces thoroughness and follow-up in cases for which medical and social data on patients may be hard to locate. The program's focus on integrated medical and social services for mothers and children allows research to be carried out in an otherwise chaotic milieu. The provision of primary care that focuses on the needs of families permits mothers, caretakers, and children to comply with the requirements of a research protocol. The reverse is also true: in the absence of integrated care, research would not be possible.

The benefits of this approach are clear, but difficulties are also present. The continuity of research funds cannot be guaranteed. Balancing the needs of mothers and children may cause conflicts. Some hospital staff, patients, and child welfare professionals tend to mistrust or fear scientific research. Many HIV-positive children are in foster custody, and social workers and others who care for those children understandably wish to protect their rights. The staff at Harlem Hospital, however, work closely with the foster care system, acknowledging the disadvantages as well as the advantages of experimental protocols. The Child Welfare Administration of New York City has developed a medical advisory board to evaluate protocols and now advises that the "best potential treatment option" may be experimental therapy. In such cases, a child's natural parents are approached for their consent. If the parents are deceased or cannot be found after diligent effort, the commissioner may grant consent for the child's entry into an experimental protocol.

In 1986 and 1987 few alternatives existed for the care of HIV-positive children outside of the households of their natural parents. Many children who were medically ready for discharge but whose natural parents could not care for them thus spent much of their lives as "boarder babies," hospitalized for want of a less institutional setting for care (Hegarty et al., 1988). Since 1988 several options have been developed. Resources have been made available to recruit foster care families willing to care for children at risk for HIV infection. New York City established the Incarnation Children's Center (ICC), a transitional unit that offers medical care and nurturing in a home-like environment. Children remain at ICC until an appropriate foster home is identified.

In contrast to the widespread assumption that HIV-positive children are often "abandoned," experience at ICC shows that only 20 percent of children come to ICC through abandonment at time of admission: 80 per cent of the children admitted to Incarnation Center during the past 2-1/2 years do have some involvement with family members. About one-third have frequent weekly visits from parents or immediate extended kin, and about one-third have occasional visits (every 2 to 4 weeks) from both male and female family members. Fathers visit children at the Center (which is located at the edge of Harlem) more often than they do at Harlem Hospital. The homelike atmosphere at ICC perhaps encourages more frequent visits, especially by older fathers who work and who have relationships with drug-addicted mothers.

A total of 190 children have so far been cared for at ICC, of whom 162 children are now in homes: 85 percent are in foster homes with nonrelatives, and 15 percent have been returned to their natural families, although they were originally slated for transfer to foster homes. As the number of infected children continues to rise, the need for additional alternate care facilities will also increase. The experience at ICC shows that the length of the children's stays in hospital can be reduced and that children and their families can be offered nurturing care that is difficult to provide in hospital settings.

There are now a number of children with HIV/AIDS in the local Harlem schools. Some were infected through blood products; others became infected through perinatal transmission. The availability of medical treatments has increased the expected lifespan of infected children, and HIV-infected children as old as 10, 11, and 12 years of age are in school. In addition to HIV-related health problems, some children manifest behavior disorders related to factors other than HIV. Fetal alcohol syndrome may be evident, as well as the long-term effects of low birthweight, lack of prenatal care, and maternal drug use during pregnancy. And some children may live with mothers who continue to take drugs or who live with men who do.

At school, HIV-infected children often face a staff that lacks the knowledge or means to confront the many problems associated with their condition. At home, for complex reasons that include fear of community reaction or the desire to protect the child from full knowledge about the illness, parents or caretakers may also avoid discussing the full dimensions of the disease. However, with earlier diagnosis and treatment that can now prolong life, there are stronger incentives to deal with the fear and prejudice that HIV infection arouses. Some experts argue that the concept of long-term, complex medical therapy should be presented to educators, caretakers, and medical staff (including physicians) and reinforced over time (Abrams and Nicholas, 1990).

RELIGION: CONFLICT OVER CONDOMS AND
AIDS EDUCATION FOR YOUNG PEOPLE

From the beginning of the HIV/AIDS epidemic, there has been a continuous conflict over the role of education about safer sex and condoms in preventing the transmission of HIV. This debate has been particularly sharp when the targets of the educational and condom distribution programs have been young people of high school age, although there has been strong resistance in the national government to condom education for persons of all ages (Specter, 1989).

The proponents of safer sex education and condom provision to youths point out that they do not necessarily approve of early sexual experimentation on the part of young people, but that large numbers of young persons are sexually active under conditions of relative ignorance about the consequences of their conduct. The decision not to provide safer sex education or condoms to young people places them in danger of the transmission of HIV and other STDs that increase the likelihood of HIV transmission. The arguments of the proponents are short term, pragmatic, and health oriented: young people are sexually active; it is unlikely that they will abstain regardless of how often they are exhorted, and they are in danger of contracting a fatal disease. The logical consequence of this position is the provision of age-appropriate sex education that includes information about same-gender sex, modes of HIV transmission and methods of prevention, as well as the provision of condoms without either mandatory counseling or parental consent.

The opponents of safer sex education and the provision of condoms stress the long term, the role of the parent and church versus the school and the state, and issues of morality. In their view, the control of the sexuality of young people properly resides with parents and the religious institutions to which parents and children belong, which emphasize chastity before marriage and fidelity afterward. The provision of safer sex education and condoms threaten these goals and appear to condone sexual experimentation. For some religious groups, such as the Roman Catholic church, condoms are a completely forbidden form of birth control.

The antagonists in New York City have been locked in a debate largely directed not at each other, but at the relatively uncommitted wider community. The immediate targets of the arguments are such decision makers, such as school board members and school administrators or those who appoint them.

When condom provision in the public senior high schools was proposed in 1986, an active coalition of religious groups, spearheaded by the Archdioceses of New York and Brooklyn, persuaded the school board to reject the proposal. In the fall of 1990 the new school chancellor asked that the members of the newly appointed school board support a plan for condom distribution (Berger, 1990b). He noted the many AIDS cases among young people and reported that 80 percent of New York City's 261,000 public high school students were having intercourse. Four of the five new members of the seven-member board reported that they favored such distribution. The plan was opposed by one board member, who said, "It sends a message to young people that we expect them to have sex" (Berger, 1990b:B4). The officials of the Roman Catholic church made their position clear by pointing out that condom provision "says that the universal value that places sexual activity as acceptable only within the context of marriage can neither be taught by our schools nor accepted by our students" (Berger, 1990b:B4).

In December 1990 the Board of Education received the chancellor's plan to distribute condoms to all students who requested them. All public high schools were to be included, and counseling or parental consent was not required (Berger, 1990d). Opponents remained adamant, and some potential supporters wanted counseling to be provided, including information on condom use and how to persuade a partner to use one. In addition, they wanted all students to be told that sexual abstinence before marriage is the best method of prevention (Berger, 1990a). Proponents of the program wished to dissociate it from pregnancy prevention—the issues were simply those of HIV disease and health. They hoped to avoid further conflict with the Roman Catholic church over birth control.

The role of the Roman Catholic church in AIDS education and prevention had already produced conflict regarding church obligations in AIDS prevention education when receiving state funds for health care services. The New York State Public Health Council voted to exempt Catholic-operated nursing homes and hospitals from the requirement that HIV/AIDS patients receive condoms, safer sex counseling, contraceptives, and abortion services. AIDS activists opposed receipt of public funds by Catholic-operated institutions unless they agreed to provide prevention information (e.g., the role of condoms in AIDS prevention), which they declined to do because it is contrary to church doctrine. The church stated that such information violates its "institutional conscience" and can be received elsewhere. In another dispute, the Archdiocese refused to lease to the Board of Education unused Catholic parochial school space for special education classes on AIDS prevention. The leases were barred unless the board waived its sex education curriculum, which includes information on forms of contraception not approved by the church. The decision was based on the evaluation of the 1984 sex education curriculum that, according to the evaluation "makes no mention of modesty, chastity, premarital sexual abstinence or even marital fidelity" (Goldman, 1991:30).

The Board of Education itself was divided on the condom plan. The four African American and Hispanic members favored it (in varying degrees), and the three white members opposed it, again in varying degrees. One of the opponents objected to the board's citation in its curriculum of literature from a gay and lesbian organization that had published a booklet that one board member considered particularly offensive, although that booklet was not used in school education (Berger, 1990c).

An open meeting conducted by the board in February 1991 attracted 277 speakers and ran from 10 a.m. until late in the evening. The division between the proponents and opponents was clear: on one side were religious groups and those whose allegiance was to traditional values; on the other side were health professionals, AIDS workers, persons with AIDS, and activist groups. The disagreements among African Americans mirrored the larger debate, with distortions born of racial discrimination: Did the provision of condoms to African American youths signal a racist lack of faith in their ability to be sexually abstinent? (This same subtext framed the needle-exchange debate: the conflict between health promotion and the danger that needle provision would simply support or expand the use of drugs in already afflicted communities.) Actual research about the utility of condoms, either in preventing HIV transmission or in influencing the sexual activity of young people, was rarely cited in the debate over condom use. The actual experiences of school districts across the country that had implemented condom programs were rarely discussed (Lewin, 1991). The complexity of the studies and the mixed results they presented seemed to limit their usefulness in public debate (Dreyfoos, 1991). A few weeks after the public meeting Mayor David Dinkins backed the condom plan without counseling or parental consent (Berger, 1991a). The board approved the plan for condom provision without parental consent by a vote of four to three, divided along racial and ethnic lines, with some discussion of a future provision for a parental option to exclude their children from the program (Berger, 1991b).

The ideological structure of the conflict and the social composition of the opposing groups were predictable and similar to conflicts over HIV/AIDS and sexuality in other communities and at the national level. Although the specific outcome in any community is unpredictable, there are constants: the relative inadequacy of scientific evidence on those questions for which science is important (e.g., if the presence of a condom provision program increases or decreases sexual activity among the young) and the irrelevance of scientific findings in settling what are ultimately conflicts between different religious and secular perspectives on the solution of social problems.

CONCLUSIONS

The panel's findings on the HIV/AIDS epidemic among gay men, intravenous drug users, and women and children in New York City reflect a highly localized epidemic that is increasingly concentrated among poor people and racial and ethnic minorities. Responding to the problem of HIV requires knowledge of the local communities and an understanding of the cultural realities of those who live there. The inner-city poor may live in New York City, but they do not live in the same New York City as those who are more affluent and better protected from the epidemic (and many other risks) by regular employment, health care insurance, and lower crime rates. Those with HIV/AIDS among the inner-city poor often live and die in invisible neighborhoods within the segregated communities of the city.

The February 1991 end of the Citizens Commission on AIDS for New York City and Northern New Jersey was an important signal of the changed political and economic context at the beginning of the second decade of the HIV/AIDS epidemic. The commission was a major example of a foundation-supported volunteer attempt to provide private-sector leadership and offer a nonpartisan influence on public policy in dealing with HIV/AIDS. Its demise, after somewhat less than 4 years of life, can be attributed to the normal processes of wear and tear on volunteer efforts, the completion of some of the original tasks set by the organization, and the declining interest of the private funding sector in supporting organizations dealing with the HIV/AIDS epidemic. Indeed, in its final report, the commission reflected on the unfinished task and what lies ahead in what may yet be the most devastating phase of the epidemic (Citizens Commission on AIDS for New York City and Northern New Jersey, 1991):

> The AIDS epidemic continues its relentless course, with no end in sight. But AIDS is fading from public concern. When the Citizens Commission on AIDS was created three and a half years ago, AIDS was an unpopular cause. It is now rapidly becoming a "post-popular" cause, without ever having truly engaged widespread public support.

Such a conclusion after the first decade of an epidemic that has taken a minimum of 30,000 lives in New York City requires an attempt to understand a catastrophe that may ultimately take nearly 200,000 lives in New York City, cost billions of dollars, and leave untold numbers of shattered lives, but will have passed through the city without fundamental impacts on the overall life of the city.

Epidemics appear to have much in common. They share a common dramaturgical form of progressive acknowledgment, collective agreement on an explanatory framework, and a negotiated public response (Rosenberg, 1989). They differ, however, according to the particular social and biological environments in which they take place. HIV disease in New York City occurs increasingly in the context of socioeconomic and ethnic deprivation, as well as among populations already suffering high levels of morbidity and mortality. The New York City epidemic is thus exceptional in certain ways, but it is not exceptional in that it is embedded in the ongoing life of the city (to some extent, in the life of Northern New Jersey and San Juan, Puerto Rico, as well). The particular impact of the HIV/AIDS epidemic can only be appreciated when one examines the complex of social and biological problems with which it constantly interacts.

Such an examination, even though only partially covered in this report, has revealed that the synergism of plagues that converges on certain areas of New York City and the people who dwell in them creates the seedbed for an epidemic that will devastate those people far more seriously than HIV/AIDS will devastate the nation at large. In those areas—as in similar areas in cities throughout the country—the social institutions that might control the spread of the disease and provide care for those who suffer from it are already overburdened or nonexistent. The panel does not believe one can generalize from New York City to the United States; at the same time, the panel suggests that monitoring the impact of HIV/AIDS, that is, attempting to see the epidemic's course in light of the social context in which it moves, will show similar patterns elsewhere.

NOTE

1. In August 1991 prisoners known to be infected with HIV were allowed to participate in the Family Reunion Program of the state prison system, which allows inmates overnight visits with their spouses. This participation had been denied to HIV-positive prisoners for 10 years, and the denial had survived court tests by prisoners rights groups in the past. The reason offered for the change in policy was that there had been an evolution in the understanding of the disease by the prison authorities over the past 10 years (Verhovek, 1991).

REFERENCES

ACT-UP/New York (1991) *ACT-UP New York: Capsule History.* New York: ACT-UP.

Abrams, E.J., and S.W. Nicholas (1990) Pediatric HIV infection. *Pediatric Annals* 19(8):482-487.

Adam, B.D. (1987) *The Rise of a Gay and Lesbian Movement.* Boston: Twayne Publishers.

Altman, L.K. (1991) New York moving to limit TB spread. *New York Times* December 8:A1.

Andrews, R., B. Preston, E. Howell, and M. Keyes (1989) *A Comparative Analysis of AIDS Service Demonstration Projects in Los Angeles, Miami, New York, and San Francisco.* Washington, D.C.: SysteMetrics/McGraw Hill, Inc.

Aral, S., and K. Holmes (1990) Epidemiology of personal behavior and sexually transmitted diseases. In K. Holmes, et al., *Sexually Transmitted Diseases.* New York: McGraw Hill.

Aral, S.O., and K.K. Holmes (1991) Sexually transmitted diseases in the AIDS era. *Scientific American* 264:62-69.

Association of the Bar of the City of New York/Joint Subcommittee on AIDS in the Criminal

Justice System (1989) *AIDS and the Criminal Justice System: A Fir Recommendations.* New York: Association of the Bar of the City of Ne

Barbacci, M.B., G.A. Dalabetta, J.T. Repke, B.L. Talbot, P. Charache, et al. (1990) immunodeficiency virus infection in women attending an inner-city prenatal clinic: ineffectiveness of targeted screening. *Sexually Transmitted Diseases* 17:122-126.

Barnes, P.F., A.B. Bloch, P.T. Davidson, and D.E. Snider (1991) Tuberculosis in patients with human immunodeficiency virus infection. *New England Journal of Medicine* 324:1644-1649.

Bayer, R. (1981) *Homosexuality and American Psychiatry: The Politics of Diagnosis.* New York: Basic Books, Inc.

Bayer, R. (1991) The dependent center: the first decade of the AIDS epidemic in New York City. Unpublished manuscript, Department of Sociological Medical Sciences, Columbia University.

Belkin, L. (1991) Top TB peril: not taking medicine. *New York Times* November 18:B1.

Berger, J. (1990a) Condom plan for schools draws criticism. *New York Times* December 6:B1.

Berger, J. (1990b) Five out of seven ask condoms in the schools: New York's chancellor backed on distribution. *New York Times* September 27:B1.

Berger, J. (1990c) New York city school board members clash on condom proposal. *New York Times* December 20:B4.

Berger, J. (1990d) Opposition to condom plan by some principals is seen. *New York Times* December 5:B3.

Berger, J. (1991a) Dinkins backs condom plan: some board members work on a compromise. *New York Times* February 26:B1.

Berger, J. (1991b) School board approves plan for condoms: rejects any provision for parental consent. *New York Times* February 28:B1.

Blumstein, P., and P. Schwartz (1983) *American Couples.* New York: William Morrow.

Brudney, K., and J. Dobkin (1991) Resurgent tuberculosis in New York City: HIV, homelessness, and the decline of tuberculosis control programs. *American Review of Respiratory Disease* 144:745-749.

Bryant, M. (1991) ACT-UP: playing the inside and the outside. *Medicine and Health Perspectives* April 1.

Buehler, J.W., R.L. Berkelman, and J.K. Stehr-Green (1992) The completeness of AIDS surveillance. *Journal of Acquired Immune Deficiency Syndromes* 5(3):257-264.

Cade, J. (1990) Status report: state prisons and the courts. *National Prison Project Journal* 22(Winter):7-8.

Carey, J.M. (1990) *AIDS in New York City.* New York: American Council on Science and Health.

Carrier, J.M. (1989) Sexual behavior and the spread of AIDS in Mexico. *Medical Anthropology* 10:129-142.

Centers for Disease Control (CDC) (1990) *HIV/AIDS Surveillance Report.* December:1-8. Atlanta, Ga.: Centers for Disease Control.

Centers for Disease Control (CDC) (1992) *HIV/AIDS Surveillance Report.* Atlanta, Ga.: Centers for Disease Control.

Chaisson, M.A., R.L. Stoneburner, D.S. Hildebrandt, W.E. Ewing, E.E. Telzak, et al. (1990) Heterosexual Transmission of HIV-1 With the Use of Smokeable Freebase Cocaine Crack. Paper presented at the Sixth International Conference on AIDS, San Francisco.

Chambre, S.M. (1991) The volunteer response to the AIDS epidemic in New York City: implications for research on voluntarism. *Nonprofit and Voluntary Sector Quarterly* 20:267-288.

Chavkin, W. (1990) Drug addiction and pregnancy: policy crossroads. *American Journal of Public Health* 80:483-487.

Citizens Commission on AIDS for New York City and Northern New Jersey (1991) *AIDS: Is There a Will to Meet the Challenge?* New York: Citizens Commission on AIDS for New York City and Northern New Jersey.

Clatts, M.C. (1992) Poverty, drug use, and AIDS: converging lines in the life stories of women in Harlem. In *Minority Women and Health: Gender and the Experience of Illness*. (In Press).

Clatts, M.C., E. Springer, and M. Washburn (1990a) Outreach to Homeless Youth in New York City: Implications for Planning and Practice in Social Services. Paper presented at the annual meeting of the American Public Health Association, New York.

Clatts, M.C., W.R. Davis, S. Deren, and S. Tortu (1990b) 1990: Sex for Crack: The Many Faces of Risk Within the Street Economy of Harlem. Paper presented at the 2nd Annual Demonstration Conference, Bethesda, Maryland.

Dao, J. (1992) New York's prisoners with AIDS ask for dignity during last days. *New York Times* March 22:A1.

Des Jarlais, D.C. (1985) AIDS Among Intravenous Drug Users: Overview and Update. Paper presented at the International Conference on AIDS, Atlanta, Georgia.

Dobie, K. (1990) Stick men and giants: inside the Rikers Island AIDS ward. *Village Voice* December 4:28-37.

Dreyfoos, J. (1991) Condoms can decrease teen-age pregnancy and AIDS risks. *New York Times* February 11:A18.

Drucker, E. (1986) AIDS and addiction in New York City. *American Journal of Drug and Alcohol Abuse* 12:165-181.

Erikson, K.T. (1976) *Everything in Its Path: Destruction of Community in the Buffalo Creek Flood*. New York: Simon and Schuster.

Fordyce, E.J., and R. Stoneburner (1990) Patterns of High Risk Sexual Behavior Among Gay and Bisexual Clients at New York City STD Clinics, 1981-1989, and Associated AIDS Morbidity Trends. Paper presented at the annual meeting of the American Public Health Association, New York.

Fordyce, E.J., S. Blum, A. Balanon, and R.L. Stoneburner (1991) A method for estimating HIV transmission rates among female sex partners of male intravenous drug users. *American Journal of Epidemiology* 130:590-598.

Franke, K.M. (1989) Discrimination Against HIV Positive Women by Abortion Clinics in New York City. Paper presented at the Fifth International Conference on AIDS, Montreal.

Gage, L.S., V.S. Weslowski, D.P. Andrulis, E. Hintz, and A.B. Campter (1991) *America's Safety Net Hospitals: The Foundation of Our Nation's Health System*. Washington, D.C.: National Association of Public Hospitals.

Gager, C.T. (1988) *Twelve Health Center Districts in Need: A Birth Atlas*. New York: Community Service Society of New York.

Gangi, R., and J. Murphy (1990) *Imprisoned Generation: Young Men Under Criminal Custody in New York State*. New York: Correctional Association of New York.

Gemson, D.H., J. Colombotos, J. Elinson, E.J. Fordyce, and R. Stoneburner (1989) *The Role of the Physician in AIDS Prevention: A Survey of Primary Care Physicians in New York City*. Final Report to the New York City Department of Health.

Goldman, A.L. (1991) Citing sex classes, bishop bars school leases. *New York Times* January 12:30.

Greenberg, A.B., R. Evans, E. Bryan, E. Lopez, and P. Thomas (1990) Completeness of AIDS Case Reporting and the Spectrum of HIV Disease Among Outpatients in New York City. Paper presented at the Sixth International Conference on AIDS, San Francisco.

Gwinn, M., M. Pappaioanou, J.R. George, W.H. Hannon, S.C. Wasser, M.A. Redus, R. Hoff,

F.G. Grady, A. Willoughby, A.C. Novello, L.R. Peterson, T.J. Dondero, and J.W. Curran (1991) Prevalence of HIV infection in childbearing women in the United States. *Journal of the American Medical Association* 265(13):1704-1708.

Hamid, A. (1990) The political economy of crack-related violence. *Contemporary Drug Problems* Spring:31-78.

Hammett, T.M., S. Moini, L. Harrold, and M. Weissberg (1989) *1988 Update: AIDS in Correctional Facilities. Issues and Practices in Criminal Justice.* Washington, D.C.: National Institute of Justice.

Hansfield, H.H. (1986) Totally safe sex or AIDS response. *American Journal of Pubic Health* 76(5):588-589.

Hansell, D. (1990) Presentation to NAS Panel on Monitory Social Impact of the AIDS Epidemic New York Study Group. April 2, 1990.

Hawkeswood, W.G. (1991) One of the Children: An Ethnography of Identity and Gay Black Men. Ph.D. dissertation. Anthropology Department, Columbia University.

Hegarty, J.D., E.J. Abrams, V.E. Hutchinson, S.W. Nicholas, M.S. Suarez et al. (1988) The medical care costs of human immunodeficiency virus-infected children in Harlem. *Journal of the American Medical Association* 260:1901-1905.

Holmes, K.K., J.M. Karon, and J. Kreiss (1990) The increasing frequency of heterosexually acquired AIDS in the United States, 1983-1988. *American Journal of Public Health* 80:858-863.

Hopper, K. (1990) The new urban niche of homelessness: New York city in the late 1980s. *Bulletin of the New York Academy of Medicine* 66:435-50.

Inciardi, J.A. (1991) King rats, chicken heads, slow necks, freaks and bloodsuckers: a glimpse at the Miami sex for drugs market. Unpublished manuscript, Department of Criminal Justice, University of Delaware.

Kenny, M., J. Mantel, N. Cortez, V. Gonzalez, and L.S. Brown (1990) HIV Prevention Among Women at Risk: An Ethnographic Analysis. Paper presented at the annual meeting of the American Public Health Association, New York.

Lambert, B. (1988a) The cool reaction to New York's "good news" on AIDS, dissent and distrust. *New York Times* July 21:B1,B2.

Lambert, B. (1988b) Halving of estimate on AIDS is raising doubts in New York. *New York Times* July 20:A1.

Lambert, B. (1988c) Number of AIDS cases in New York still varies. *New York Times* September 23:B3.

Lambert, B. (1988d) Puzzling questions are raised on statistics on AIDS epidemic. *New York Times* July 24:B4.

Lambert, B. (1990a) AIDS travels New York-Puerto Rico "air bridge." *New York Times* June 15:B1.

Lambert, B. (1990b) AIDS war shunned by many doctors. *New York Times* April 23:A1.

Lessner, L. (1991) Projection of AIDS incidence in women in New York. *American Journal of Public Health* 81(Suppl.: The New York State HIV Seroprevalence Project):30-34.

Levine, M.P. (1979) Gay ghetto. *Journal of Homosexuality* 4:363-377.

Levine, M.P. (1989) The Impact of AIDS on the Homosexual Clone Community in New York City. Paper presented at the Fifth International Conference on AIDS, Montreal.

Lewin, T. (1991) Studies on teen age sex cloud condom issue. *New York Times* February 8:A14.

Loomis, K. (1989a) AIDS: The numbers game. *New York* March 6:44-49.

Loomis, K. (1989b) Voodoo statistics: the health department's mess. *Village Voice* April 4:33-34.

Marotta, T. (1981) *The Politics of Homosexuality.* Boston, Mass.: Houghton Mifflin Co.

Martin, J.L., M.A. Garcia, and S. T. Beatrice (1989) Sexual behavior changes and HIV antibody in a cohort of New York City gay men. *American Journal of Public Health* 79(4):501-503.

McFadden, R.D. (1992) A drug-resistant TB results in 13 deaths in New York prisons. *New York Times* November 16:A1.

Menendez-Bergad, S., E. Drucker, S.H. Vermund, R.R. Castano, R.R. Perez-Agosto, et al. (1990) AIDS mortality among Puerto Ricans and other Hispanics in New York City, 1981-1987. *Journal of Acquired Immune Deficiency Syndromes* 3:644-648.

Miller, H.G., C.F. Turner, and L.E. Moses (1990) *AIDS: The Second Decade.* Committee on AIDS Research and the Behavioral, Social, and Statistical Sciences, National Research Council. Washington, D.C.: National Academy Press.

Morse, D.L., L. Lessner, M.G. Medvesky, D.M. Glebatis, and L.F. Novick (1991) Geographic distribution of newborn HIV seroprevalence in relation to four sociodemographic variables. *American Journal of Public Health* 81(Suppl.: The New York State HIV Seroprevalence Project):25-29.

Musto, D. (1987) *The American Disease: Origins of Narcotic Control.* New York: Oxford University Press.

Navarro, M. (1991) Dated AIDS definition keeps benefits from many patients. *New York Times* July 8:A1,B5.

Navarro, M. (1992) AIDS patients, facing TB, now fear even the hospital. *New York Times* March 15:A1.

New York City Commission on Human Rights (1989) The Extent and Impact of HIV-Related Discrimination in New York City—A Survey of PWAS and Service Providers. Unpublished draft report, AIDS Division, New York City Commission on Human Rights.

New York City Department of Health (1989a) *City Health Information* 8(4).

New York City Department of Health (1989b) *City Health Information* 8(7).

New York City Department of Health (1990a) Cases of AIDS in Your Neighborhood: The Bronx. Cumulative Adult AIDS Case by Race, Gender, Age and Risk Factor. August 1990. AIDS Program Services, New York City Department of Health.

New York City Department of Health (1990b) Cases of AIDS in Your Neighborhood: Brooklyn. Cumulative Adult AIDS Case by Race, Gender, Age and Risk Factor. August 1990. AIDS Program Services, New York City Department of Health.

New York City Department of Health (1990c) Cases of AIDS in Your Neighborhood: Manhattan. Cumulative Adult AIDS Case by Race, Gender, Age and Risk Factor. August 1990. AIDS Program Services, New York City Department of Health.

New York City Department of Health (1990d) Cases of AIDS in Your Neighborhood: Queens. Cumulative Adult AIDS Case by Race, Gender, Age and Risk Factor. August 1990. AIDS Program Services, New York City Department of Health.

New York City Department of Health (1990e) Cases of AIDS in Your Neighborhood: Staten Island. Cumulative Adult AIDS Case by Race, Gender, Age and Risk Factor. August 1990. AIDS Program Services, New York City Department of Health.

New York City Department of Health (1991) *City Health Information* 10(3).

New York State Department of Health (1988) *AIDS in New York State.* Albany: New York State Department of Health.

New York State Department of Health (1989) *AIDS in New York State.* Albany: New York State Department of Health.

New York State Department of Health, New York AIDS Institute (1989) Management of HIV Infection in New York State Prisons.

New York State Department of Health (1990) *AIDS in New York State.* Albany: New York State Department of Health.

New York Times (1989) Crack: a disaster of historic dimension, still growing. *New York Times* May 28:E14.

Novick, L.F., D.M. Glebatis, R.L. Stricof, P.A. MacCubbin, L. Lessner, et al. (1991) Newborn seroprevalence study: methods and results. *American Journal of Public Health* 81(suppl.):15-21.

Oppenheimer, G.M., and R.A. Padgug (1991) AIDS and the crisis of health insurance. In F. Reamer, ed., *AIDS and Ethics*. New York: Columbia University Press.

Pivnick, A., A. Jacobson, K. Eric, M. Hsu, M. Mulvihill, and E. Drucker (1991) Reproductive decisions among HIV-infected, drug-using women: the importance of mother-child coresidence. *Medical Anthropology Quarterly* 5(2);153-169.

Potler, C. (1988) *AIDS in Prison: A Crisis in New York State Corrections*. New York: The Correctional Association of New York.

Purdum, T.S. (1990) Nominee for health commissioner loses vital backing. *New York Times* January 19:B1.

Raab, S. (1991) New York State to install 3000 more prison beds. *New York Times* December 8:52.

Ricardo, M. (1990) Differences in AIDS-Related Knowledge and Beliefs About Condom Use Among Black and Hispanic Women of U.S. and Non-U.S. Origin. Paper presented at the IV International Conference on AIDS Education, San Juan, Puerto Rico.

Rosenberg, C.E. (1989) What is an epidemic—AIDS in historical perspective. *Daedalus* 118(2):1-17.

Rosenthal, E. (1990) Health problems of inner city poor reach crisis point. *New York Times* December 24:1.

Rothman, D.J., E.A. Tynan, and the New York City Task Force on Single-Disease Hospitals (1990) Advantages and disadvantages of special hospitals for patients with HIV infection: a report by the New York City Task Force on Single-Disease Hospitals. *New England Journal of Medicine* 323:764-768.

Russell, M. (1990) Impediments to Accessing Services for Black Gay and Bisexual Men Who Choose Not to be "Gay Identified." Paper presented at the Sixth International AIDS Conference, San Francisco.

Schoenbaum, E.E., D. Hartel, P.A. Selwyn, R.S. Klein, K. Davenny, et al. (1989) Risk factors for human immunodeficiency virus infection in intravenous drug users. *New England Journal of Medicine* 321:874-879.

Selwyn, P.A., R.J. Carter, E.E. Schoenbaum, V.J. Robertson, R.S. Klein, et al. (1989a) Knowledge of HIV antibody status and decisions to continue or terminate pregnancy among intravenous drug users. *Journal of the American Medical Association* 261:3567-3571.

Selwyn, P.A., E.E. Schoenbaum, K. Davenny, V.J. Robertson, A.R. Feingold et al. (1989b) Prospective study of human immunodeficiency virus infection and pregnancy outcomes in intravenous drug users. *Journal of the American Medical Association* 261:1289-1294.

Siegel, K., and M. Glassman (1989) Individual and aggregate level change in sexual behavior among gay men at risk for AIDS. *Archives of Sexual Behavior* 18(4):335-348.

Smith, P.F., J. Mikl, B.I. Truman, L. Lessner, J.S. Lehman, et al. (1991) HIV infection among women entering the New York state correctional system. *American Journal of Public Health* 81(Suppl.: The New York State HIV Seroprevalence Project):35-40.

Specter, M. (1989) HHS aide blocks publication of pamphlet on condom use: action on AIDS-education brochure angers officials. *Washington Post* October 7:A2.

Stall, R., M. Ekstrand, L. Pollack, L. McKusick, and T.J. Coates (1990) Relapse from safer sex: the next challenge for AIDS prevention efforts. *Journal of Acquired Immune Deficiency Syndrome* 3:1181-1187.

Stoneburner, R.L., D.C. DesJarlais, D. Benezra, L. Gorelkin, J.L. Sotheran, et al. (1988) A larger spectrum of severe HIV-1-related disease in intravenous drug users in New York City. *Science* 242:916-919.

Taylor (1990) AIDS guerrillas. *New York Magazine* November 12:62-73.

Tierney, J. (1990) Newark's spiral of drugs and AIDS. *New York Times* December 16:A1,A23.

Trafford, A. (1988) The AIDS numbers game: body counts, on paper, are the latest political battleground. *Washington Post* (health section) July 26:WH6.

Turner, B., T. Fanning, M. Keyes, and L. Markson (1989) New York Medicaid AIDS Patients: Trends in Hospital Use and Mortality Rates. Paper presented at the Fifth International AIDS Conference, Montreal.

U.S. General Accounting Office (1989) *AIDS Forecasting: Undercount of Cases and Lack of Key Data Weaken Estimates.* GAO/FMED-89-13. Washington, D.C.: U.S. General Accounting Office.

Verhovek, S.H. (1991) Spouse visits for inmates with HIV. *New York Times* August 5:B1.

Wallace, R. (1988) A synergism of plagues: "planned shrinkage," contagious housing destruction and AIDS in the Bronx. *Environmental Research* 47:1-33.

Wasserman, G.A., V.A. Rauh, S.A. Brunelli, M. Garcia-Castro, and B. Necos (1990) Psychosocial attributes and life experiences of disadvantaged minority mothers: age and ethnic variations. *Child Development* 61(2):566-580.

Weinberg, M.S., and C.J. Williams (1974) *Male Homosexuals.* New York: Oxford University Press.

Williams, T.M., C.E. Sterk, S.R. Friedman, C.E. Dozier, and J.L. Sotheran (1988) Crack Use Puts Women at Risk for Heterosexual Transmission of AIDS. Paper presented at Fourth International Conference on AIDS, Stockholm, Sweden.

Worth, D. (1989) Sexual decision-making and AIDS: Why condom promotion among vulnerable women is likely to fail. *Studies in Family Planning* 20:297-307.

APPENDIXES

A

Biographical Sketches

ALBERT R. JONSEN is professor of ethics in medicine at the School of Medicine, University of Washington, where he has taught since 1987. Prior to that he had been chief of the Division of Medical Ethics at the University of California at San Francisco since 1972. In 1969-1972 he was president of the University of San Francisco, where he taught in the departments of philosophy and theology. He has been a member of the Institute of Medicine since 1980. He served as a member of the National Commission for the Protection of Human Subjects of Biomedical and Behavioral Research in 1974-1978 and on the President's Commission for the Study of Ethical Problems in Medicine in 1979-1982. His major publications include *The New Medicine and the Old Ethics* (Harvard University Press, 1990), *The Abuse of Casuistry* (coauthored with Stephen Toulmin, University of California, 1988), *Clinical Ethics*, 3rd ed. (coauthored with Mark Siegler and William Winslade, MacMillan, 1992), and *Ethics Consultation in Health Care* (coedited with John Fletcher and Norman Quist, Health Administration Press, 1989). He holds a Ph.D. in religious studies from Yale University.

RONALD BAYER is professor at the Columbia University School of Public Health. Previously, he was at the Hastings Center. His interests center on questions of justice and health care, occupation health, and controversies in science and technology, and for the past several years his work has increasingly concerned the AIDS epidemic. He has authored and edited several books and several dozen articles on ethical and political controversies in medicine, including *Private Acts, Social Consequences: AIDS and the Politics of Public Health* (Rutgers University Press, 1991) and *AIDS in the Industrialized Democracies: Passions, Politics and Policies* (coedited with David Kirp, Rutgers University Press, 1992). He received a B.A. degree from the University of New York at Binghamton and M.A. and Ph.D. degrees from the University of Chicago.

ALLAN M. BRANDT is Amalie Moses Kass professor of the history of medicine at Harvard Medical School and professor of the history of science at Harvard University where he is a member of the Department of Social Medicine and the Department of the History of Science. Previously he taught social medicine and history at the University of North Carolina at Chapel Hill. As an historian, his work has focused on social and cultural responses to epidemic disease. He is the author of *No Magic Bullet: A Social History of Venereal Disease in the United States Since 1880* (Oxford, 1985), as well as several articles on the HIV/AIDS epidemic in historical perspective. He received a B.A. degree from Brandeis University and a Ph.D. in American history from Columbia University.

DAVID L. CHAMBERS is the Wade H. McCree, Jr., professor of law at the University of Michigan, where he has taught since 1969. He serves also as the codirector of the AIDS Policy Clinic of the University of Michigan Law School. He teaches and writes primarily in the field of family law. From September 1985 to August 1991 he served as a member of the National Research Council's Committee on Child Development Research and Public Policy. He has also served as president of the Society of American Law Teachers. He received a B.A. from Princeton University and an L.L.B. from Harvard Law School.

DEBORAH COTTON is assistant professor of medicine at the Harvard Medical School and assistant professor of health policy and management at the Harvard School of Public Health. She is a coinvestigator in the Statistical and Data Analysis Center at the Harvard School of Public Health and in the Harvard AIDS Clinical Trials Unit, a component of the AIDS Clinical Trials Group, for which she chairs the Protocol Evaluation Subcommittee. Previously, she was a clinical associate in the Laboratory of Clinical Investigation at the National Institute for Allergy and Infectious Diseases and then senior staff fellow in the clinical oncology program at the National Cancer Institute. She also served as clinical director for AIDS at the Beth Israel Hospital in Boston, one of the first hospitals in the country to create such a position. Her current interests include the design of HIV clinical trials, alternatives to clinical trials, and the dissemination of clinical trial results. She received an A.B. degree from Brandeis University, an M.D. degree from Boston University School of Medicine, and an M.P.H. degree in epidemiology from Johns Hopkins University.

JOHN H. GAGNON is presently professor of sociology and psychology at the State University of New York at Stony Brook, where he has been on the faculty since 1968. During this time he has also been an overseas fellow at Churchill College, Cambridge University, and a visiting professor at the Graduate School of Education, Harvard University, the University of Essex, England, and Princeton University. Previously, he was research sociologist and trustee of the Institute for Sex Research at Indiana University. His research has focused on sexual learning of children, sociosexual development in adolescence and young adulthood, same gender sexual relations, and sexual theory. Since 1987 he has been working primarily on issues related to the HIV/AIDS epidemic and conducting collaborative research on sexuality and HIV disease. His major publications include *Sex Offenders* (coauthored with P.H. Gebhard, W.B. Pomeroy, and C.V. Christensen; Harper and Row, New York, 1965) and *Sexual Conduct* (coauthored with W. Simon; Aldine, Chicago, 1973). He received his B.A. and Ph.D. from the University of Chicago.

SHIRLEY LINDENBAUM is professor of anthropology at the Graduate Center of the City University of New York. Her research and publications have been concerned with the transmission and impact of epidemic disease—cholera in Bangladesh, Kuru in Papua New Guinea, and AIDS in New York City—and she has worked as a consultant for several international groups concerned with diarrheal disease, including the Harvard Institute for International Development's Applied Diarrheal Disease Research and with AIDS, including Family Health International. She was president of the Society for Medical Anthropology in 1990-1992 and is a member of the editorial boards for a number of publications in the field of social science and medicine.

EARL E. SHELP is executive director and a senior fellow in theological ethics, at the Foundation for Interfaith Research and Ministry. Prior to this appointment, he taught medical ethics at Baylor College of Medicine and at the Institute of Religion and ethics as visiting professor in the Department of Religion at Dartmouth College. He is a member of the AIDS Vaccine Trials Data and Safety Monitoring Board at the National Institutes of Health and two professional societies—the American Academy of Religion and the Society of Christian Ethics. His publications include five books on HIV/AIDS for religious readers and numerous articles about the epidemic for professional readers. He has been active in mobilizing religious congregations in Houston and elsewhere to address the needs of people with HIV/ AIDS. He received a B.S.C. from the University of Louisville and an M.Div. and a Ph.D. from the Southern Baptist Theological Seminary in Louisville, Kentucky.

MARK D. SMITH is vice president of the Henry J. Kaiser Family Foundation and oversees the foundation's Poverty and Health Program and national initiatives in health promotion. Prior to joining the Kaiser Family Foundation, he was associate director of the AIDS Service and assistant professor of medicine and of health policy and management at Johns Hopkins University. He served as special advisor on AIDS to Pennsylvania Governor Robert P. Casey and was executive director of the Philadelphia Commission on AIDS. He has published and lectured on AIDS and health care financing, ethical issues and the impact of AIDS on minorities, and AIDS screening, public education, and research. He has an undergraduate degree in Afro-American studies from Harvard College, an M.D. degree from the University of North Carolina School of Medicine, Chapel Hill, and an M.B.A. degree from the Wharton School, University of Pennsylvania. He trained in internal medicine at the University of California at San Francisco and the University of Pennsylvania.

JEFF STRYKER, who served as the panel study director, is on the staff of the Center for AIDS Prevention Studies at the University of California at San Francisco. Previously, he was on the staffs of the National Commission on AIDS, the President's Commission for the Study of Ethical Problems in Medicine, the Congressional Office of Technology Assessment, the National Leadership Commission on Health Care, and the Institute of Medicine. His interests are in health policy and medical ethics, and he serves as a consultant on AIDS policy to the Henry J. Kaiser Family Foundation. He received a B.A. degree from the University of Pennsylvania.

JAMES TRUSSELL is professor of economics and public affairs at Princeton University, associate dean of the Woodrow Wilson School of Public and International Affairs, and director of the university's Office of Population Research. He is the author or coauthor of more than 100 publications, primarily in the areas of demographic methodology and reproductive health. He received a B.S. degree in mathematics from Davidson College in 1971, an M.Phil. in economics from Oxford University in 1973, and a Ph.D. in economics from Princeton University in 1975. He is currently a member of the Committee on Population of the National Research Council.

B

Participants in Panel Activities

This appendix lists the many experts invited to speak and participate at panel meetings, case study group meetings in New York City, Miami, and Sacramento, and informal meetings in San Francisco, as well as others who contributed their insight and expertise at various points in the process of this report. The panel extends its appreciation to all and apologizes for any inadvertent omissions. Affiliations are for identification purposes only and are current as of the individual's appearance before the panel.

JEAN ALEXIS, Haitian American Community Action of Dade County, Miami
VICKI ANDERSON, The Effort, Inc., Sacramento
LISA BAILEY, Family Health Center, Inc., Miami
HARRY BAIRD, Health Crisis Network, Miami
MICHAEL BAXTER, Special Programs for Youth, San Francisco Department of Public Health
MARY BAYLESS, Health Council of South Florida, Miami
NATASHA BERRY, University of California, San Francisco
PATTY BLOMBERG, Sacramento AIDS Foundation
SAM BLUM, Health Crisis Network, Miami
PAM BRADLEY, California Children's Services, Sacramento
CYNTHIA BURNETT, Women's Civic Improvement Club, Sacramento
ANN CARTER, Comprehensive AIDS Program, University of Miami

CAROL CASSADY, Chemical Dependency Center for Women, Sacramento

MARCIA CESSAY, Agricultural Workers Health Center, Sacramento

SUSAN CHAMBRE, Departments of Sociology and Anthropology, Baruch College

DALE CHITWOOD, Department of Psychiatry, University of Miami School of Medicine

LYNELL CLANCY, Chemical Dependence Center for Women, Sacramento

GEORGE COOKE, Health Council of South Florida, Miami

MOLLY COOKE, University of California, San Francisco

ELLEN COOPER, Food and Drug Administration, U.S. Department of Health and Human Services, Rockville, Maryland

SEMA COPPERSMITH, Children's Home Society, Miami

MELINDA CUTHBERT, Department of Social and Behavioral Sciences, University of California, San Francisco

THE REVEREND RODNEY DE MARTINI, Office of AIDS Education, Archdiocese of San Francisco

ERNEST DRUCKER, Montefiore Medical Center, New York City

MICHELIN DUCENA, Haitian American Community Action of Dade County, Miami

ABIGAIL ENGLISH, National Youth Law Center, San Francisco

SHARON FARLEY-ARANAGA, Sacramento Urban Indian Health Project, Inc.

DOUGLAS FELDMAN, Department of Epidemiology and Public Health, University of Miami School of Medicine

NEIL FLYNN, Medical Center, University of California, Davis

SUSAN FOLKMAN, University of California, San Francisco

ANA GARCIA, Department of Pediatrics, University of Miami School of Medicine

THE REVEREND JAMES J. GARDINER, SA, Friars of the Atonement, New York City

JACOB GAYLE, Centers for Disease Control, U.S. Department of Health and Human Services, Atlanta, Ga.

ERIC GOOSBY, San Francisco General Hospital

THE REVEREND ANDREW GREELEY, National Opinion Research Center, Chicago

JUDY GREENSPAN, National Prison Project, Washington, D.C.

JOHN GRIGGS, United Hospital Fund, New York City

MARIO GUTIERREZ, Sierra Foundation, Rancho Cordova, California

ANSLEY HAMIB, John Jay College of Criminal Justice, New York City

TED HAMMETT, Abt Associates, Cambridge, Mass.

DAVID HANSELL, Gay Men's Health Crisis, New York City

DONALD HARDIMAN, Office of AIDS Education, Archdiocese of San Francisco
FATHER JOHN HEALY, Archdiocese of Sacramento
GREGORY HEREK, University of California, Davis
AMBER HOLLIBAUGH, New York City Commission on Human Rights
KIM HOPPER, New School for Social Research, New York City
MITCHELL HORWICH, Horwich & Zagar, Attorneys at Law, Miami
RICHARD IACINO, Center on Adult Development and Aging, Miami
PAMELA JENNINGS, AIDS Education and Prevention Unit, Sacramento County Health Department
RICHARD JOHNSON, Health Services Jail, Sacramento
RONALD JOHNSON, Minority Task Force on AIDS, New York City
FRANKLIN KAKIES, AIDS Response Programming, Lambda Community Center, Sacramento
LARRY KESSLER, AIDS Action Committee, Boston
MARC KEYSER, AIDS Action League, Sacramento
GIOK KHOE, Sacramento County Health Department
DAVID KIRP, University of California, Berkeley
REBECCA KNODT, Agricultural Workers Health Center, Sacramento
BARBARA KOENIG, Hastings Center, San Francisco
HAROLD KOODEN, New York City
SALVADOR LANDEROS, Mexican American Alcoholism Program, Sacramento
ROGER LANE, Health Crisis Network, Miami
PETER LEE, National AIDS Network, Washington, D.C.
MARTIN LEVINE, Department of Sociology and Social Psychology, Florida Atlantic University
THE REVEREND TIMOTHY LITTLE, Medical Center, University of California, Davis
CATHY LYNCH, Health Crisis Network, Miami
CATHIE LYONS, United Methodist Church, New York City
TERRY MASTRUCCI, Department of Pediatrics, University of Miami School of Medicine
SISTER ELIZABETH McMILLAN, Catholic Health Association, St. Louis
NAT MILLER, Community Outreach Prevention and Education, Inc. (COPE), Miami
THE REVEREND CURTIS MITCHELL, Antioch Progressive Baptist Church, Sacramento
OLOMIDE OGUNLANO, Family Health Center, Inc., Miami
FRANK OLDHAM, New York City Department of Health
CATHERINE O'NEILL, Legal Action Center, New York
ROBERT PADGUG, Empire Blue Cross and Blue Shield, New York
J. BRYAN PAGE, Biopsychosocial Center on AIDS, University of Miami

JAN PARKS, Mayor's Office for the Lesbian and Gay Community, New York City
WENDY PARMET, Northeastern University Law School
CHRISTINE PERILLO, The Effort, Inc., Sacramento
RABBI REX PERLMETER, Temple Israel, Miami
ROBIN PHILIPS, Options for Recovery, Sacramento
LARRY PIERRE, Center for Haitian Studies, Miami
ANITRA PIVNIK, Montefiore Hospital, New York City
THE REVEREND MICHAEL PLACE, Archdiocese of Chicago
CATHY POTLER, Correctional Association of New York, New York City
LINDA QUICK, Health Council of South Florida, Miami
THE REVEREND LAURIE REED, Hospice, Inc., Miami
DAVID RIGG, Health Crisis Network, Miami
MIM SCHOFIELD, Dade County Department of Health, Miami
THE REVEREND ED SHERRIFF, Hope House, Sacramento
SONIA SINGLETON, Community Outreach Prevention and Education, Inc. (COPE), Miami
THE REVEREND FREDA SMITH, Metropolitan Community Church, Sacramento
MARK STARR, Sacramento County Health Department
RABBI RICHARD STERNBERGER, Union of American Hebrew Congregations, Washington, D.C.
RAND STONEBURNER, New York City Department of Health
SUE STRONG, Center for AIDS Research and Education Services (CARES), Sacramento
MERCER SULLIVAN, New School for Social Research, New York City
IDA SUSSER, New York City
MICHAEL SYMONETTE, Covenant Missionary Baptist Church and Family Health Center, Miami
KATY TAYLOR, New York City Commission on Human Rights
LAURIE THOMAS, California Children's Services, Sacramento
GUILLERMO VASQUEZ, Gay Men's Health Crisis, New York City
MANUEL VEGA, Hispanic League Against AIDS, Miami
PAUL VOLBERDING, San Francisco General Hospital
MONSIGNOR BRIAN WALSH, Catholic Community Services, Miami
DENNIS WEBB, California State Office of AIDS, Sacramento
DAVID WILLIS, Milbank Quarterly, Milbank Memorial Fund, New York City
DAVID WITHUM, State Health and Rehabilitative Services, Dade County District Office, Miami
BONNIE WOLBRIDGE, Alta California Regional Center, Sacramento
RICHARD ZIMMERMAN, Departments of Sociology and Psychiatry, University of Miami

Index

A

Abortion, 287-288

Abrams, Donald, 100

Academic medicine, 57, 99-100

Acer, David J., 62

Activism, *see* Advocacy and activist groups

ACT-UP, 92, 94, 96, 119, 166-168, 264-265

Adoption, 208, 209-210

Advocacy and activist groups, 8, 14
cancer patients, 99
and drug development and approval, 89-92, 95-97, 101-102, 104, 107-108, 167-168
in New York City, 263-265
see also ACT-UP; Community-based organizations; Gay Men's Health Crisis

African Americans, 42, 171-172
churches, 123, 142-143, 149-150
and clinical research, 87, 104-105
gay men, 265-266
incarceration of, 16, 178, 179, 281
in New York City, 251-252, 275

AIDS Clinical Trials Group (ACTG), 92, 94, 95-97, 98, 102, 105-107

AIDS Coalition to Unleash Power, *see* ACT-UP

AIDS/HIV Experimental Treatment Directory, 101, 110

AIDS National Interfaith Network, 140

AIDS-related complex, 16, 91, 92

AIDS Treatment News, 101, 110

Aid to Families with Dependent Children (AFDC), 212, 213-214

Almarez, Rudolph, 61

Alternative therapies, 90, 99

American Foundation for AIDS Research, 101, 110

American Medical Association, 28, 32

Amphotericin B, 49

Antibody testing, *see* Testing and screening

ARC, *see* AIDS-related complex

Asymptomatic HIV-positive population, 21, 24, 29, 92
in prisons, 16, 186-187